Man-Chung Han and Chu-Wan Kim

SECTIONAL HUMAN ANATOMY

Transverse, Sagittal and Coronal Sections
Correlated with
Computed Tomography and Magnetic Resonance Imaging

Second Edition

ILCHOKAK   Seoul
IGAKU-SHOIN   New York · Tokyo

Authors' address

Man-Chung Han, M.D.
Professor of Radiology
Department of Diagnostic Radiology,
College of Medicine,
Seoul National University
28, Yeongun-Dong, Chongro-Ku,
Seoul, Korea

Chu-Wan Kim, M.D.
Professor and Chairman
Department of Diagnostic Radiology,
College of Medicine,
Seoul National University
28, Yeongun-Dong, Chongro-Ku,
Seoul, Korea

ISBN 0-89640-165-0 (NEW YORK)
4-260-14165-1 (TOKYO)

Copyright © 1989 by the Authors. First Edition 1985.
All the rights, including that of translation, reserved.
No part of this publication may be reproduced, stored in retrieval system, or transmitted in any other form or by any means, electronic, mechanical, recording, or otherwise, without the prior written permission of the authors.

Printed by Pyung Hwa Dang Printing Co., Ltd., Seoul, Korea

PREFACE TO THE SECOND EDITION

Since the first edition of this book was published three years ago, we have witnessed an ever increasing clinical application of sectional imaging modalities. The most dramatic appearance seems to be the development and propagation of "State of the Art" quality MR imaging units.

The main purpose of this second edition is to integrate MR images with anatomy color plates and CT images. This rearrangement offers side by side correlation of all three images in two pages and readers will have more comprehensive understanding of correlated anatomy.

We also upgraded MR images using a 2.0 tesla superconductive magnet system developed by Professor Zang-Hee Cho and his colleagues.

Finally, anatomy color plates of sagittal sections of the brain with corresponding MR images have been added.

Consequently there are now three segmental anatomic parts; Brain · Head & Neck, Chest and Abdomen & Pelvis. Each consists of anatomic color plates, CT and MR images in smaller scales.

We believe this second edition to be one step forward in a continuous effort, as our old saying correctly pointed out "the beginning is a half success".

April, 1989
                                                                                          Man-Chung Han, M.D.
Chu-Wan Kim, M.D.

제 2 판 머 리 말

 새로운 단면영상진단방법이 임상진료에 널리 이용되어 인체단면해부학 서적의 필요성이 높아지고, 이에 따라 『Sectional Human Anatomy, Correlated with CT and MRI』가 발간된 지 3년여가 지났다.

 이 책은 1985년도 북미방사선의학회 학술대회에서의 전시를 계기로 미국의 Igaku-Shoin과 해외판매권의 계약을 맺을 수 있게 되었고, 미국 및 일본을 비롯한 해외에 수출도 되었다.

 그동안 국내 여러분의 서평 및 의견과 日本醫學放射線學會雜誌, Radiology, American Journal of Roentgenology 및 British Journal of Radiology 등의 해외학술지에 게재된 서평을 참고로 하였으며, 또한 저자들이 불만스럽게 생각하였던 점을 보완하고, 몇 군데 오기를 바로잡아서 여기에 제 2 판을 출간하게 되었다.

 제 2 판의 특징은 원색 해부단면상과 전산화단층촬영상(CT) 및 자기공명영상(MRI)을 좌우면에 나란히 배치한 점이다. 따라서 모든 영상의 배치가 상하좌우가 동일하고 해부학명 기술의 방향과 같아서 보기에 편리하도록 하였다. 이를 위하여 원색 해부단면상은 약간, CT 및 MRI 상은 상당히 축소되었다. 해부단면상에서 뇌의 시상단면상을 추가하였으며, 뇌 및 복부의 시상단면상은 MRI 만 대비하였다. 또한 두부 CT상 중에서 그 대조도나 질이 낮은 것은 대체하였다. 따라서 원색 인체해부단면상은 90개가 되었고, CT상 69개, MRI 상 90개 총 249개를 수록하였다.

 제 2 판에 사용된 MRI 장치는 한국과학원 조장희 교수팀이 개발하고 금성의료기주식회사가 제작한 2.0 tesla 초전도형 자기공명영상장치이며, 제 2 판에서의 상전도식장치보다 영상의 질이 월등히 높아졌음은 특기할 만하다.

 이 책이 최근 급속히 보급되고 있는 단면영상진단의 기본적인 해부학 교과서로서 국내외에서 널리 이용되었으면 하는 바람이다.

 다시 한번 본교실 교직원 여러분에게 감사하며 이번에도 모든 정성을 쏟아주신 서울대학교병원 심영보 의학사진실장의 노고를 치하하고 인내로써 협조하여 주신 일조각 여러분에게 감사한다.

1989년 4월 일

한 만 청
김 주 완

PREFACE TO THE FIRST EDITION

With the advent of new diagnostic modalities including ultrasonography, computed tomography and magnetic resonance imaging, there has been a steadily growing demand for atlases which display the human body in multidirectional section.

It is no longer only the anatomists who deal with pictures of sections of the human body on a daily basis. Today, clinicians in ever increasing numbers must do the same.

The purpose of this book is to provide a detailed depiction of sectional anatomy for medical students, residents, and practitioners of radiology, medicine and surgery.

The color photos of the anatomic specimens in this atlas have the advantage of being more realistic than previously used schematic drawings or black and white photos. Each anatomical structure is labeled directly on the photos for quick review, but not every structure is labeled in every illustration. Since each anatomic section is sequential, an unlabeled structure can be identified by its position in preceding or subsequent sections.

For easy understanding, segmental anatomy has been organized into three parts; head and neck, chest, and abdomen and pelvis. Each part consists of sequential anatomic sections and corresponding CT images, except in sagittal sections. In part four, magnetic resonance images are presented so that they can be compared with the anatomic and CT sections.

To make the information contained in this book accessible to a large audience the index terms are written in English, Chinese, and Korean.

We are deeply grateful to the many people whose assistance was invaluable in compiling this atlas. We would like to express our special thanks to the faculty of the Department of Anatomy for their assistance in preparing the cadavers. This atlas would not have been completed without help from the residents of our Department of Diagnostic Radiology, under the guidance of Dr. Jung-Gi Im, one of the contributors, who devoted his time and effort to this project.

We owe a special debt of gratitude to Professor Zang-Hee Cho, Korea Advanced Institute of Science and Technology, for his kind assistance in obtaining the magnetic resonance imaging.

We would also like to extend our thanks to Department of Radiology, Korea General Hospital, for the help in collecting CT images and to Mr. Young-Bo Shim for his excellent color photographs.

Finally, we would like to express our deep appreciation to our publisher, Ilchokak, whose understanding, patience and advice was of invaluable help.

September, 1985

Man-Chung Han, M.D.
Chu-Wan Kim, M.D.

제1판 머리말

　최근 의학부문에 초음파촬영, 전산화단층촬영 및 자기공명영상촬영 등의 새로운 진단방법이 개발되어 임상에 이용됨에 따라, 인체의 단면해부학에 관한 지식은 해부학분야에서는 물론 일상 진료에 임하는 모든 임상의사에게도 필수적인 것이 되었다.

　이러한 추세에 따라 외국에서는 단면해부학서적이 이미 발간되어 왔으나 인체단면이 흑백으로만 인쇄되었거나, 천연색상인 경우에도 상이 불분명하거나, 각 구조물을 표기하는데 있어서 간결하지 못한 점이 있어 아쉬움을 느끼고 있었다. 한편으로는 한국인을 위한 해부학서적은, 한국인 사체를 사용하여 제작되는 것이 바람직하다는 생각도 평소에 가지고 있었다. 이러한 이유로 하여 저자들은 3년 전부터 이 책의 발간준비를 시작하게 되었다.

　이 책은 의과대학 학생을 비롯하여 전공의·내과계·외과계 및 방사선과학분야의 전문의를 위하여 제작되었으며, 인체의 단면과 해당부위의 전산화단층촬영영상을 대비시켰고 더 나아가서 일부분은 자기공명영상도 삽입하여 해부학 자체만이 아닌 임상진료에 이용될 수 있는 해부도보가 되도록 노력하였다.

　인체의 85개의 각 단면을 모두 천연색상으로 인쇄하였으며, 단면에 나타난 각각의 구조물은 독자로 하여금 쉽게 파악할 수 있도록 단면사진에 직접 약어로 된 문자로 표기하였다. 모든 구조물을 표기하려고 노력하였으나, 앞뒤로 중복되는 구조물인 경우는 생략된 경우도 있다. 한편 색인은 영문, 한문 및 한글을 차례로 기술하여 해부학적 구조물 표기에 일관성이 있도록 하였다.

　우리나라 의학교육 및 의료계의 현실에 따라 부득이 영문학명 위주로 표기하였으며 이에 따라 이 책이 외국인에게도 널리 애용될 수 있으리라 믿는다.

　이 책에 게재된 자기공명영상은 한국과학기술원에서 개발한 0.15 tesla의 상온도자석 자기공명영상장치로 촬영한 것으로 그 의의가 크다고 할 수 있다.

　이 책에 사용된 사체의 고정 및 보관과 색인정리에 적극적인 협력과 지도를 아끼지 않았던 서울대학교 의과대학 해부학교실 교수진에게 감사를 드리고 자기공명영상을 수록할 수 있도록 협조하여 주신 한국과학기술원의 조장희교수 및 대학원생 여러분과 전산화단층촬영사진 수집에 협력해 주신 고려병원 방사선과에 감사의 말씀을 드린다.

　선명한 천연색 및 흑백사진을 얻기 위하여 열과 성을 다하였던 서울대학교병원 사진실 십영보씨의 노고를 치하하고 아울러 본 저서의 출간이 가능하도록 헌신적인 노력을 하여 준 서울대학교 의과대학 진단방사선과학교실 교수 전원 및 의국원들에게 감사하며 특히 사체절단에서부터 출판과정의 세부사항까지 일선에서 일을 관장한 임정기교수의 노고는 특기하여야만 할 것이다. 끝으로 이해와 인내를 가지고 꾸준히 협조를 아끼지 않았던 일조각 여러분에게 감사한다.

1985년 9월   일

한　만　청
김　주　완

INTRODUCTION

An excellent way to understand the three dimensional anatomical structure of the human body is by studying multidirectional sections of a cadaver with corresponding radiographic images. The ultimate objective of this atlas is to portray normal sectional anatomy and anatomical relationships in basic three dimensional form.

A. Preparation of the Cadavers

Immediately after the cadavers were brought to the Department of Anatomy they were embalmed by injecting a preserving fluid, consisting of 10% formalin and glycerine, through one of the femoral arteries. The cadavers were then placed in the embalming machine for one month, which facilitates fixation of the tissue with the aid of high atmospheric pressure.

The major arterial and venous channels were filled with red and blue dye, respectively, for the sake of artificial accentuation of the vascular trees. Dye was injected through the femoral artery and vein with application of 300mmHg and 200mmHg pressure. Some of the dye extravasated through unidentified routes to the extravascular potential spaces of the pleura, pericardium and peritoneum. Though this was an unintended side effect, it demonstrates clearly the potential spaces or fascial planes. The mixture of gelatin solution and water soluble dye provides excellent solidification of the dye in the vascular space, thus preventing leakage and intrusion to adjacent structures during saw cutting of the cadaver.

After the period of fixation and dye infusion, the cadavers were placed in horizontal position on the cabinet of the freezing room. With an additional application of dry ice around the cadaver, the body was maintained in anatomical position for a complete freezing period of 48 hours. Complete freezing of the body provided uniform hardness of the tissue so as to present uniform resistence to the progression of the band saw.

B. Section and Preparation of Anatomical Slices

All anatomical specimens in this book were cut by using a rotating band saw, except sagittal sections of the brain. For ease of handling, extremities were removed. The head was cut into slices with a reference plane of orbitomeatal line in transverse section. The adjustable guiding plate parallel to the saw blade was tightly attached to the surface of each slice in order to obtain uniform thickness. The planes of reference in the transverse section of the chest, abdomen and pelvis were both nipples and the anterior superior iliac spine, respectively. The thickness of each slice varies according to the location, ranging from 1cm to 1.5cm. Immediately after sectioning, each slice was placed on a glass plate and the surface of the slice was cleaned with running water and a gauze. Then, another glass plate was placed on the exposed side and the slice was turned over. The cleaned slices were covered with cloth and glass plate to prevent excessive wetness and dryness of the surface. They were then stored in the cold morgue for not more than 48 hours. Before photographing, some of the extravasated dye and contents of the natural cavities were removed.

C. Photography

The photographic equipment for the cadaver consists of a Mamiya RB 67 Camera with Sekkor 90mm 3.8 lens. Exposure time was 1/60 sec with the aperture set at 8. Two 500W lamps were placed 1.5m away from the specimen at a 45 degree angle. Kodak CII films (70×60mm) were used.

Pictures were taken of both sides of each slice. Photographs of the transverse section of the head and neck are of real size, while sagittal sections of the body are reduced to 0.75 times their natural size. Transverse sections of the body are reduced ranging from 0.5 to 0.75 times to their real size.

The photographs had been chosen and arranged to a large extent on the basis of their clinical importance. So, transverse sections were viewed from the bottom side. The sagittal section of the chest is arranged with the anterior chest at the reader's left side because of its familiarity. The abdominal and pelvic sagittal sections are arranged in reversed order for the convenience of ultrasonogram interpretation.

Sagittal slices of the body were obtained as a single piece from lower neck to upper thigh. However, for anatomical detail and systematic arrangement the chest and the abdomen(including the pelvis), they were photographed separately.

CT scans were obtained with a GE CT/T 9800 scanner(General Electric, Milwaukee, Winsconsin). Though we tried to select identical pictures for comparison with corresponding anatomic slices, this was not possible in all cases because the location of internal organs varies.

Magnetic resonance images were obtained on a Goldstar Spectro-20,000 machine operating at 2.0 tesla (Goldstar, Seoul, Korea). For clarity of anatomic detail, all MR images in this book were obtained with spin-echo pulse sequences with a TR/TE of 500msec/30msec for brain, head & neck, and abdomen & pelvis. All chest images were obtained with ECG-gating, gated to every heart beat, and TE of 30msec.

D. Labelling

A great effort has been made to label the structures as much as possible. Abbreviations were placed directly on the photographs to allow prompt recognition. For a single word, the abbreviation consists of the first two or three letters, and for multiple words, the first letter of each word is used in capital letters. For the sake of clarity, each abbreviation corresponds to only one structure.

Jung-Gi Im, M.D.

CONTENTS

PREFACE TO THE SECOND EDITION iii
PREFACE TO THE FIRST EDITION v
INTRODUCTION vii

		Plate number	*Page*
PART ONE	BRAIN, HEAD and NECK		
	Transverse (Cadaver, CT & MRI)	1-19	3
	Coronal (Cadaver, CT & MRI)	20-28	43
	Sagittal (Cadaver & MRI)	29-33	63
PART TWO	CHEST		
	Transverse (Cadaver, CT & MRI)	34-42	77
	Sagittal (Cadaver & MRI)	43-48	97
PART THREE	ABDOMEN and PELVIS		
	Transverse (Cadaver, CT & MRI)	49-80	113
	Sagittal (Cadaver & MRI)	81-90	179

INDEX 201

CONTRIBUTORS

From   Department of Diagnostic Radiology
College of Medicine,
Seoul National University
Seoul, Korea

Kee-Hyun Chang, M.D.
Associate Professor

Byung-Ihn Choi, M.D.
Associate Professor

Man-Chung Han, M.D.
Professor

Moon-Hee Han, M.D.
Instructor

Jung-Gi Im, M.D.
Assistant Professor

Heung-Sik Kang, M.D.
Assistant Professor

Chu-Wan Kim, M.D.
Professor and Chairman

In-One Kim, M.D.
Assistant Professor

Seung-Hyup Kim, M.D.
Assistant Professor

Jae-Hyung Park, M.D.
Associate Professor

Kyung-Mo Yeon, M.D.
Associate Professor

PART 1
BRAIN, HEAD AND NECK

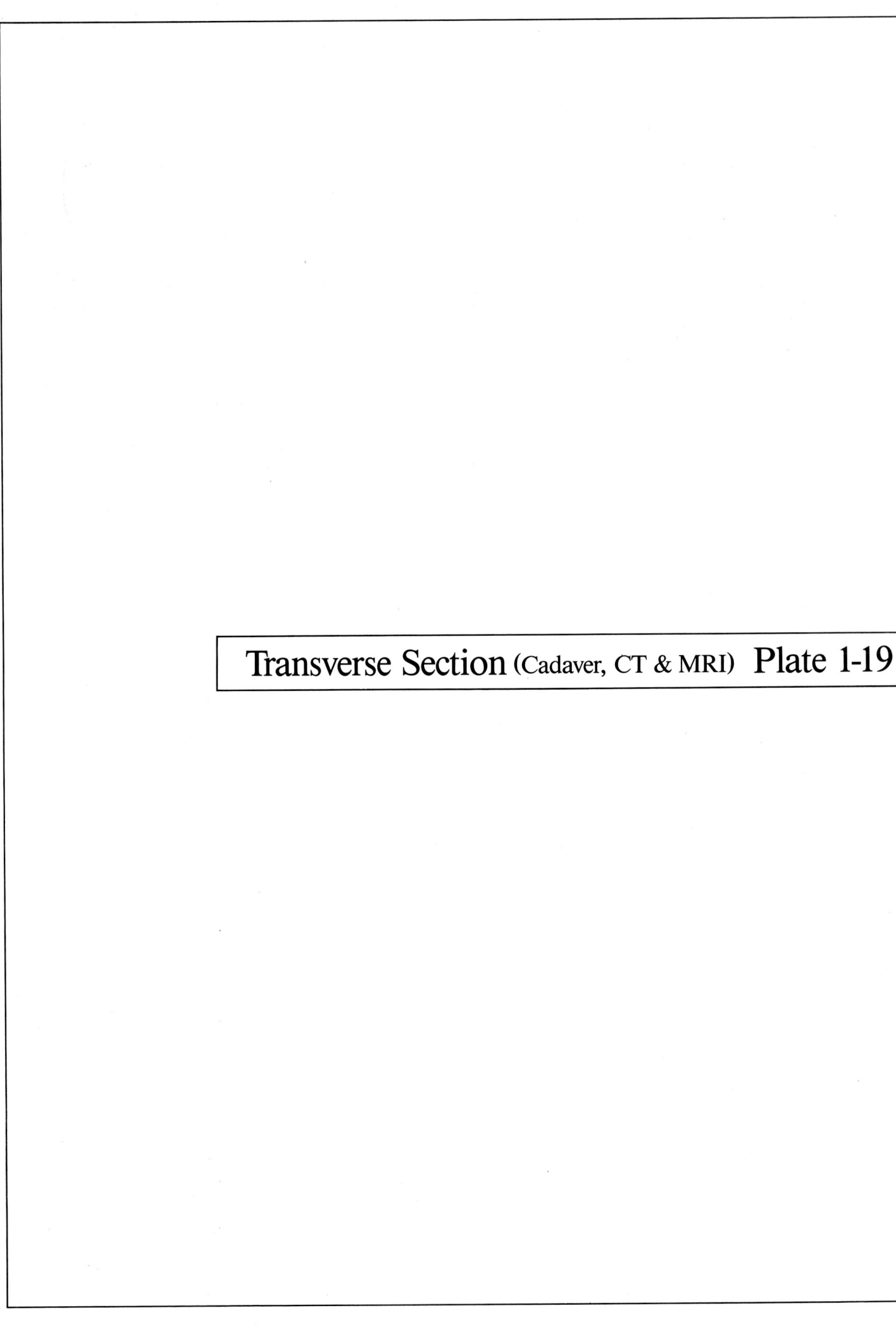

Transverse Section (Cadaver, CT & MRI) Plate 1-19

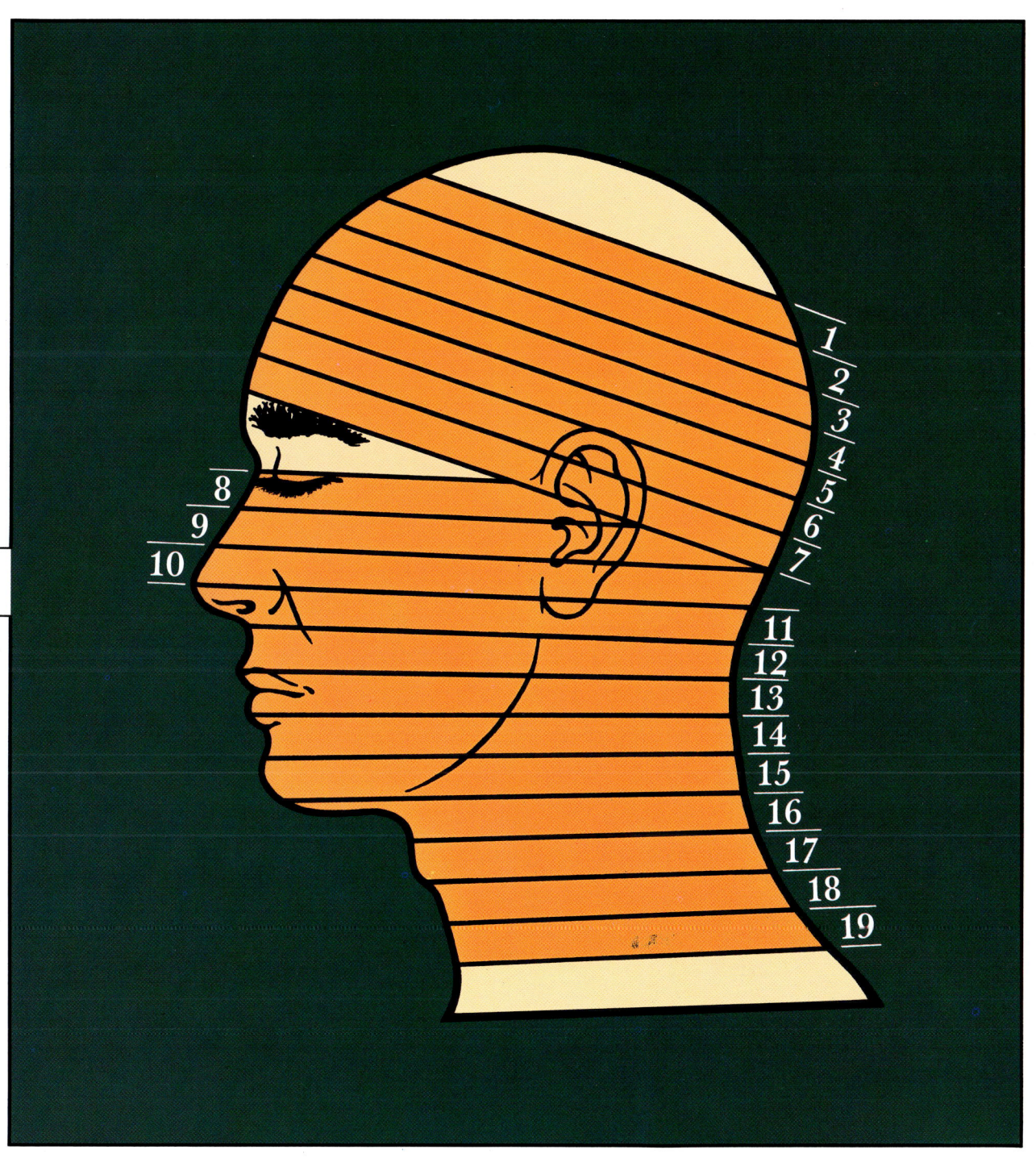

Plate 1. TRANSVERSE BRAIN

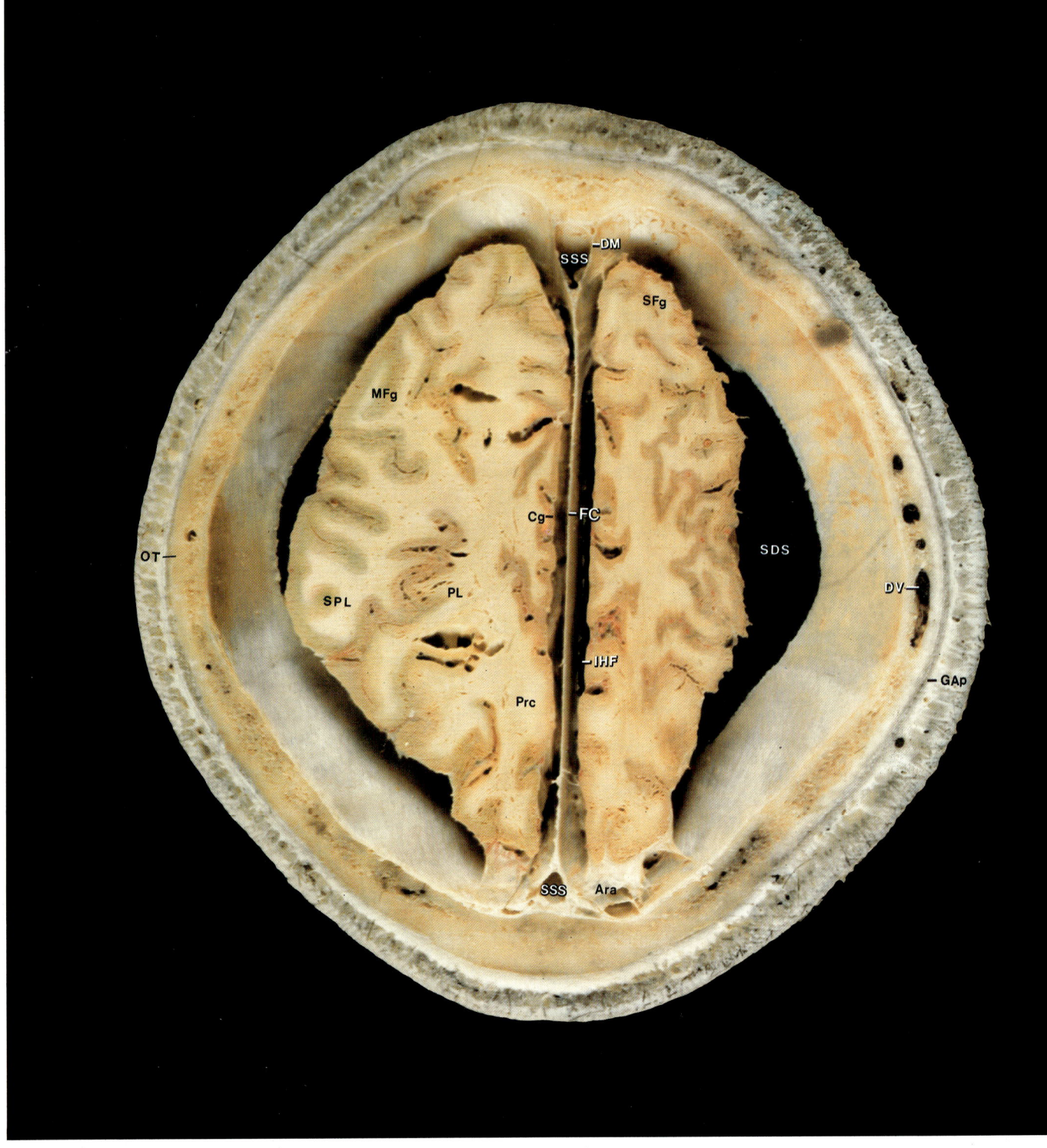

Ara	Arachnoid membrane
Cg	Cingulate gyrus
DM	Dura matter
DV	Diploic vein
FC	Falx cerebri
FL	Frontal lobe
GAp	Galea aponeurotica
IHF	Interhemispheric fissure
MFg	Middle frontal gyrus
OT	Outer table of calvarium
PL	Parietal lobe
Pal	Paracentral lobule
Pog	Postcentral gyrus
Prc	Precuneus
Prg	Precentral gyrus
SDS	Subdural space
SFg	Superior frontal gyrus
SPL	Superior parietal lobule
SSS	Superior sagittal sinus

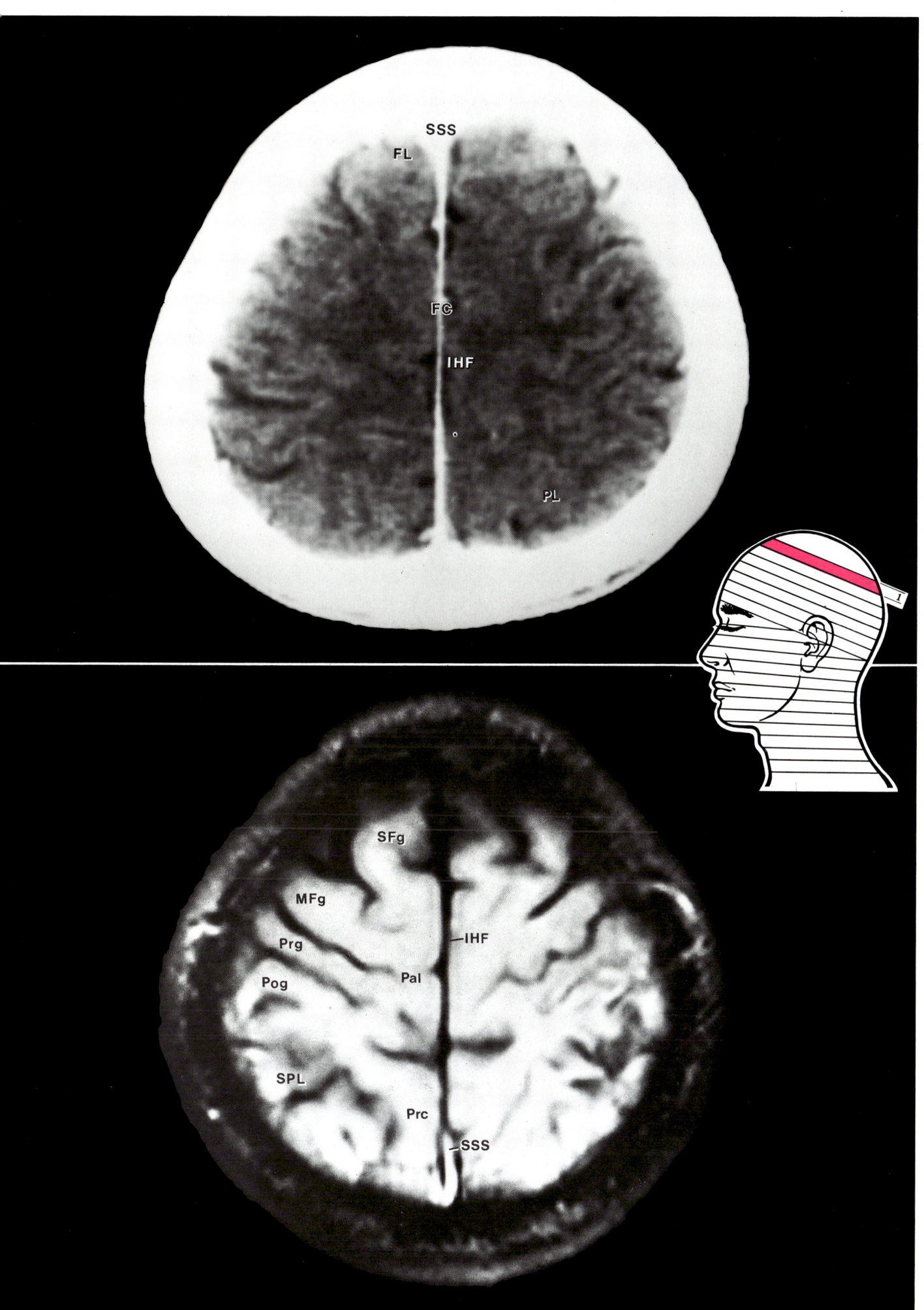

Plate 2. Transverse BRAIN

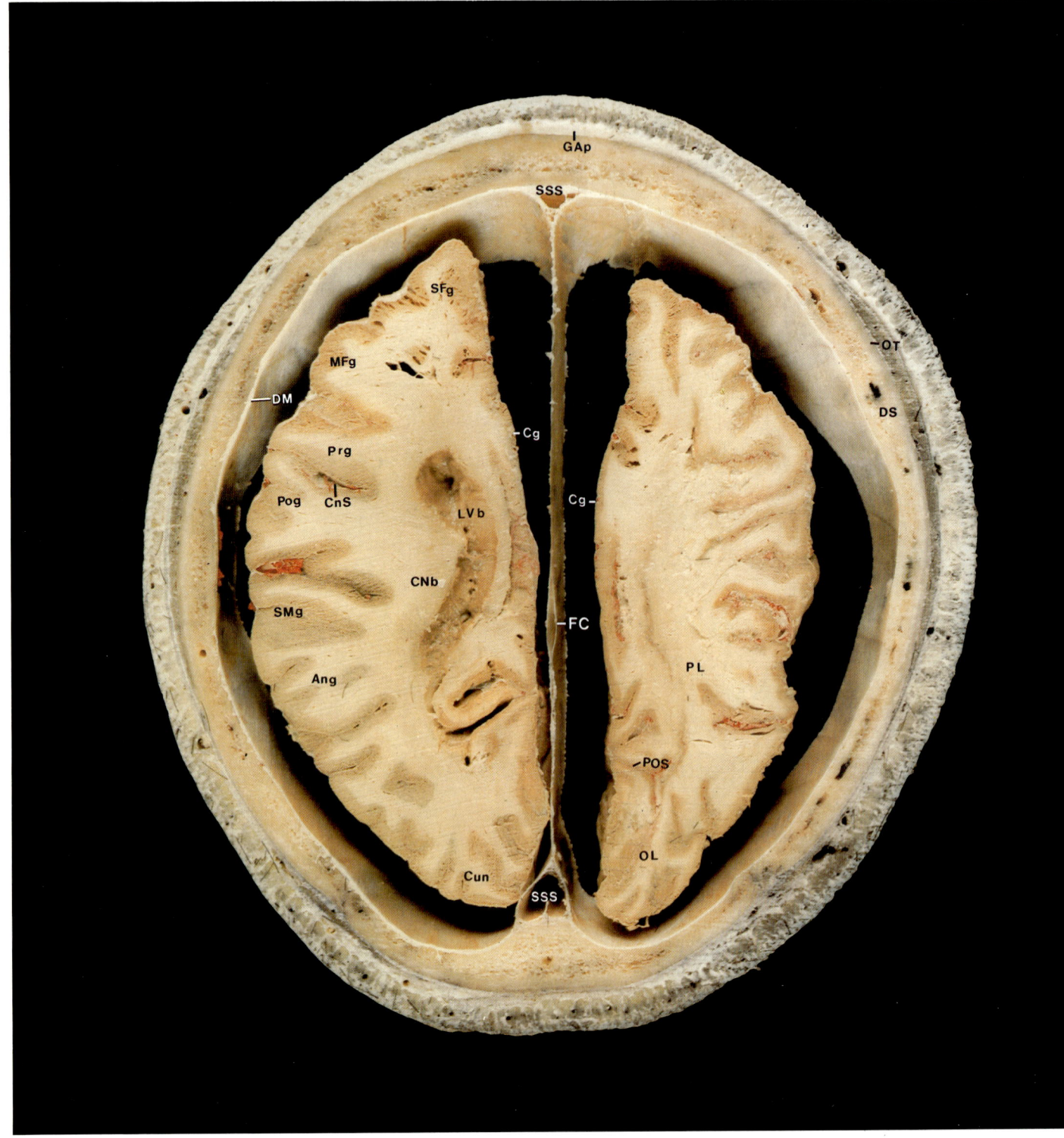

Ang	Angular gyrus	Prc	Precuneus
CNb	Caudate nucleus, body	Prg	Precentral gyrus
Cg	Cingulate gyrus	SFg	Superior frontal gyrus
CnO	Centrum ovale	SMg	Supramarginal gyrus
CnS	Central sulcus	SSS	Superior sagittal sinus
Cun	Cuneus		
DM	Dura matter		
DS	Diploic space		
FC	Falx cerebri		
FL	Frontal lobe		
GAp	Galea aponeurotica		
LVb	Lateral ventricle, body		
MFg	Middle frontal gyrus		
OL	Occipital lobe		
OT	Outer table of calvarium		
PL	Parietal lobe		
POS	Parieto-occipital sulcus		
Pog	Postcentral gyrus		

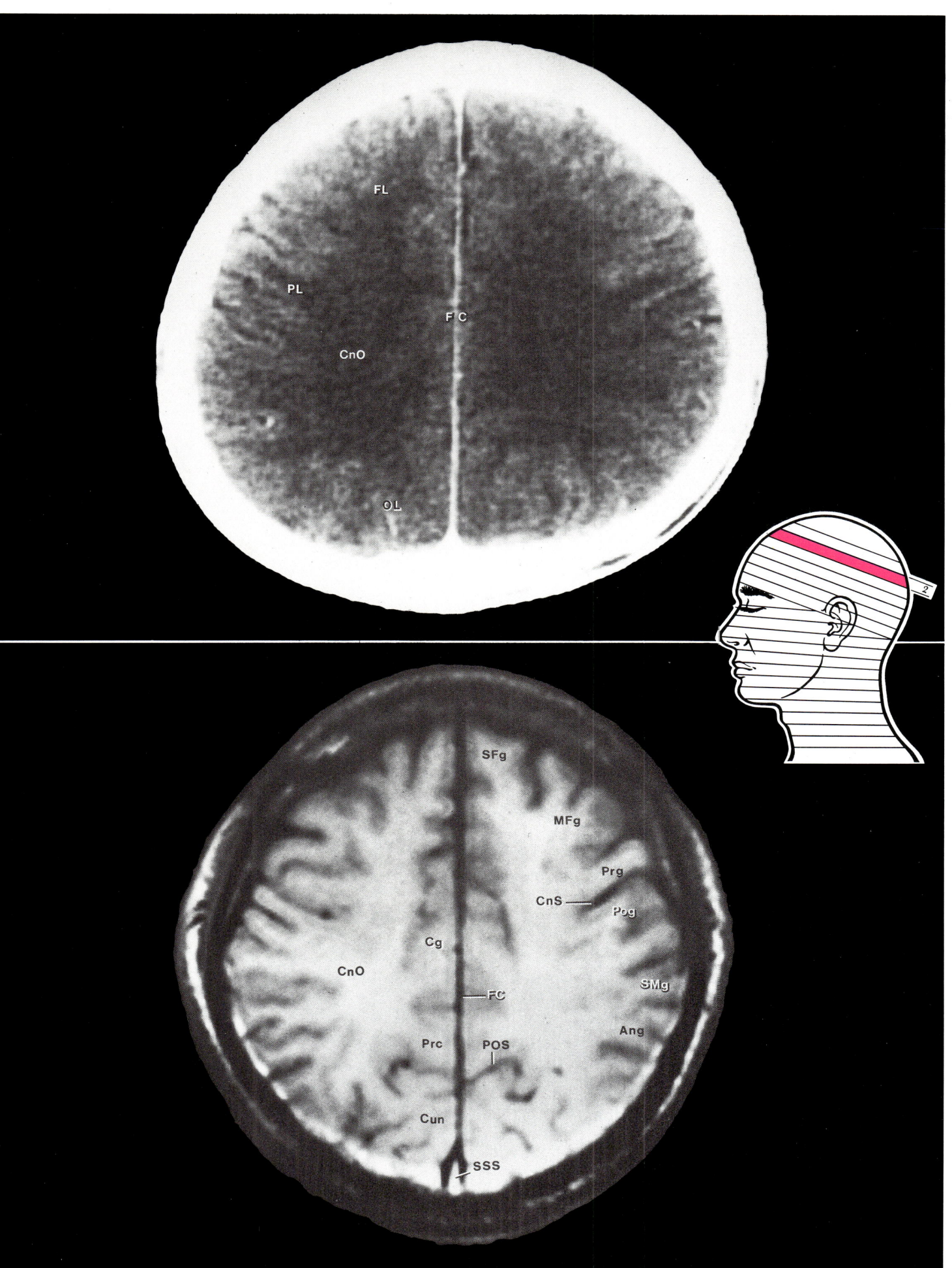

Plate 3. Transverse BRAIN

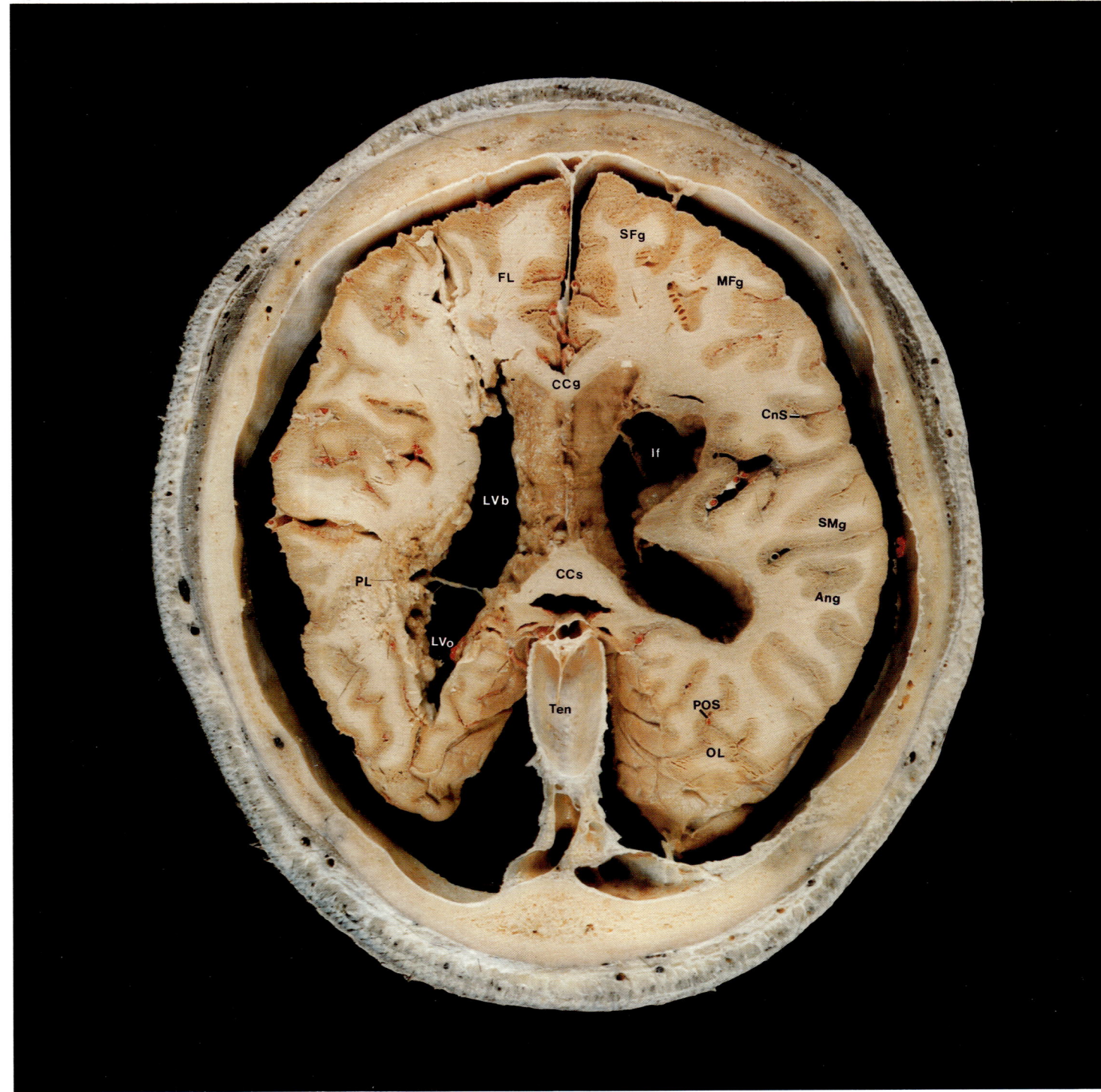

Ang	Angular gyrus	Pog	Postcentral gyrus
CCg	Corpus callosum, genu	Prg	Precentral gyrus
CCs	Corpus callosum, splenium	SFg	Superior frontal gyrus
CR	Corona radiata	SMg	Supramarginal gyrus
Cg	Cingulate gyrus	SSS	Superior sagittal sinus
CnS	Central sulcus	Ten	Tentorium cerebelli
Cun	Cuneus		
FC	Falx cerebri		
FL	Frontal lobe		
IFg	Inferior frontal gyrus		
If	Old infarct		
LVb	Lateral ventricle, body		
LVo	Lateral ventricle, occipital horn		
MFg	Middle frontal gyrus		
MTg	Middle temporal gyrus		
OL	Occipital lobe		
PL	Parietal lobe		
POS	Parieto-occipital sulcus		

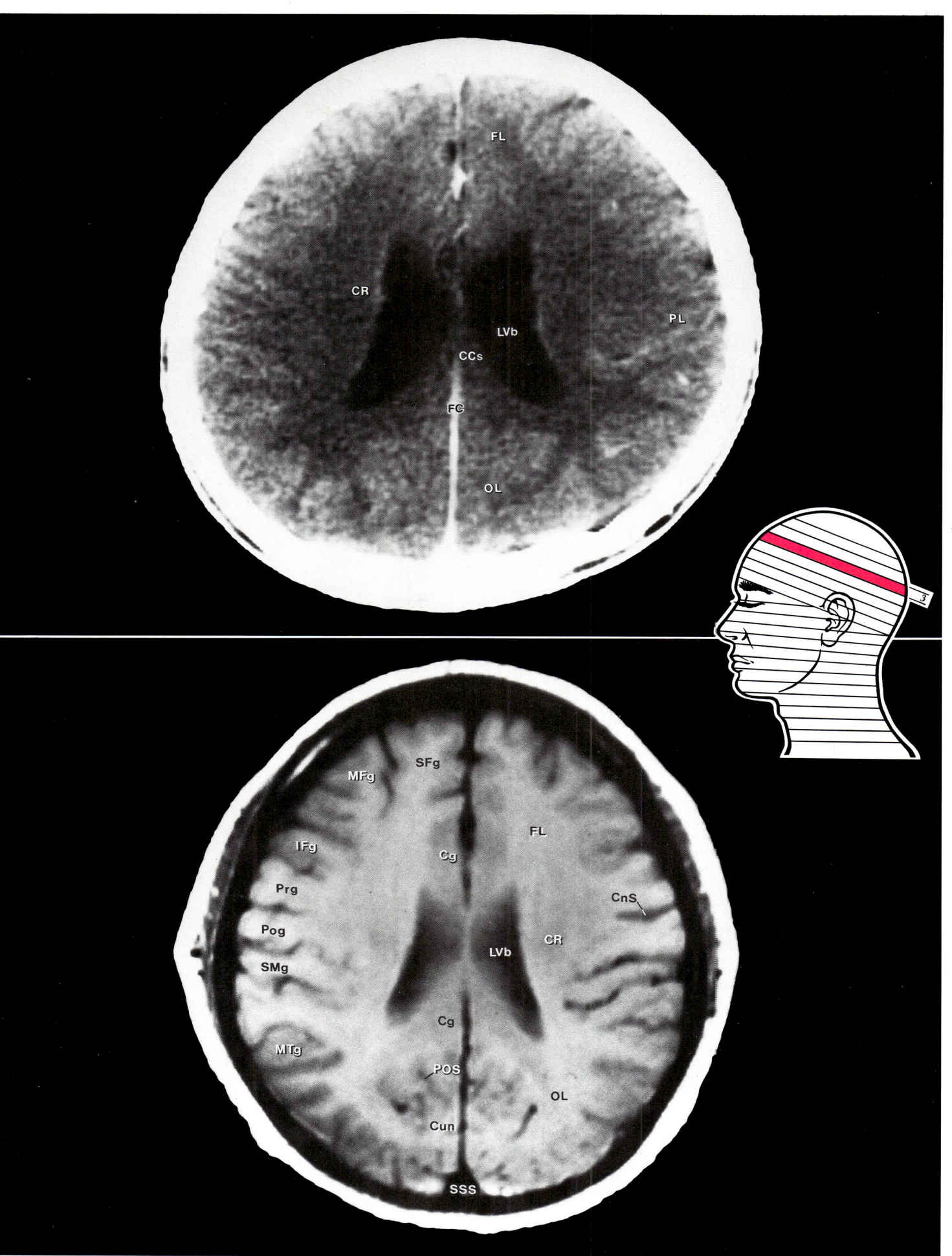

Plate 4. Transverse BRAIN

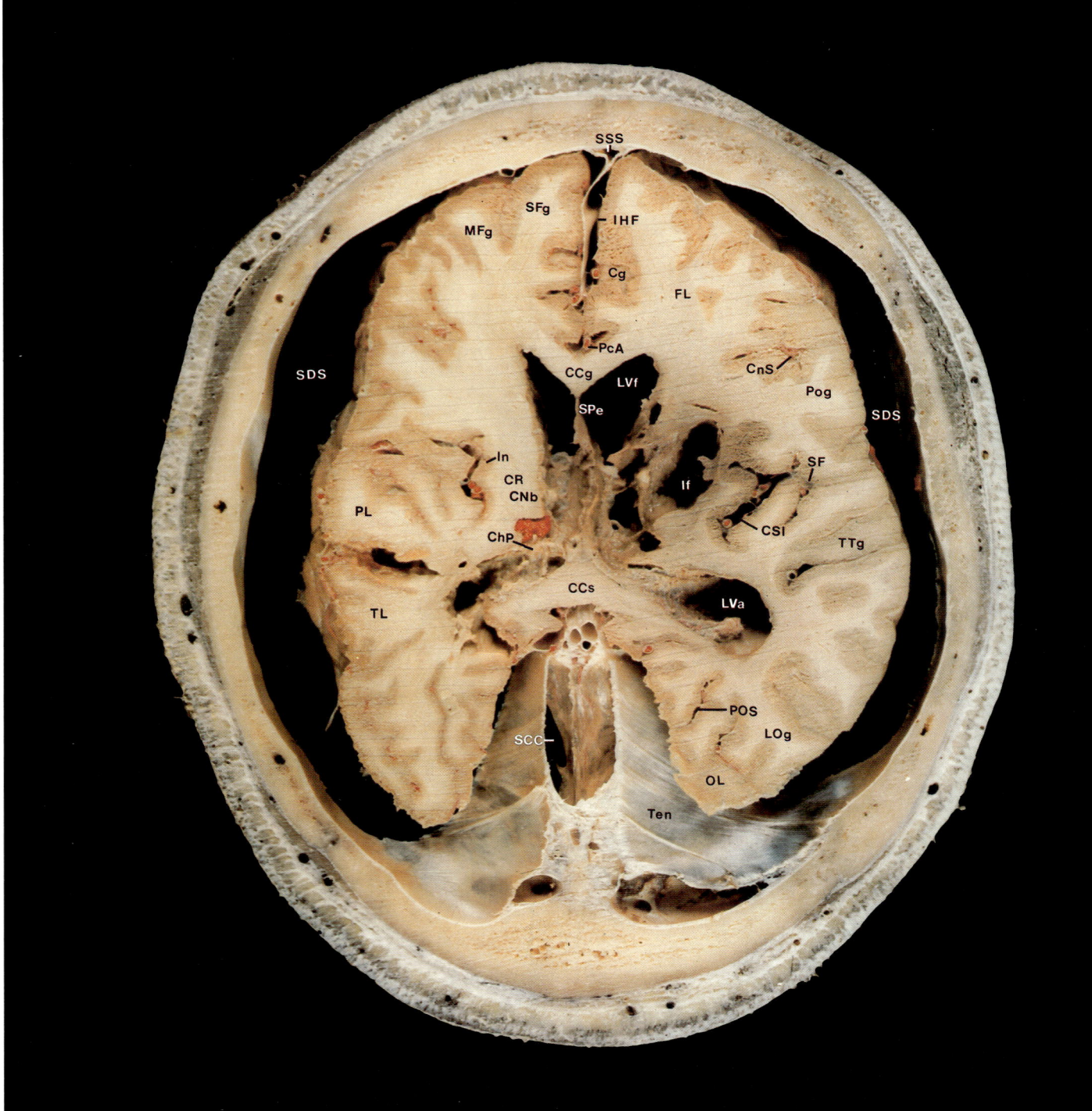

CCg	Corpus callosum, genu	LOg	Lateral occipital gyrus	SPe	Septum pellucidum
CCs	Corpus callosum, splenium	LVa	Lateral ventricle, antrum	SSS	Superior sagittal sinus
CNb	Caudate nucleus, body	LVb	Lateral ventricle, body	STg	Superior temporal gyrus
CNh	Caudate nucleus, head	LVf	Lateral ventricle, frontal horn	StS	Straight sinus
CR	Corona radiata	LVo	Lateral ventricle, occipital horn	TL	Temporal lobe
CSI	Circular sulcus of insula	MFg	Middle frontal gyrus	TTg	Transverse temporal gyrus
CaS	Calcarine sulcus	MTg	Middle temporal gyrus	Ten	Tentorium cerebelli
Cg	Cingulate gyrus	OL	Occipital lobe		
ChP	Choroid plexus of lateral ventricle	OpR	Optic radiation		
CnS	Central sulcus	PL	Parietal lobe		
Cun	Cuneus	POS	Parieto-occipital sulcus		
FC	Falx cerebri	PcA	Pericallosal artery		
FL	Frontal lobe	Pog	Postcentral gyrus		
ICV	Internal cerebral vein	Prg	Precentral gyrus		
IFg	Inferior frontal gyrus	SCC	Superior cerebellar cistern		
IHF	Interhemispheric fissure	SDS	Subdural space		
If	Old infarct	SF	Sylvian fissure		
In	Insula	SFg	Superior frontal gyrus		

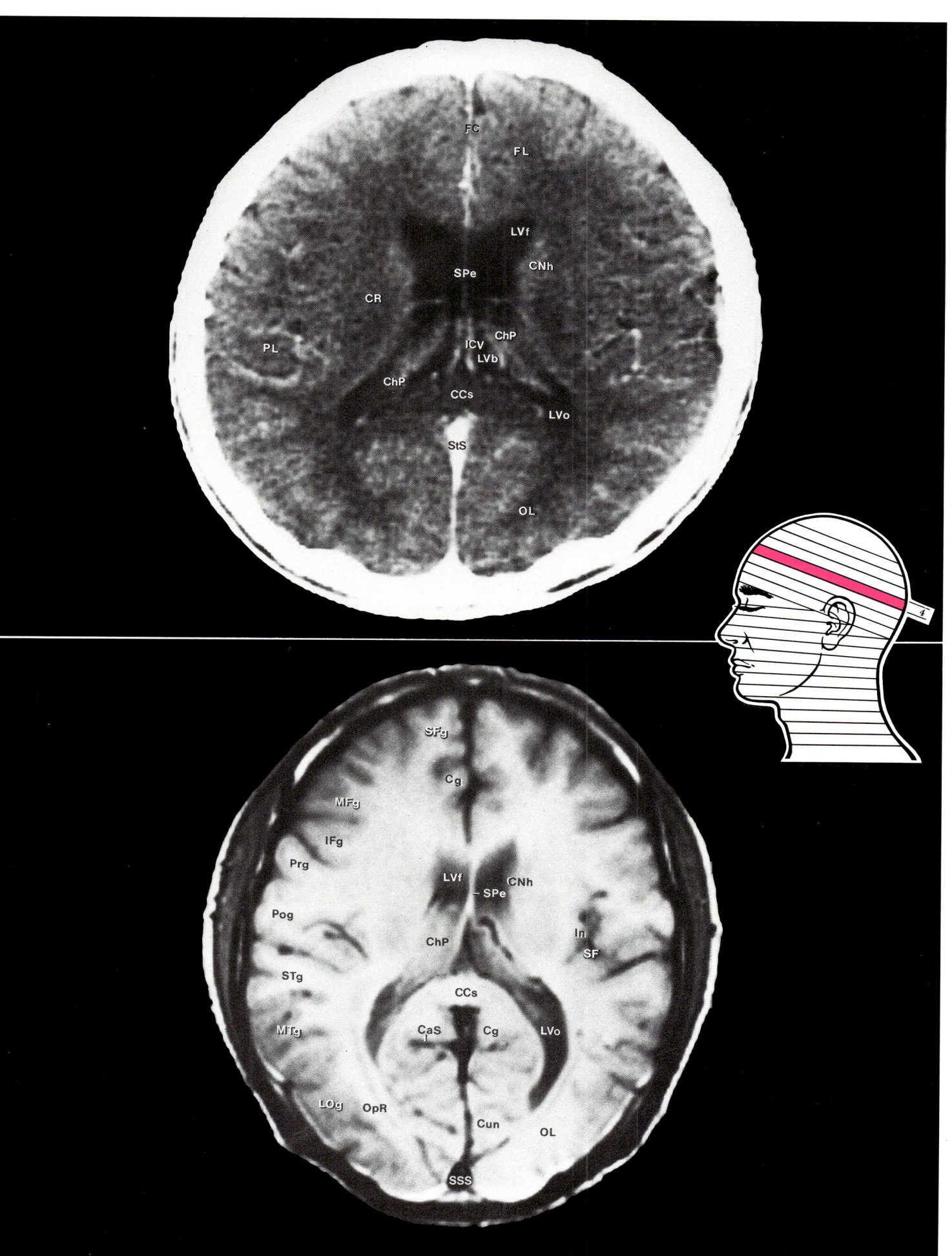

Plate 5. Transverse BRAIN

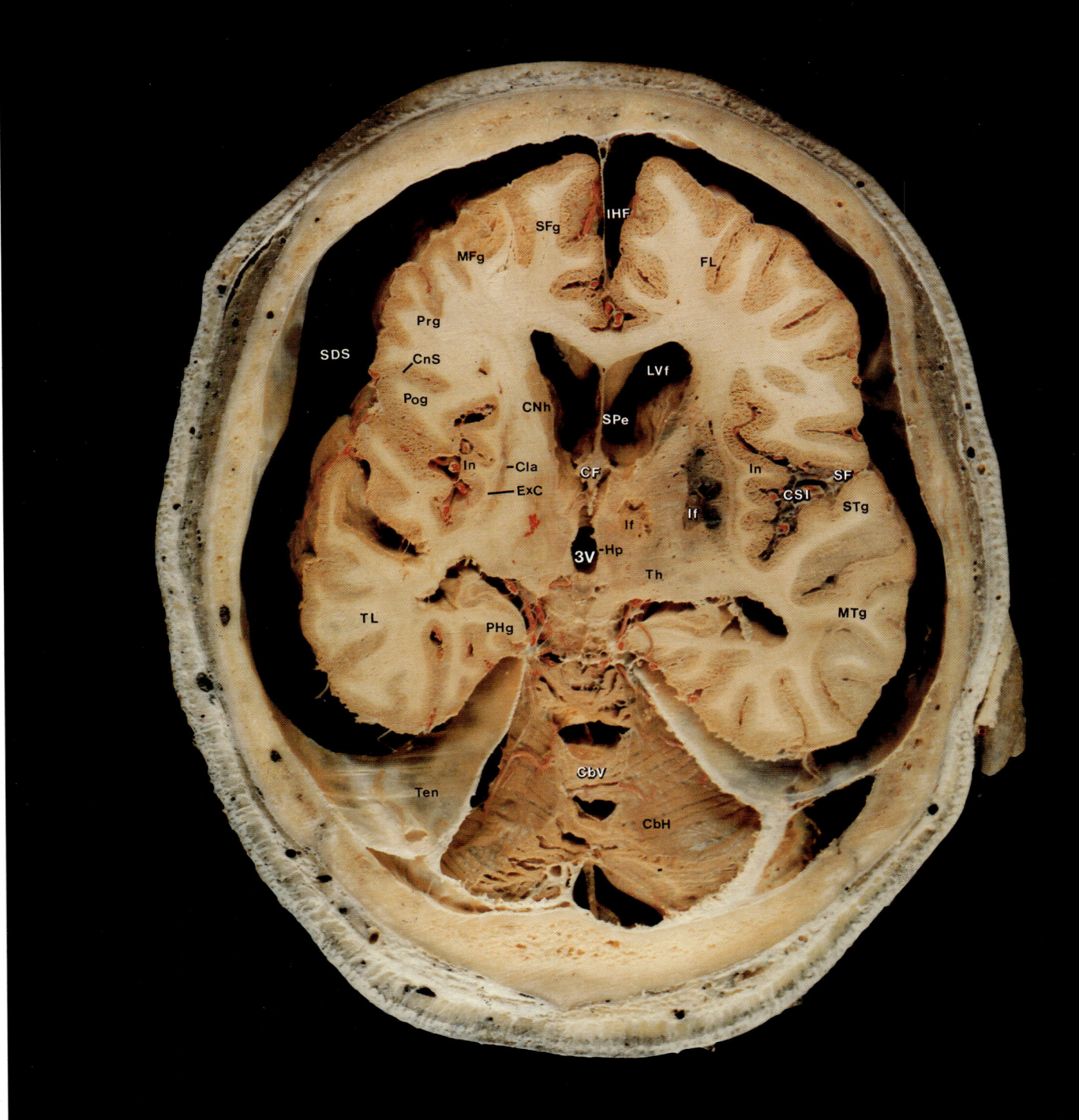

3V	3rd ventricle	ICa	Internal capsule, anterior limb	SDS	Subdural space
CCb	Corpus callosum, body	ICp	Internal capsule, posterior limb	SF	Sylvian fissure
CF	Column of fornix	IFg	Inferior frontal gyrus	SFg	Superior frontal gyrus
CNh	Caudate nucleus, head	IHF	Interhemispheric fissure	SPe	Septum pellucidum
CSI	Circular sulcus of insula	ITg	Inferior temporal gyrus	STg	Superior temporal gyrus
CbH	Cerebellar hemisphere	If	Old infarct	TL	Temporal lobe
CbV	Cerebellar vermis	In	Insula	Ten	Tentorium cerebelli
Cg	Cingulate gyrus	LVf	Lateral ventricle, frontal horn	Th	Thalamus
Cla	Claustrum	MFg	Middle frontal gyrus		
CnS	Central sulcus	MOTg	Medial occipitotemporal gyrus		
EC	External capsule	MTg	Middle temporal gyrus		
ExC	Extreme capsule	OL	Occipital lobe		
FC	Falx cerebri	PHg	Parahipocampal gyrus		
FL	Frontal lobe	PnG	Pineal gland		
GP	Globus pallidus	Pog	Postcentral gyrus		
Hi	Hippocampus	Prg	Precentral gyrus		
Hp	Hypothalamus	Pu	Putamen		
ICV	Internal cerebral vein	QC	Quadrigeminal cistern		

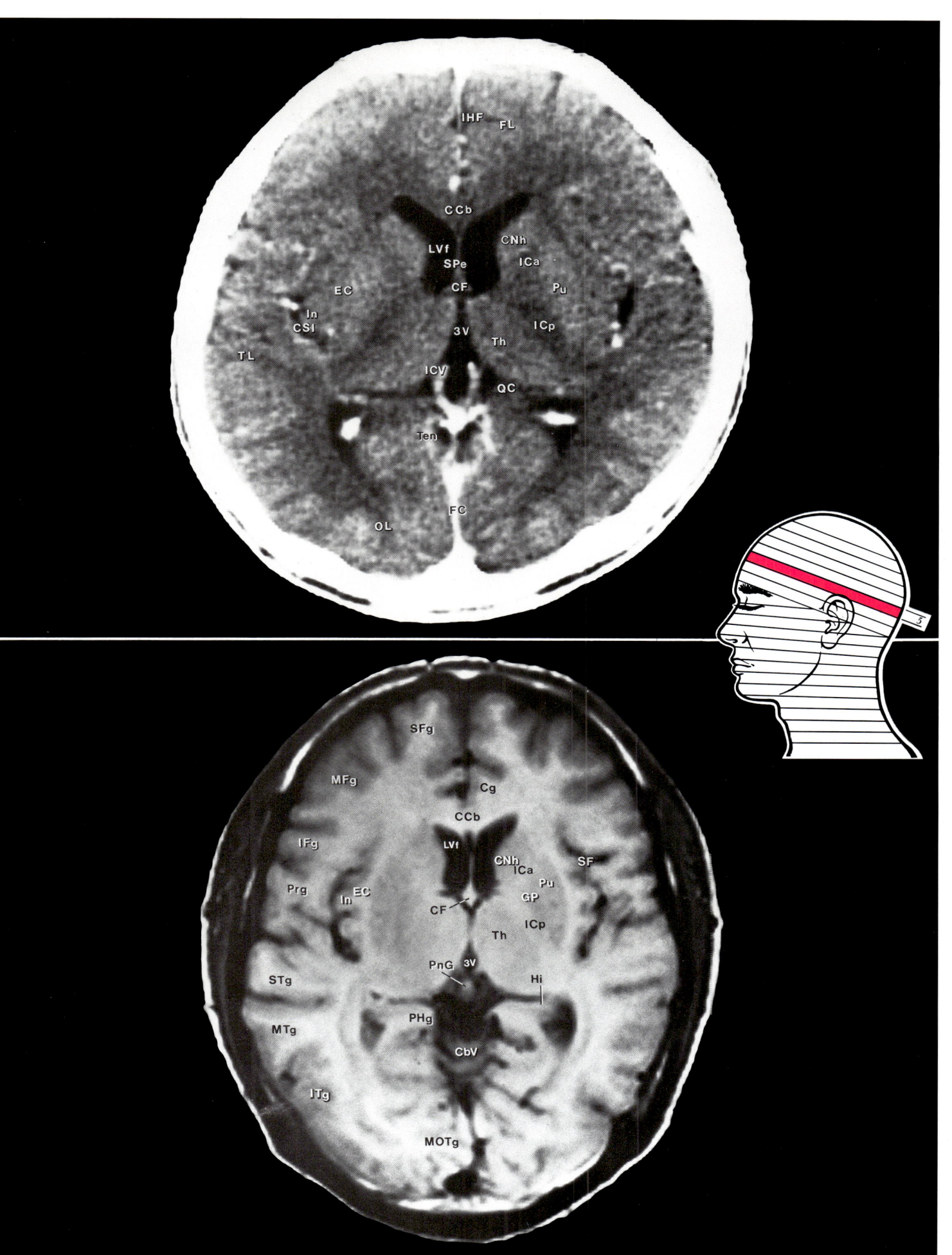

Plate 6. Transverse BRAIN

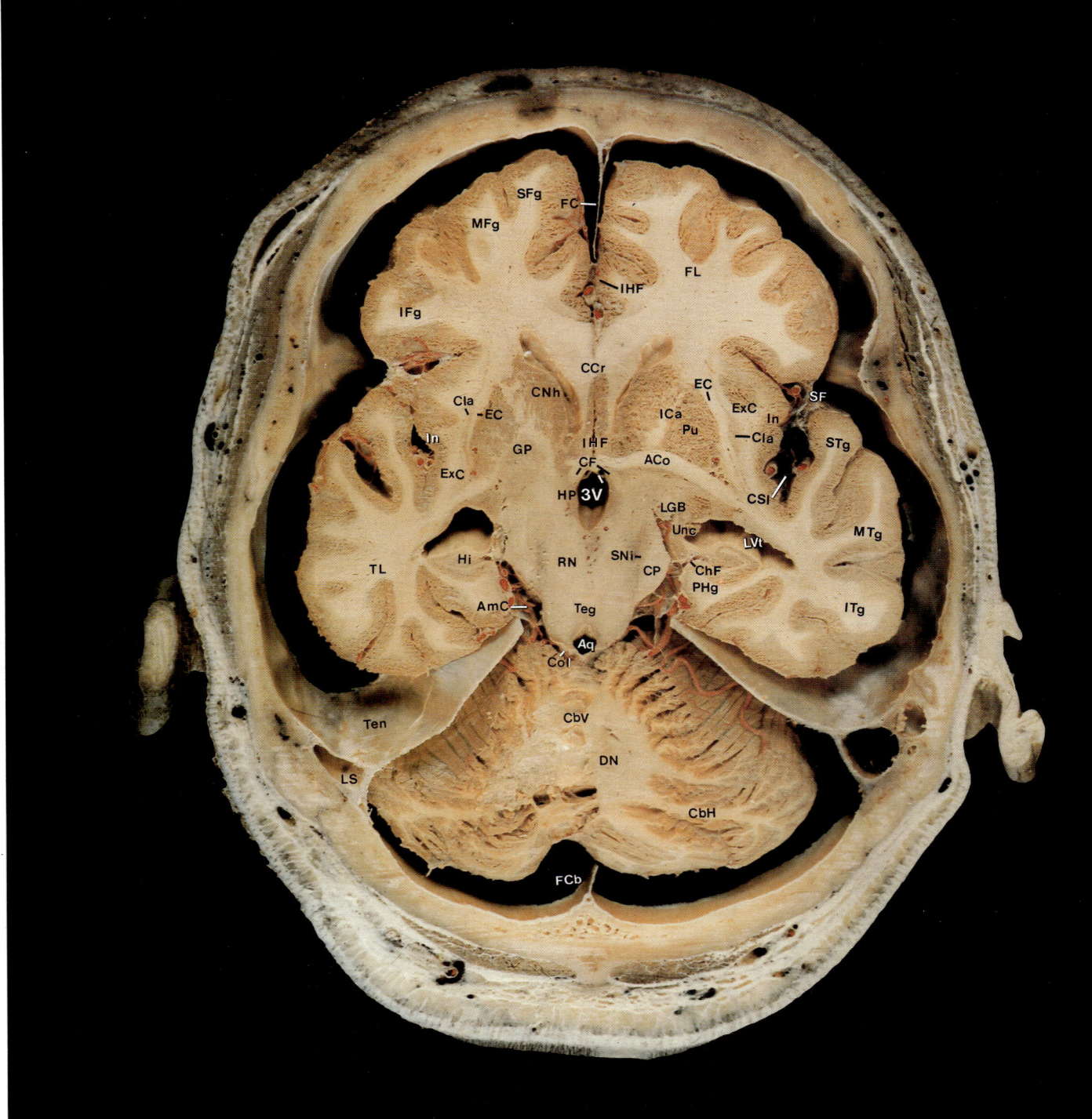

3V	3rd ventricle	ExC	Extreme capsule	MTg	Middle temporal gyrus
ACo	Anterior commissure	FC	Falx cerebri	Mi	Midbrain
AmC	Ambient cistern	FCb	Falx cerebelli	PHg	Parahipocampal gyrus
Aq	Cerebral aqueduct	FL	Frontal lobe	PcA	Pericallosal artery
CCg	Corpus callosum, genu	GP	Globus pallidus	Pu	Putamen
CCr	Corpus callosum, rostrum	Hi	Hippocampus	QC	Quadrigeminal cistern
CF	Column of fornix	Hp	Hypothalamus	RN	Red nucleus
CNh	Caudate nucleus, head	ICa	Internal capsule, anterior limb	SF	Sylvian fissure
CP	Cerebral peduncle	IFg	Inferior frontal gyrus	SFg	Superior frontal gyrus
CSI	Circular sulcus of insula	IHF	Interhemispheric fissure	SNi	Substantia nigra
CSP	Cavum septum pellucidum	ITg	Inferior temporal gyrus	STg	Superior temporal gyrus
CbH	Cerebellar hemisphere	In	Insula	TL	Temporal lobe
CbV	Cerebellar vermis	LGB	Lateral geniculate body	Teg	Tegmentum, midbrain
ChF	Choroidal fissure	LS	Lateral sinus	Ten	Tentorium cerebelli
Cla	Claustrum	LVf	Lateral ventricle, frontal horn	Unc	Uncus
Col	Colliculi (Quadrigeminal plate)	LVt	Lateral ventricle, temporal horn		
DN	Dentate nucleus	MCA	Middle cerebral artery		
EC	External capsule	MFg	Middle frontal gyrus		

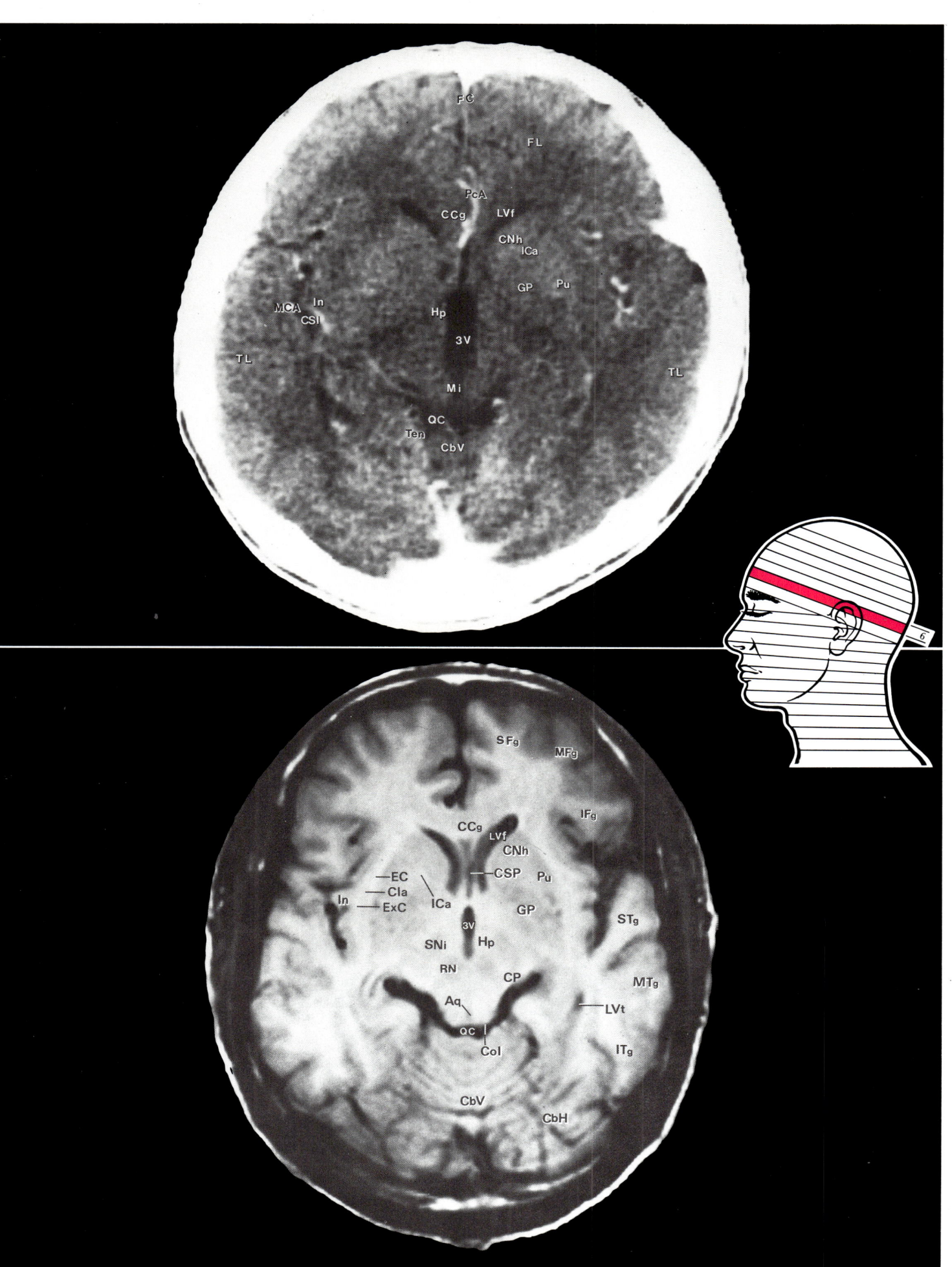

Plate 7. Transverse BRAIN

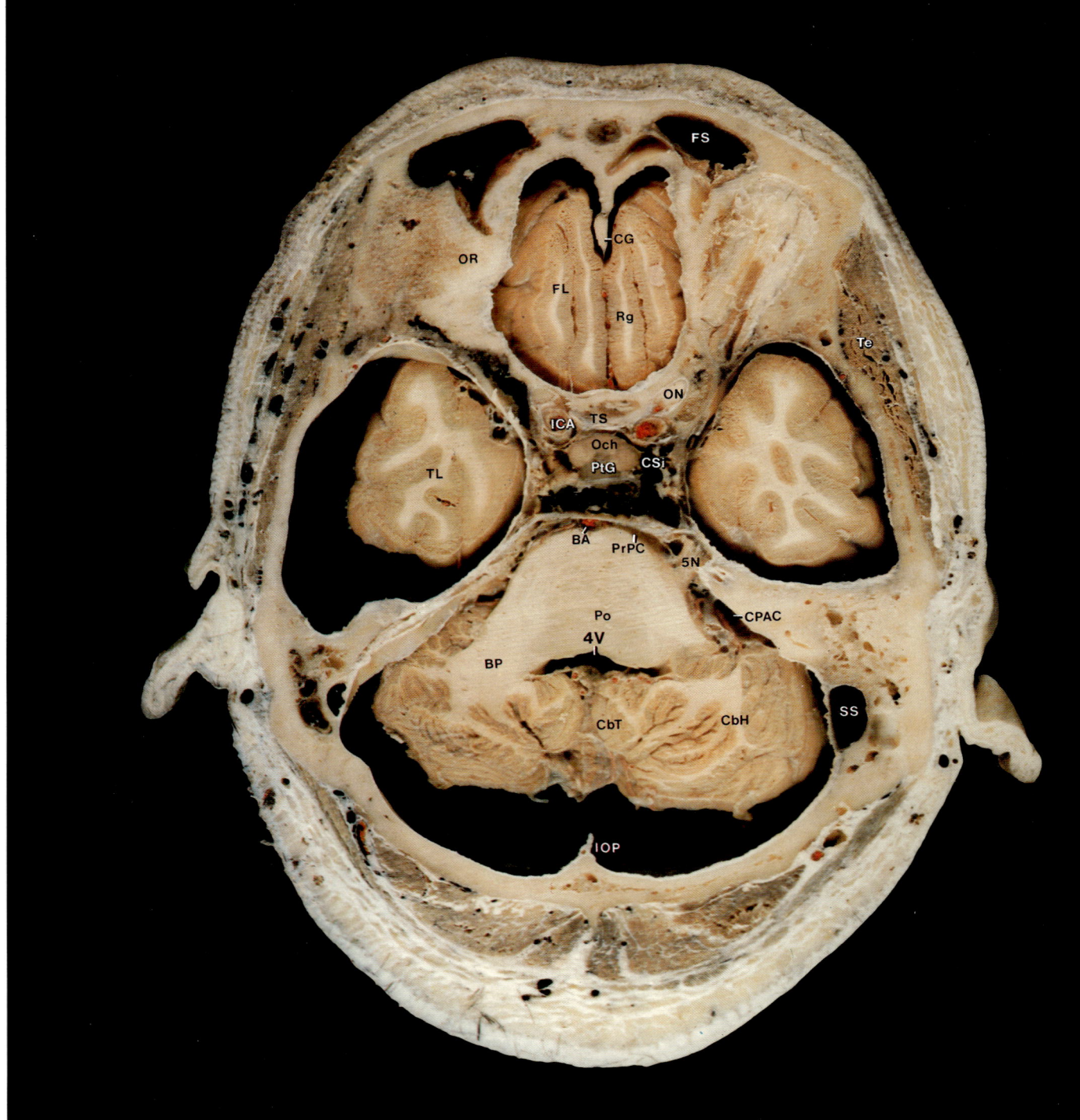

4V	4th ventricle	ITg	Inferior temporal gyrus	SuSC	Suprasellar cistern
5N	5th cranial nerve	LVt	Lateral ventricle, temporal horn	TL	Temporal lobe
ACA	Anterior cerebral artery	MAC	Mastoid air cells	TS	Tuberculum sellae
BA	Basilar artery	MCA	Middle cerebral artery	Te	Temporalis muscle
BP	Brachium pontis	MTg	Middle temporal gyrus	Unc	Uncus
CG	Crista galli	ON	Optic nerve		
CPAC	Cerebellopontine angle cistern	OR	Orbital roof		
CSi	Cavernous sinus	Och	Optic chiasm		
CbH	Cerebellar hemisphere	Og	Orbital gyrus		
CbT	Cerebellar tonsil	PCA	Posterior cerebral artery		
CbV	Cerebellar vermis	PHg	Parahippocampal gyrus		
DN	Dentate nucleus	Po	Pons		
FC	Falx cerebri	PrPC	Pre-pontine cistern		
FL	Frontal lobe	PtG	Pituitary gland		
FS	Frontal sinus	PtS	Pituitary stalk		
ICA	Internal carotid artery	Rg	Rectal gyrus		
IHF	Interhemispheric fissure	SS	Sigmoid sinus		
IOP	Internal occipital protuberance	STg	Superior temporal gyrus		

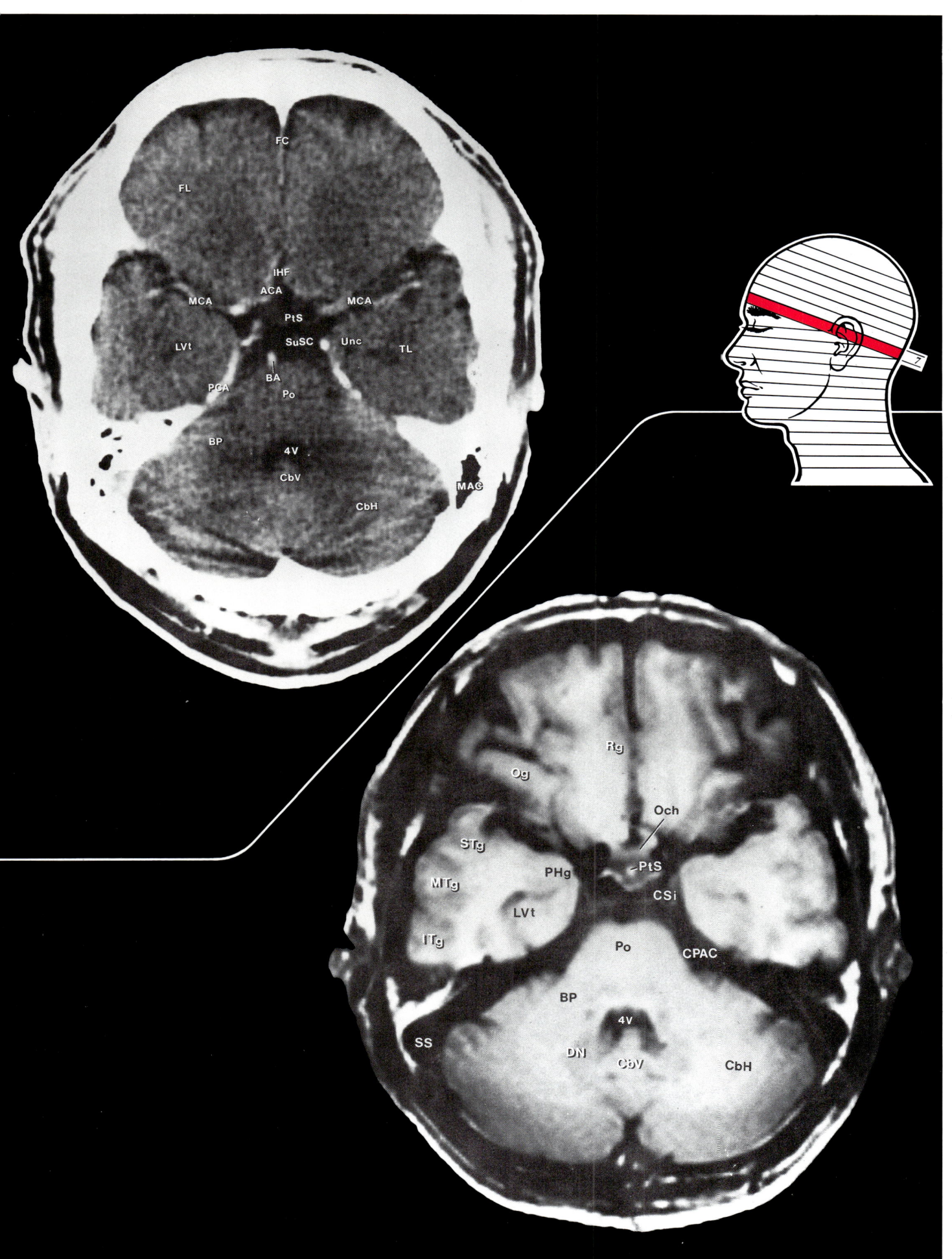

— 17 —

Plate 8. Transverse Head and Neck

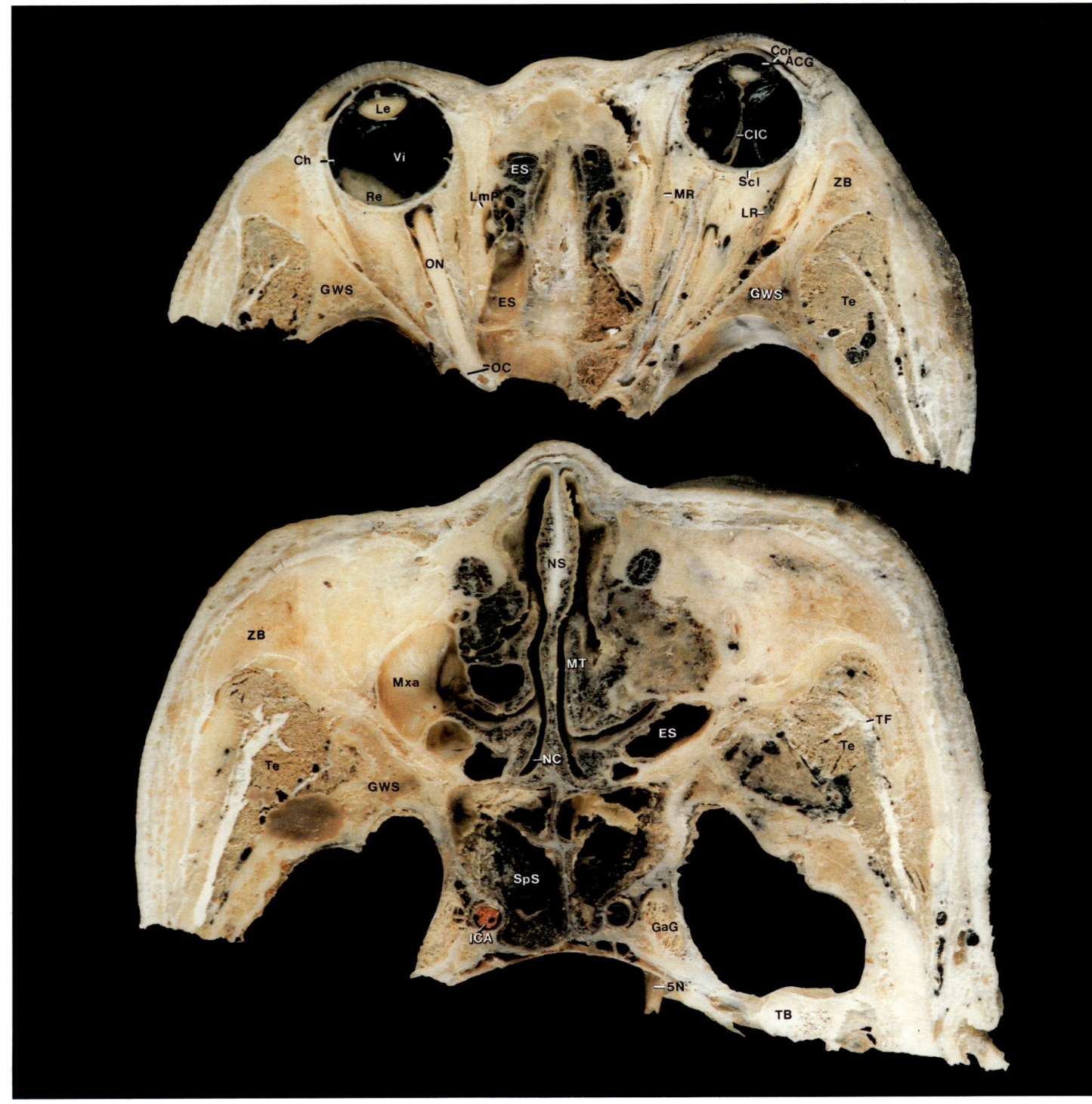

5N	5th cranial nerve	NS	Nasal septum
ACG	Anterior chamber of globe	OC	Optic canal
ClC	Cloquet canal	ON	Optic nerve
Ch	Choroid	Re	Retina
Cor	Cornea	Scl	Sclera
ES	Ethmoid sinus	SpS	Sphenoid sinus
Ey	Eyeball	TB	Temporal bone
GWS	Greater wing of sphenoid	TF	Temporalis fascia
GaG	Gasselian ganglion	TL	Temporal lobe
ICA	Internal carotid artery	Te	Temporalis muscle
LR	Lateral rectus muscle	Vi	Vitreous
Le	Lens	ZB	Zygomatic bone
LmP	Lamina papiracea		
MR	Medial rectus muscle		
MT	Middle turbinate		
Mxa	Maxillary sinus, antrum		
NC	Nasal cavity		
NLD	Nasolacrimal duct		

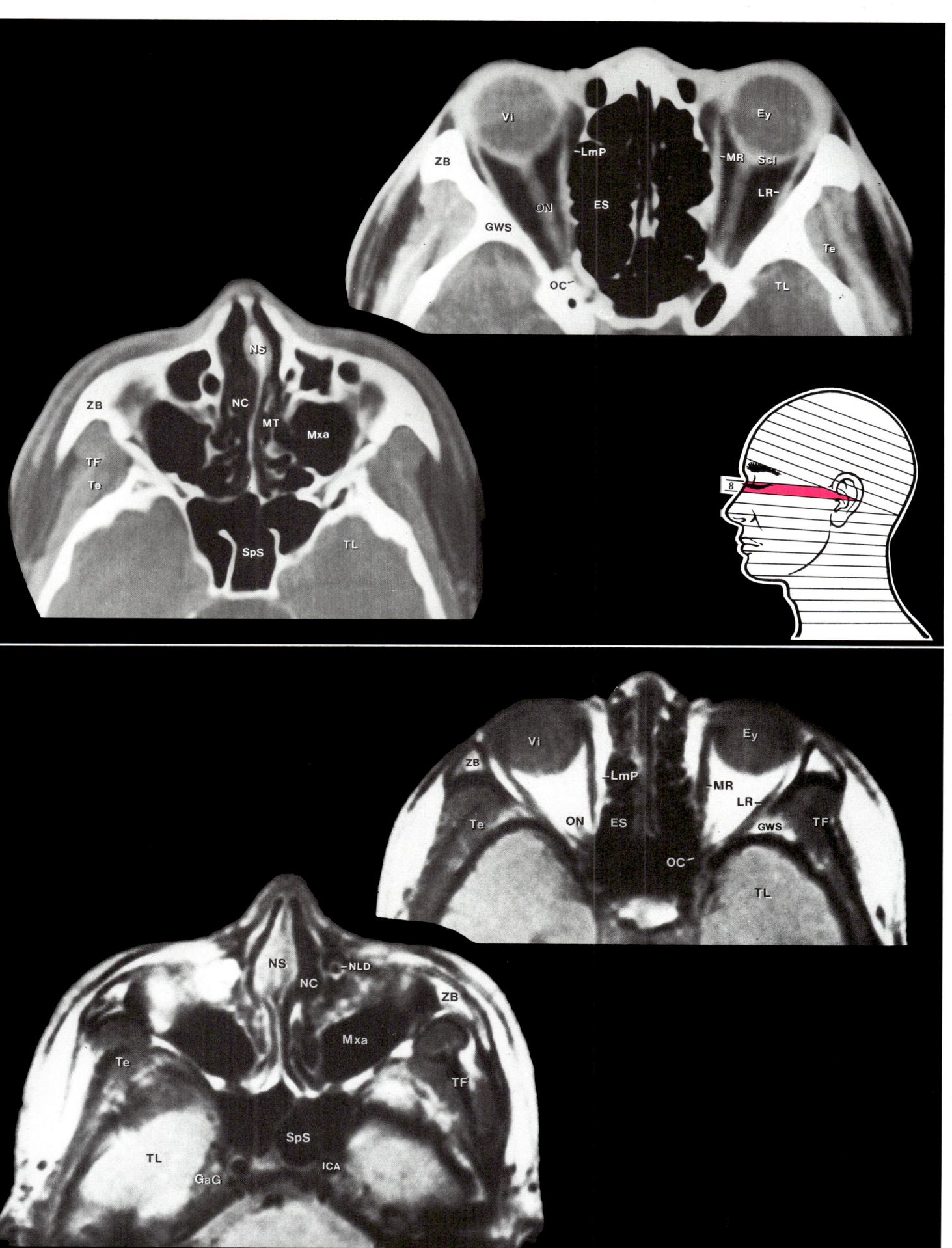

— 19 —

Plate 9. TRANSVERSE HEAD AND NECK

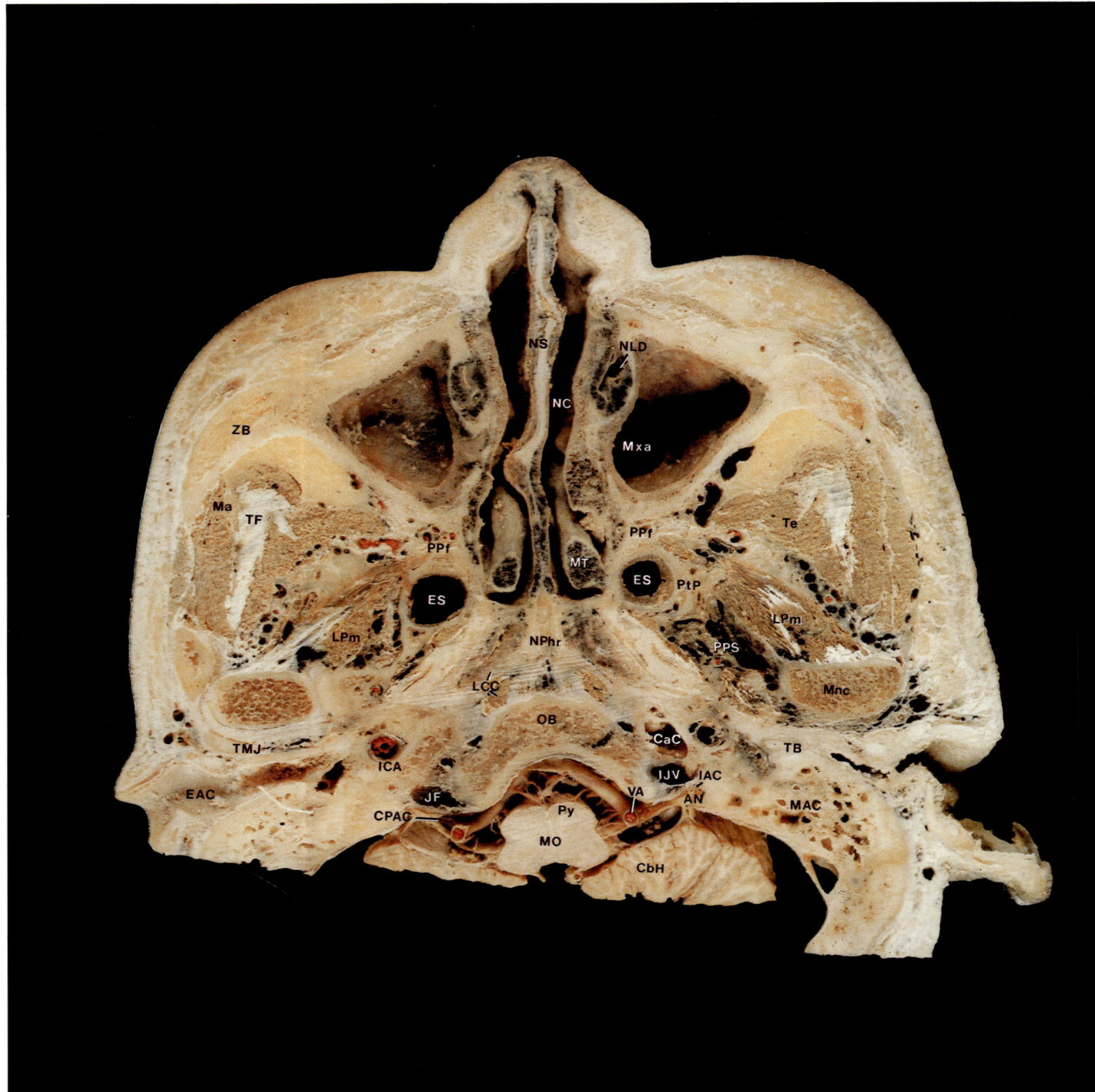

AN	Acoustic nerve	NC	Nasal cavity
CPAC	Cerebellopontine angle cistern	NLD	Nasolacrimal duct
CaC	Carotid canal	NPh	Nasopharynx
CbH	Cerebellar hemisphere	NPhr	Nasopharynx, roof
EAC	External auditory canal	NS	Nasal septum
ES	Ethmoid sinus	OB	Occipital bone
IAC	Internal auditory canal	PPS	Parapharyngeal space
ICA	Internal carotid artery	PPf	Pterygopalatine fossa
IJV	Internal jugular vein	PtP	Pterygoid plate
JF	Jugular foramen	Py	Pyramid
LCC	Longus capitis & colli muscle	TB	Temporal bone
LPm	Lateral pterygoid muscle	TF	Temporalis fascia
MAC	Mastoid air cells	TMJ	Temporomandibular joint
MO	Medulla oblongata	Te	Temporalis muscle
MT	Middle turbinate	VA	Vertebral artery
Ma	Masseter muscle	ZB	Zygomatic bone
Mnc	Mandible, condylar process		
Mxa	Maxillary sinus, antrum		

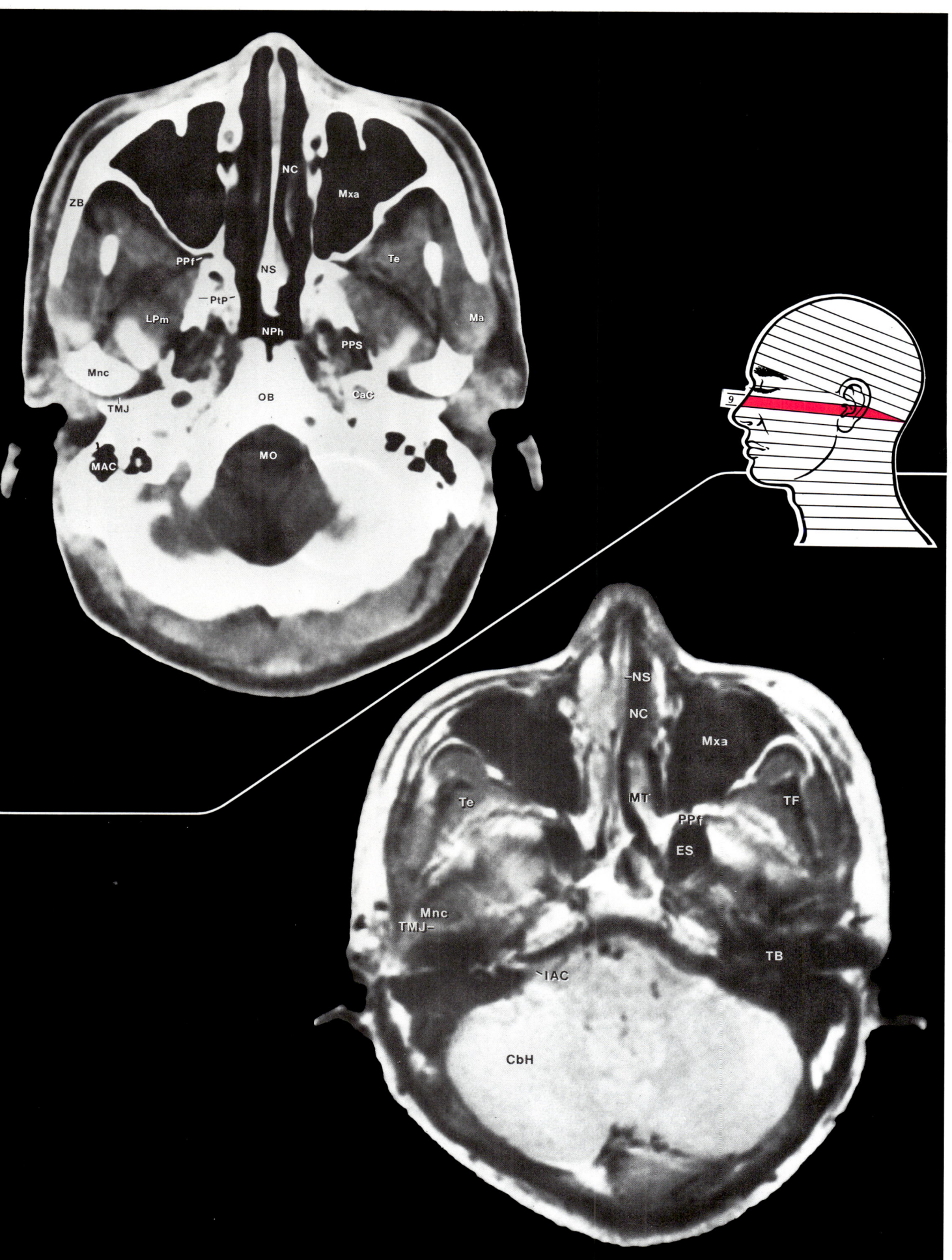

Plate 10. TRANSVERSE HEAD AND NECK

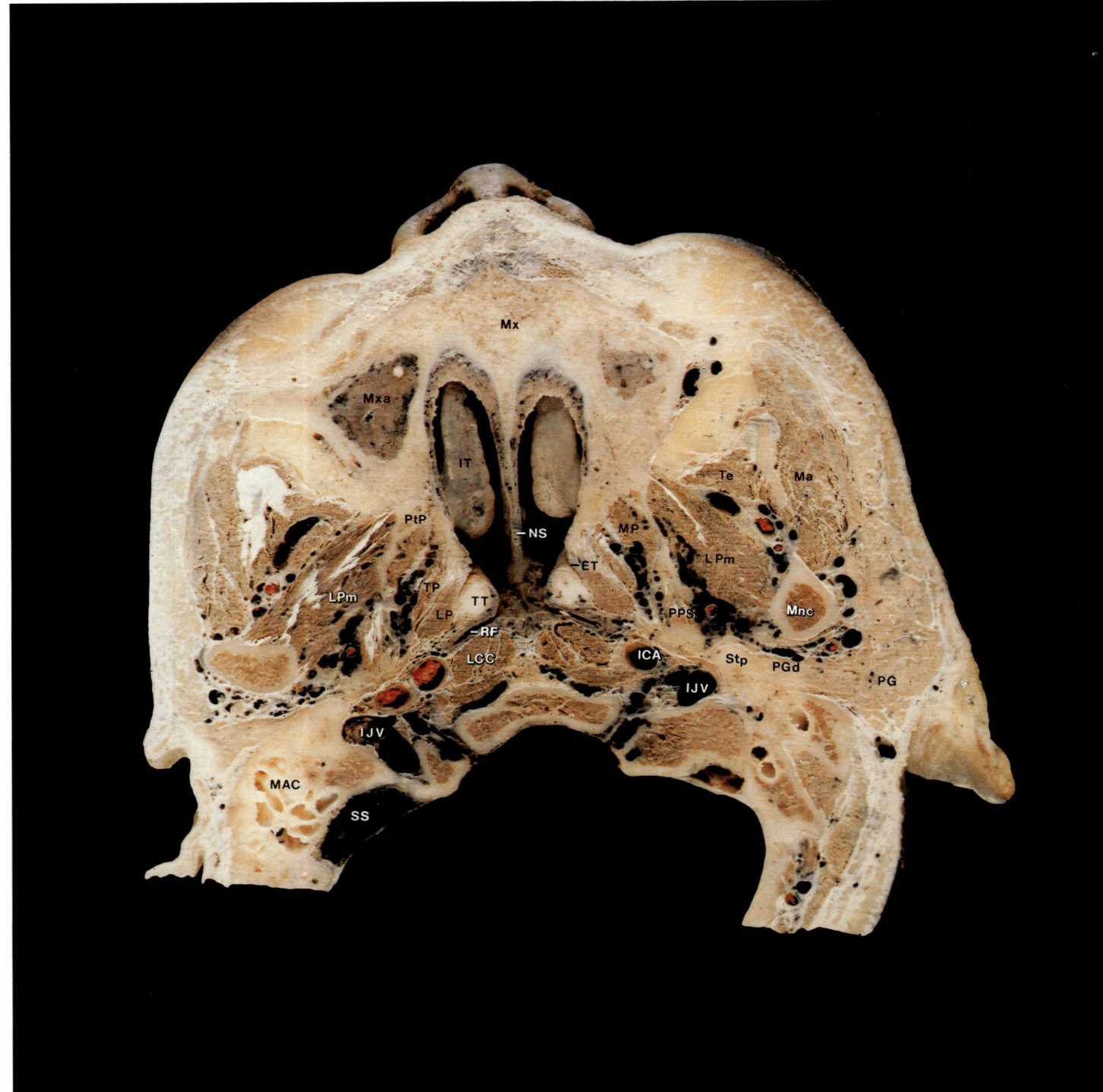

CbH	Cerebellar hemisphere	PG	Parotid gland
ET	Eustachian tube	PGd	Parotid gland, deep lobe
ICA	Internal carotid artery	PPS	Parapharyngeal space
IJV	Internal jugular vein	PtP	Pterygoid plate
IT	Inferior turbinate	RF	Rosenmuller fossa
LCC	Longus capitis & colli muscle	RMV	Retromandibular vein
LP	Levator palati muscle	SS	Sigmoid sinus
LPm	Lateral pterygoid muscle	Stp	Styloid process
MAC	Mastoid air cells	TP	Tensor palati muscle
MO	Medulla oblongata	TT	Torus tubarius
MP	Medial pterygoid muscle	Te	Temporalis muscle
Ma	Masseter muscle		
Mnc	Mandible, condylar process		
Mnr	Mandible, ramus		
Mx	Maxilla		
Mxa	Maxillary sinus, antrum		
NS	Nasal septum		
NPh	Nasopharynx		

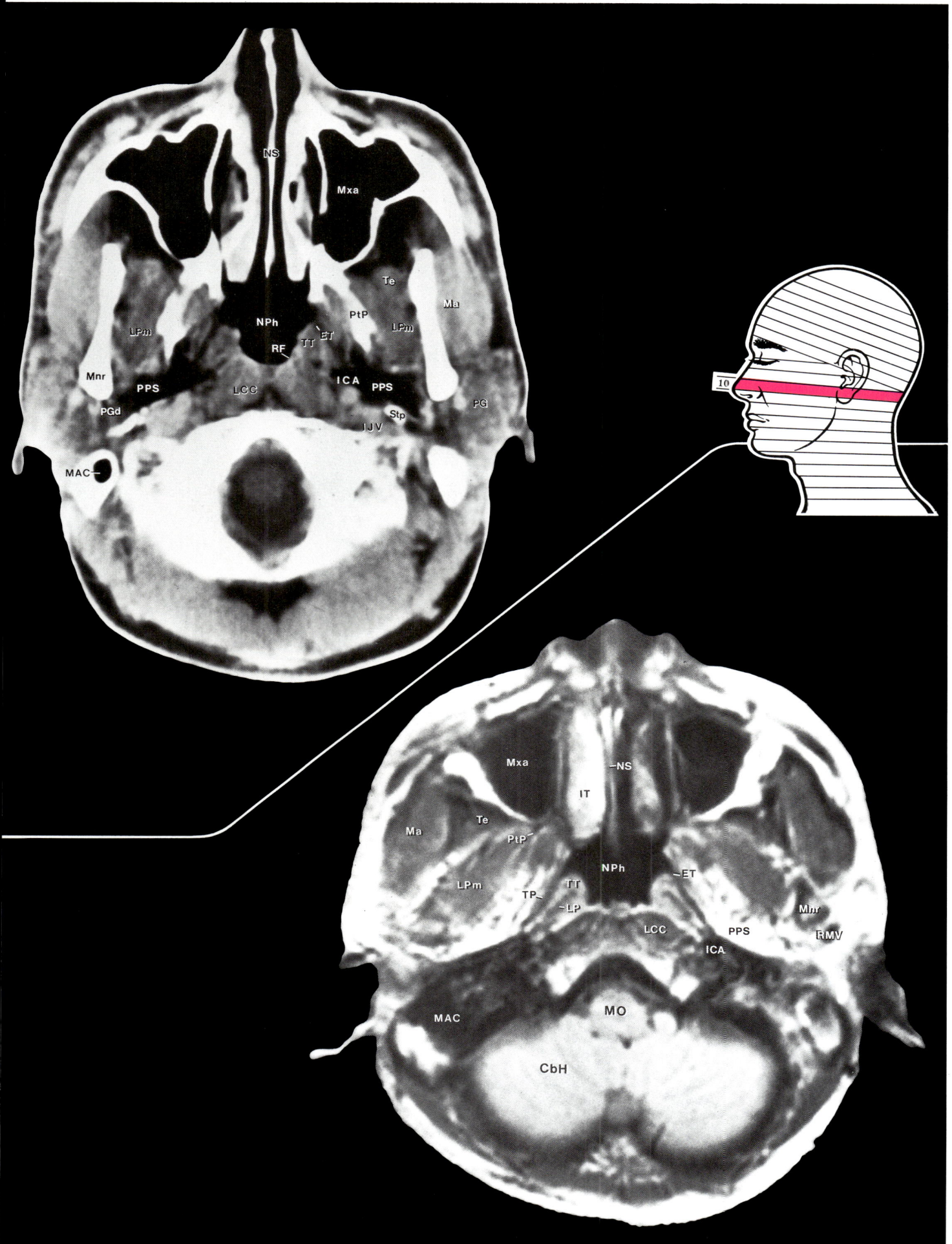

Plate 11. Transverse HEAD and NECK

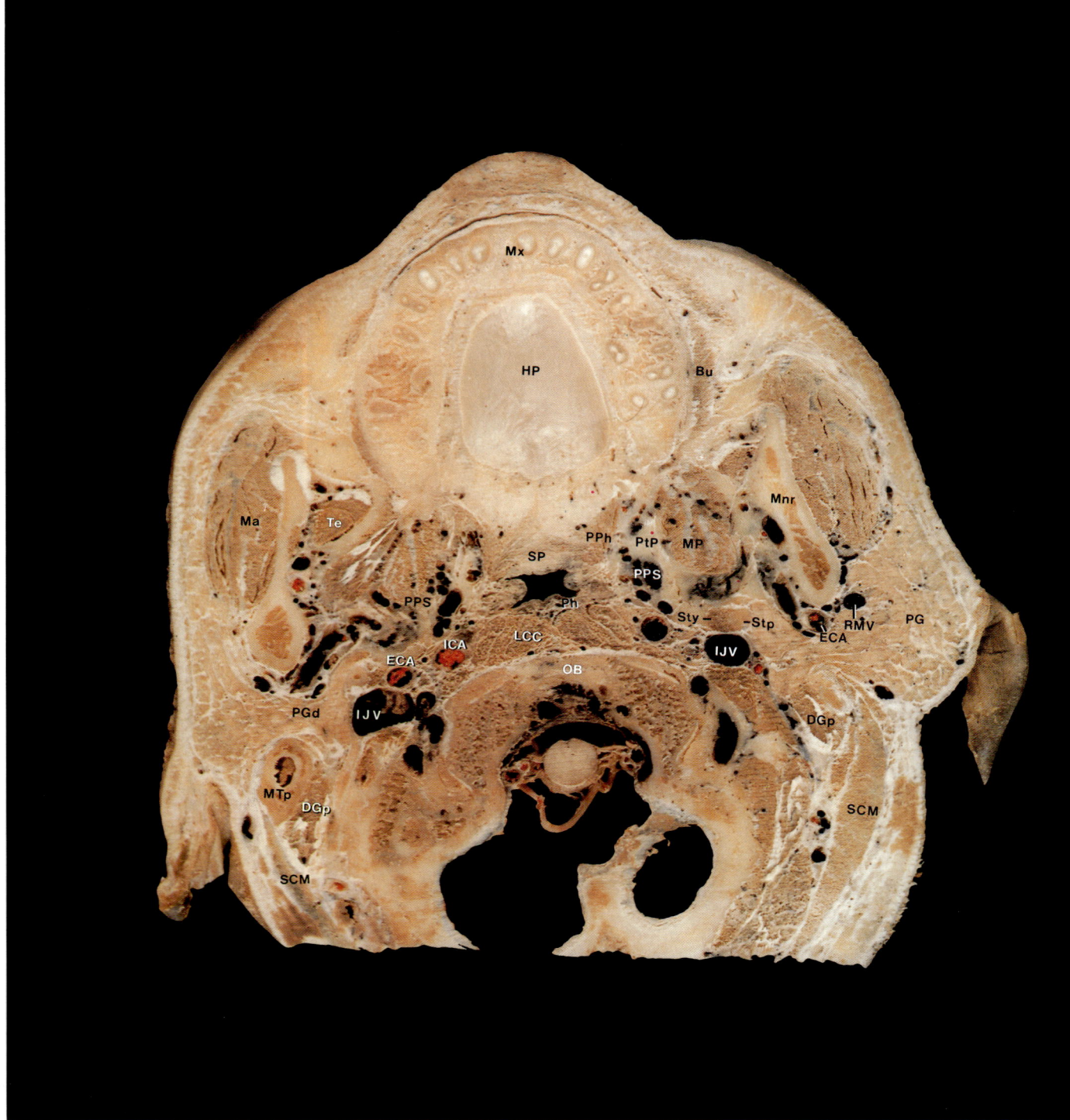

Bu	Buccinator muscle	Ph	Pharyngeal muscles
DGp	Digastric muscle, posterior belly	PtP	Pterygoid plate
ECA	External carotid artery	RMV	Retromandibular vein
HP	Hard palate	SCM	Sternocleidomastoid muscle
ICA	Internal carotid artery	SP	Soft palate
IJV	Internal jugular vein	Stp	Styloid process
LCC	Longus capitis & colli muscle	Sty	Styloid muscle
MP	Medial pterygoid muscle	Te	Temporalis muscle
MTp	Mastoid tip	VA	Vertebral artery
Ma	Masseter muscle		
Mnr	Mandible, ramus		
Mx	Maxilla		
NPh	Nasopharynx		
OB	Occipital bone		
PG	Parotid gland		
PGd	Parotid gland, deep lobe		
PPS	Parapharyngeal space		
PPh	Palatopharyngeus muscle		

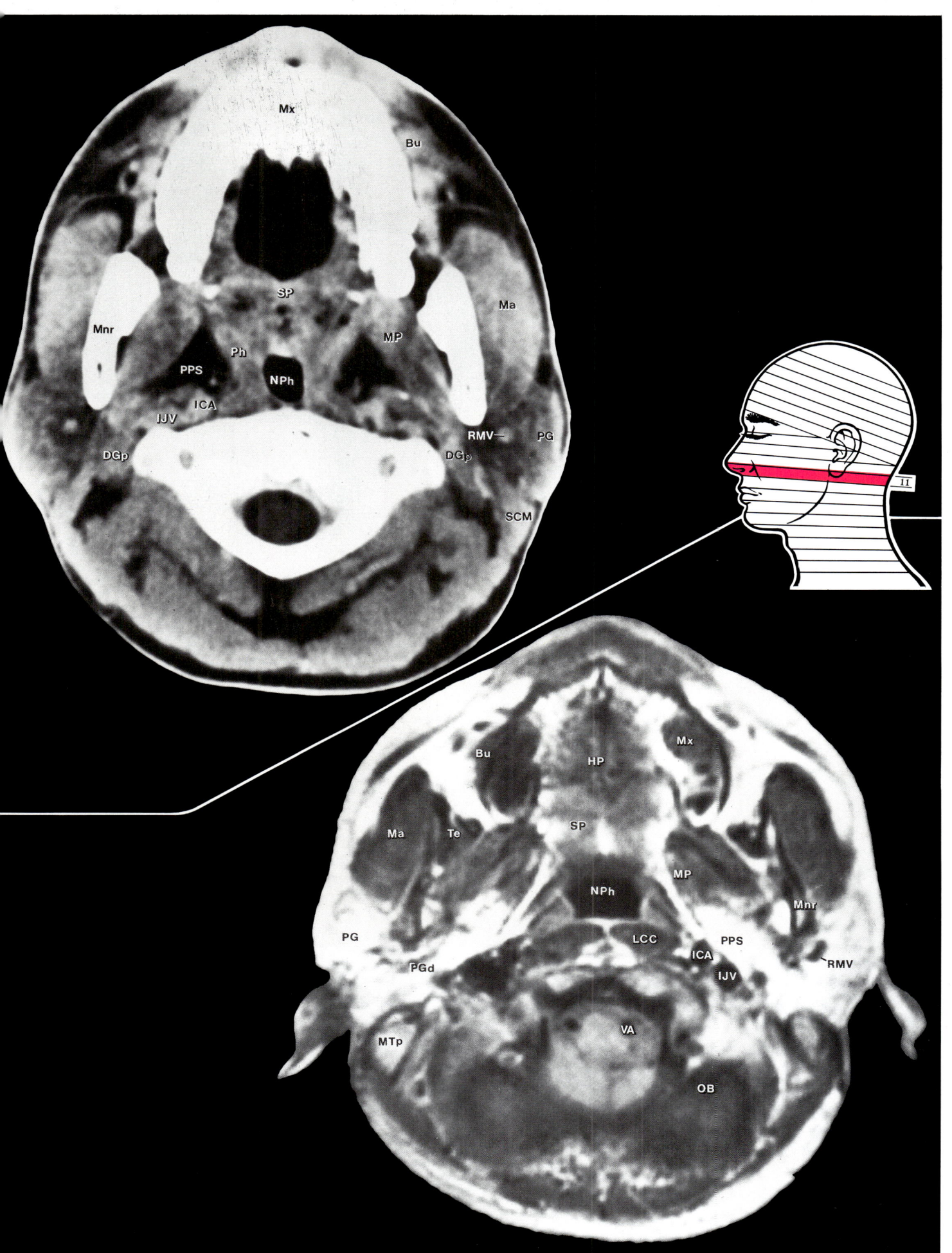

Plate 12. Transverse HEAD AND NECK

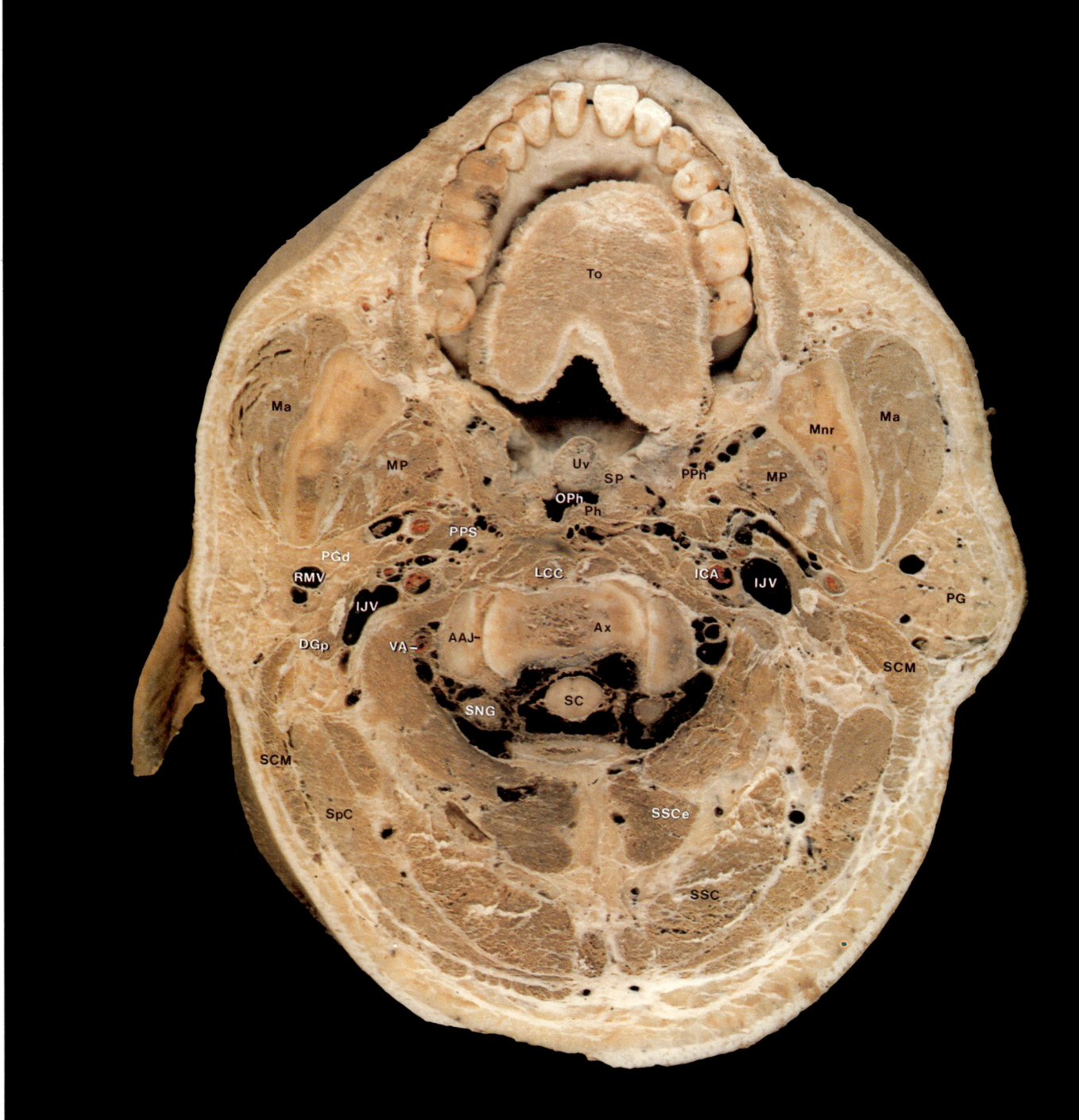

AAJ	Atlantoaxial joint
Ax	Axis
Bu	Buccinator muscle
DGp	Digastric muscle, posterior belly
ICA	Internal carotid artery
IJV	Internal jugular vein
LCC	Longus capitis & colli muscle
MP	Medial pterygoid muscle
Ma	Masseter muscle
Mnr	Mandible, ramus
OPh	Oropharynx
PG	Parotid gland
PGd	Parotid gland, deep lobe
PPS	Parapharyngeal space
PPh	Palatopharyngeus muscle
Ph	Pharyngeal muscles
RMV	Retromandibular vein
SAS	Subarachnoid space
SC	Spinal cord
SCM	Sternocleidomastoid muscle
SNG	Spinal nerve ganglion
SP	Soft palate
SSC	Semispinalis capitis muscle
SSCe	Semispinalis cervicalis muscle
SpC	Splenius capitis muscle
To	Tongue
Uv	Uvula
VA	Vertebral artery

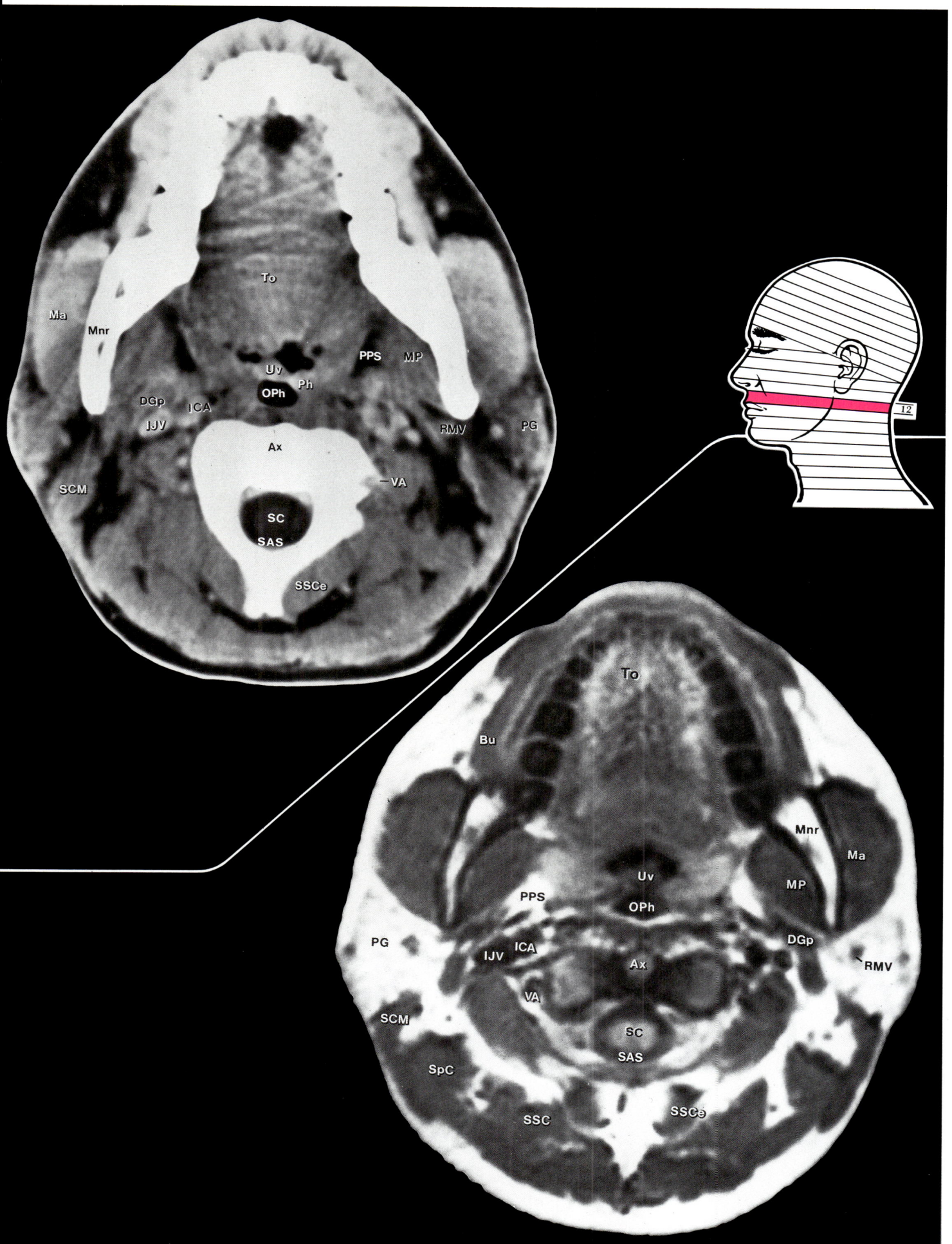

Plate 13. TRANSVERSE HEAD AND NECK

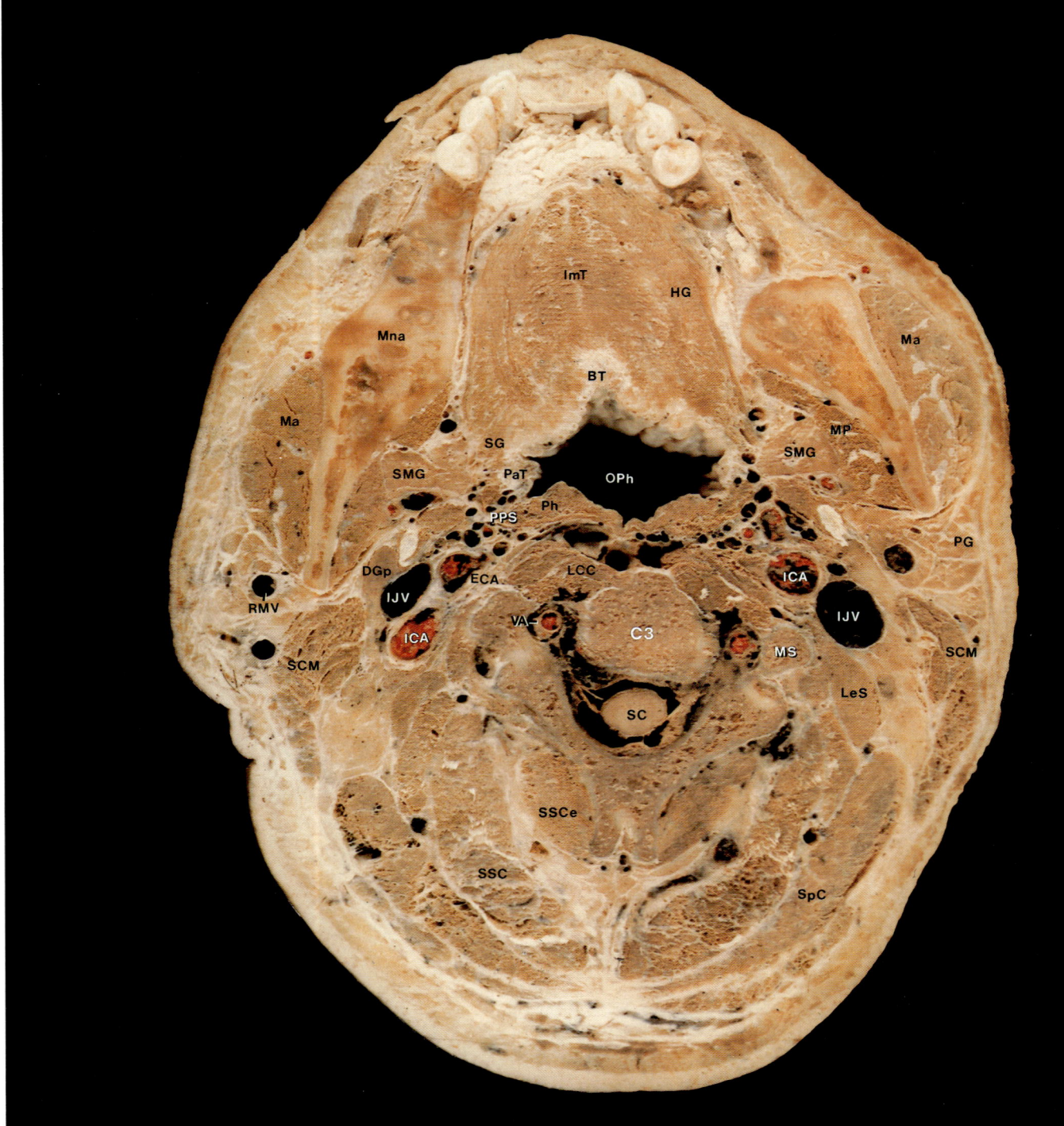

BT	Base of tongue	PPS	Parapharyngeal space
C3	C3 vertebral body	PaT	Palatine tonsil
DGp	Digastric muscle, posterior belly	Ph	Pharyngeal muscles
ECA	External carotid artery	RMV	Retromandibular vein
HG	Hyoglossus muscle	SAS	Subarachnoid space
ICA	Internal carotid artery	SC	Spinal cord
IJV	Internal jugular vein	SCM	Sternocleidomastoid muscle
ImT	Intrinsic muscle of tongue	SG	Styloglossus muscle
LCC	Longus capitis & colli muscle	SMG	Submandibular gland
LeS	Levator scapularis muscle	SSC	Semispinalis capitis muscle
MP	Medial pterygoid muscle	SSCe	Semispinalis cervicalis muscle
MS	Middle scalene muscle	SpC	Splenius capitis muscle
Ma	Masseter muscle	VA	Vertebral artery
Mna	Mandible, angle		
Mnb	Mandible, body		
OPh	Oropharynx		
PG	Parotid gland		
PGd	Parotid gland, deep lobe		

— 28 —

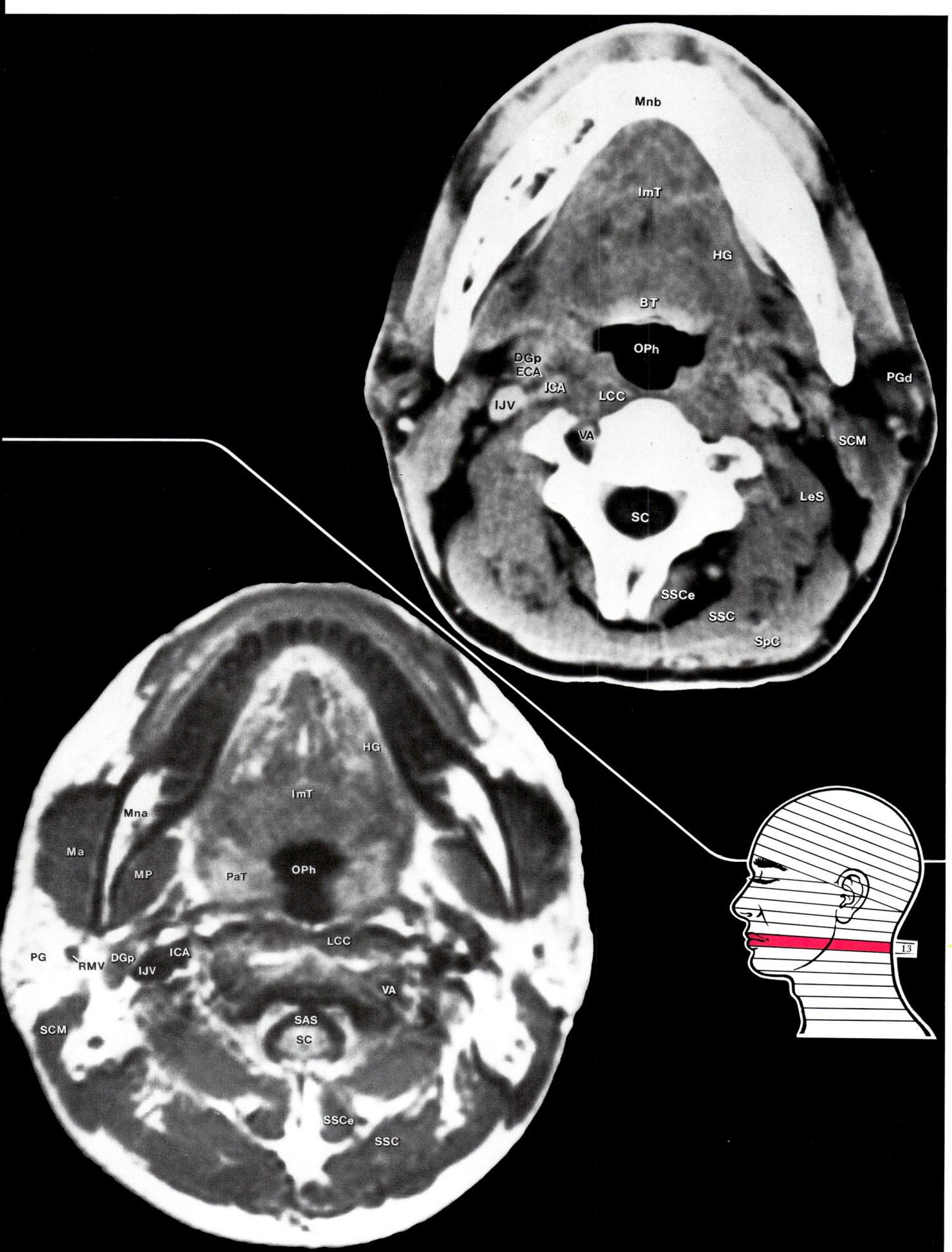

Plate 14. Transverse HEAD AND NECK

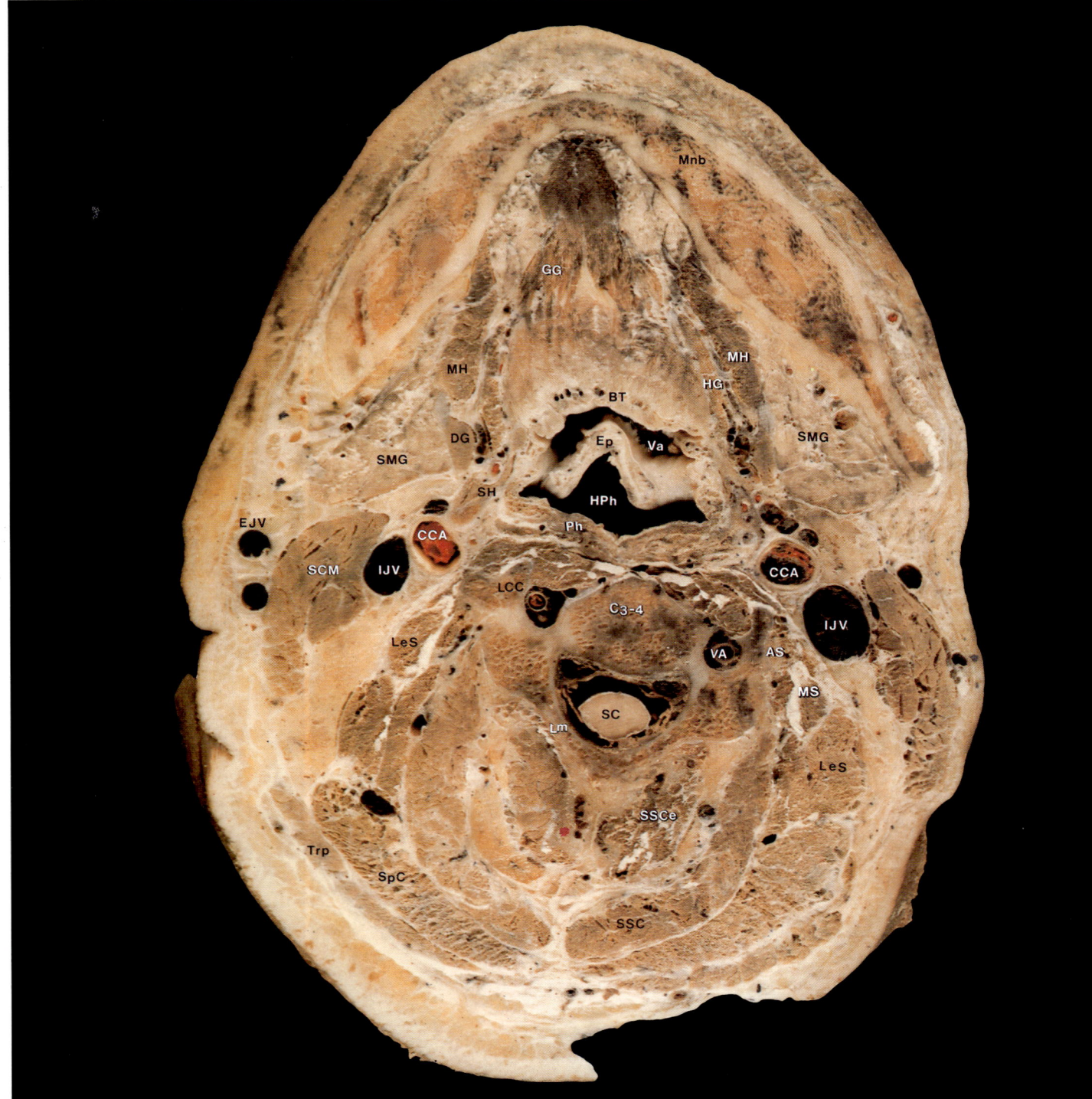

AS	Anterior scalene muscle	Mnb	Mandible, body
BT	Base of tongue	PPS	Parapharyngeal space
C3-4	C3-4 intervertebral disc	Ph	Pharyngeal muscles
CCA	Common carotid artery	SC	Spinal cord
DG	Digastric muscle	SCM	Sternocleidomastoid muscle
ECA	External carotid artery	SH	Stylohyoid muscle
EJV	External jugular vein	SMG	Submandibular gland
Ep	Epiglottis	SSC	Semispinalis capitis muscle
GG	Genioglossus muscle	SSCe	Semispinalis cervicalis muscle
HG	Hyoglossus muscle	SpC	Splenius capitis muscle
HPh	Hypopharynx	Trp	Trapezius muscle
ICA	Internal carotid artery	VA	Vertebral artery
IJV	Internal jugular vein	VB	Vertebral body
LCC	Longus capitis & colli muscle	Va	Vallecula
LeS	Levator scapularis muscle		
Lm	Lamina		
MH	Mylohyoid muscle		
MS	Middle scalene muscle		

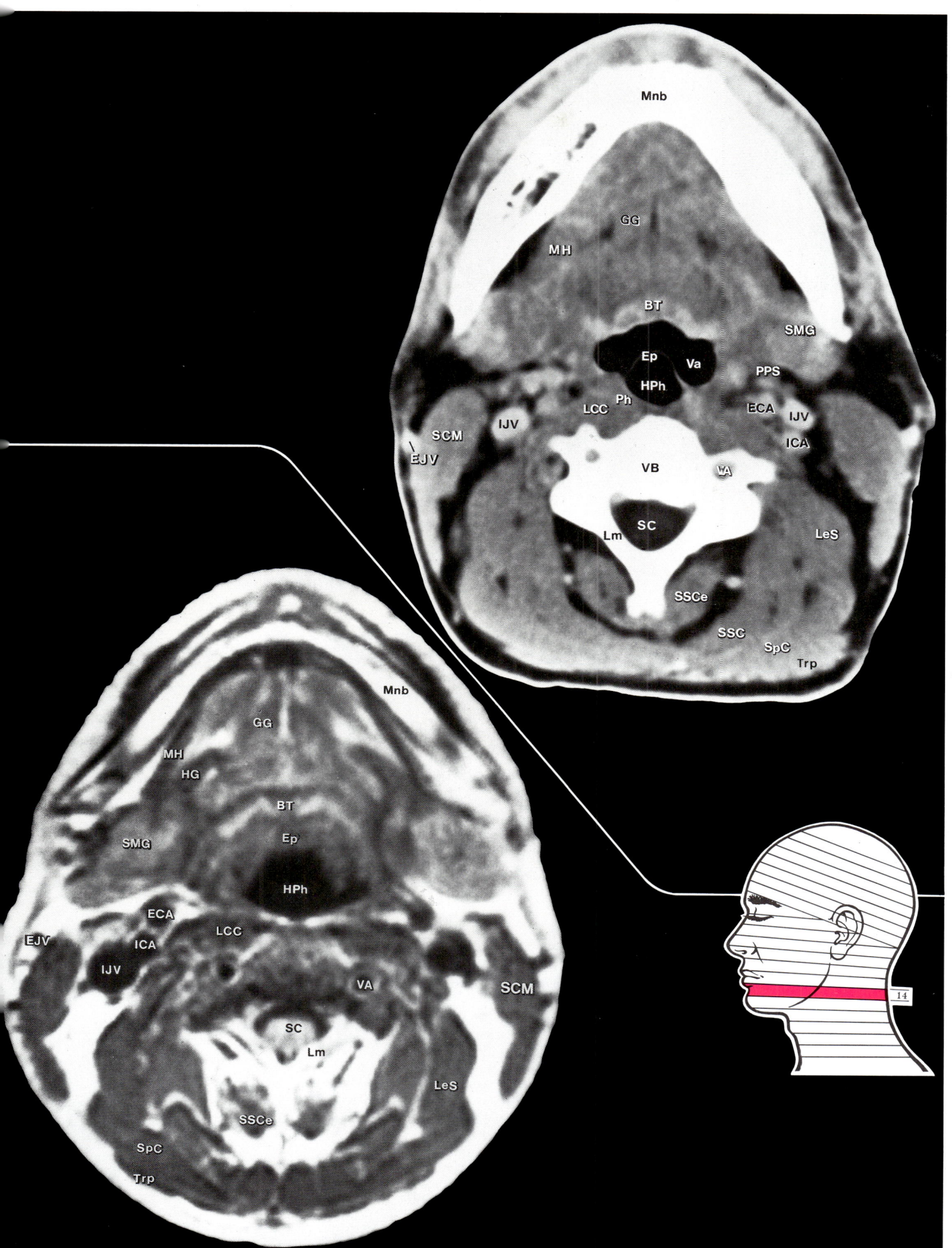

Plate 15. Transverse HEAD AND NECK

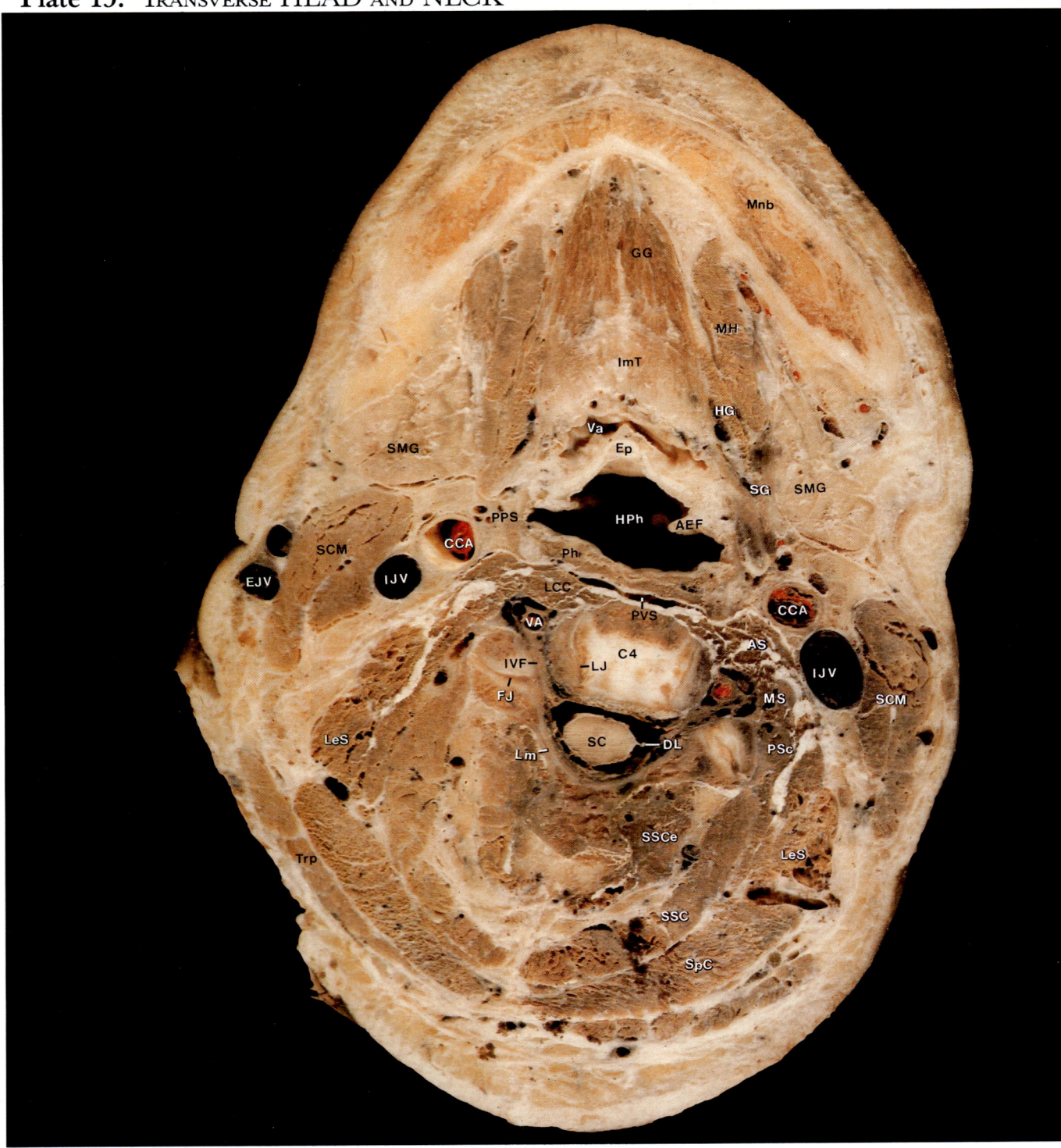

AEF	Aryepiglottic fold	LJ	Luschka joint	VA	Vertebral artery
AS	Anterior scalene muscle	LeS	Levator scapularis muscle	Va	Vallecula
C4	C4 vertebral body	Lm	Lamina		
CCA	Common carotid artery	MH	Mylohyoid muscle		
DL	Dentate ligament	MS	Middle scalene muscle		
ECA	External carotid artery	Mnb	Mandible, body		
EJV	External jugular vein	PPS	Parapharyngeal space		
Ep	Epiglottis	PSc	Posterior scalane muscle		
FJ	Facet joint of cervical spine	PVS	Prevertebral space		
GG	Genioglossus muscle	Ph	Pharyngeal muscles		
HB	Hyoid bone	SC	Spinal cord		
HG	Hyoglossus muscle	SCM	Sternocleidomastoid muscle		
HPh	Hypopharynx	SG	Styloglossus muscle		
ICA	Internal carotid artery	SMG	Submandibular gland		
IJV	Internal jugular vein	SSC	Semispinalis capitis muscle		
IVF	Intervertebral foramen	SSCe	Semispinalis cervicalis muscle		
ImT	Intrinsic muscle of tongue	SpC	Splenius capitis muscle		
LCC	Longus capitis & colli muscle	Trp	Trapezius muscle		

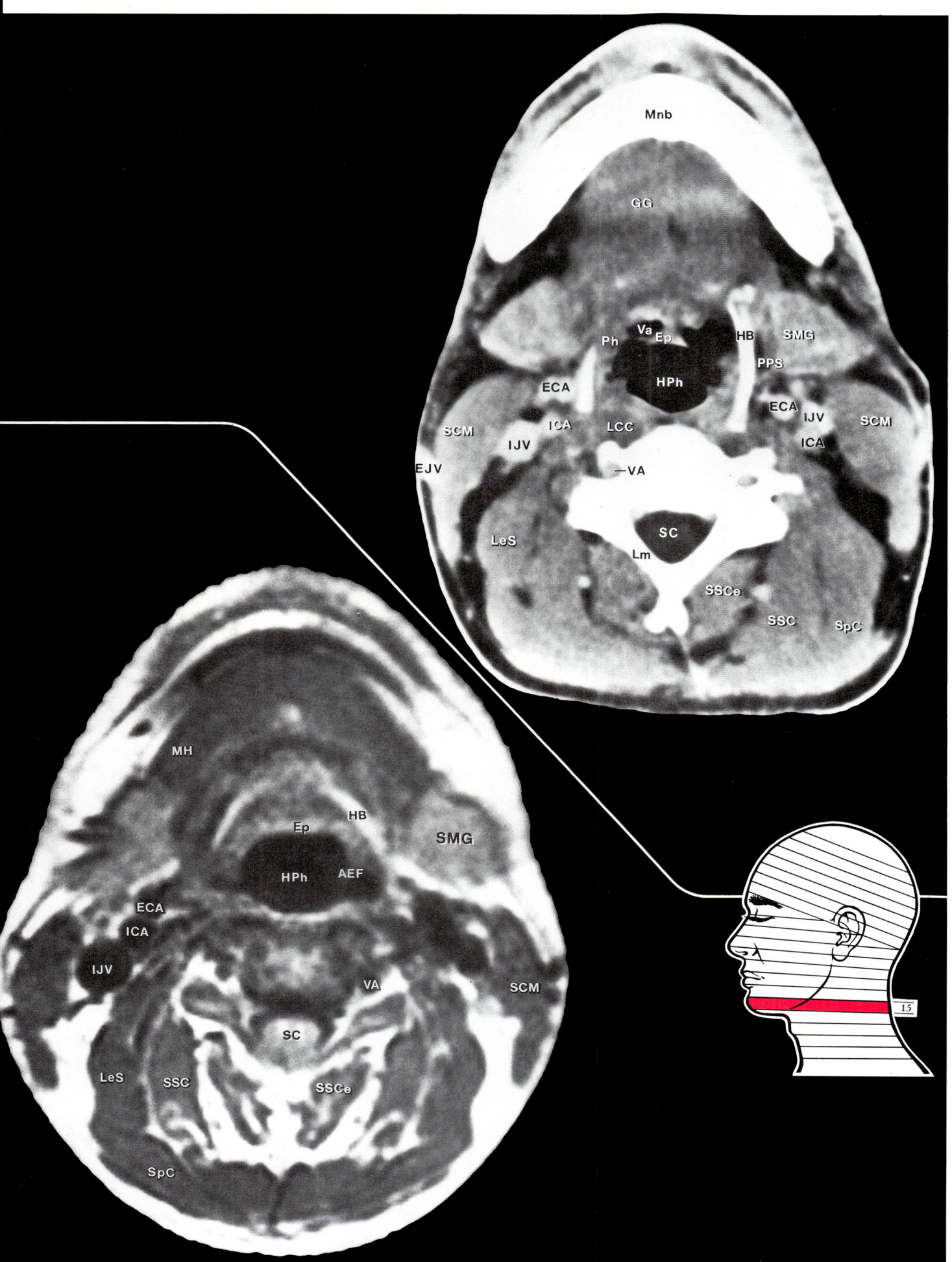

Plate 16. Transverse HEAD and NECK

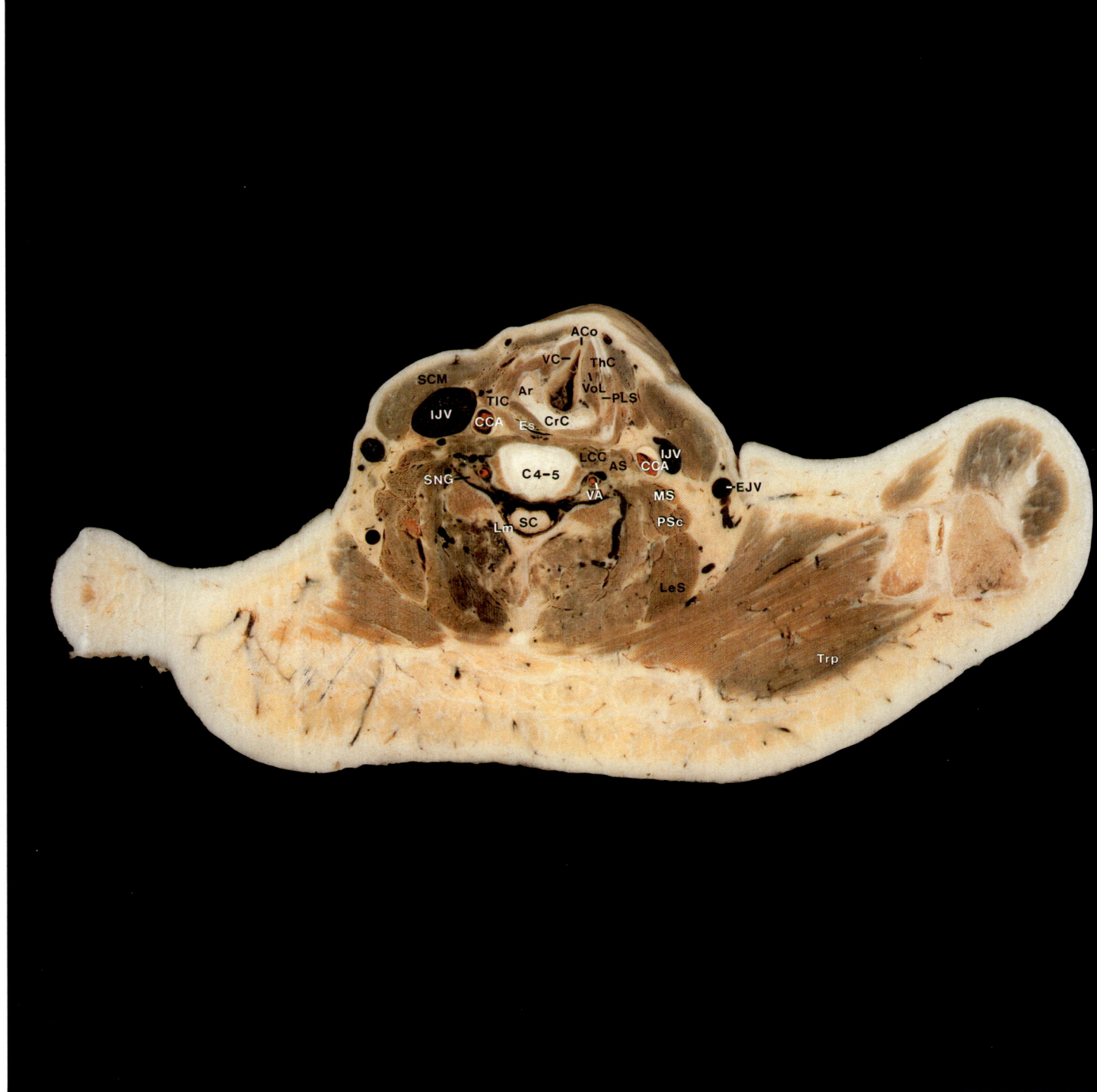

ACo	Anterior commissure of larynx	SNG	Spinal nerve ganglion
AS	Anterior scalene muscle	TIC	Thyroid cartilage, inferior cornu
Ar	Arytenoid	ThC	Thyroid cartilage
C4-5	C4-5 intervertebral disc	TrF	Transverse foramen
CCA	Common carotid artery	Trp	Trapezius muscle
CrC	Cricoid cartilage	VA	Vertebral artery
EJV	External jugular vein	VB	Vertebral body
Es	Esophagus	VC	Vocal cord
IJV	Internal jugular vein	VoL	Vocal ligament
LCC	Longus capitis & colli muscle		
LeS	Levator scapularis muscle		
Lm	Lamina		
MS	Middle scalene muscle		
PLS	Paralaryngeal space		
PSc	Posterior scalane muscle		
SC	Spinal cord		
SCM	Sternocleidomastoid muscle		
SCe	Spinalis cervicalis muscle		

— 34 —

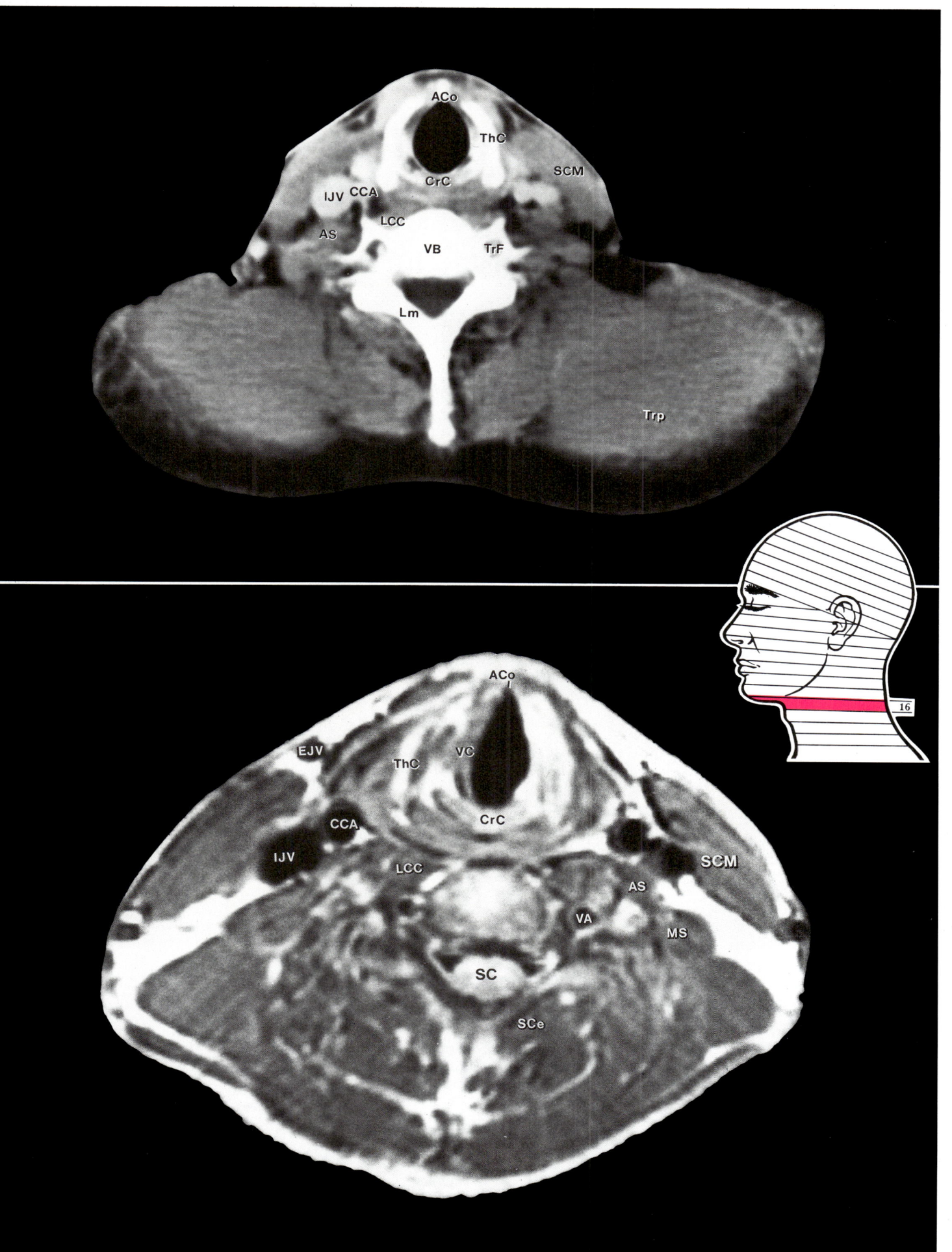

Plate 17. Transverse HEAD AND NECK

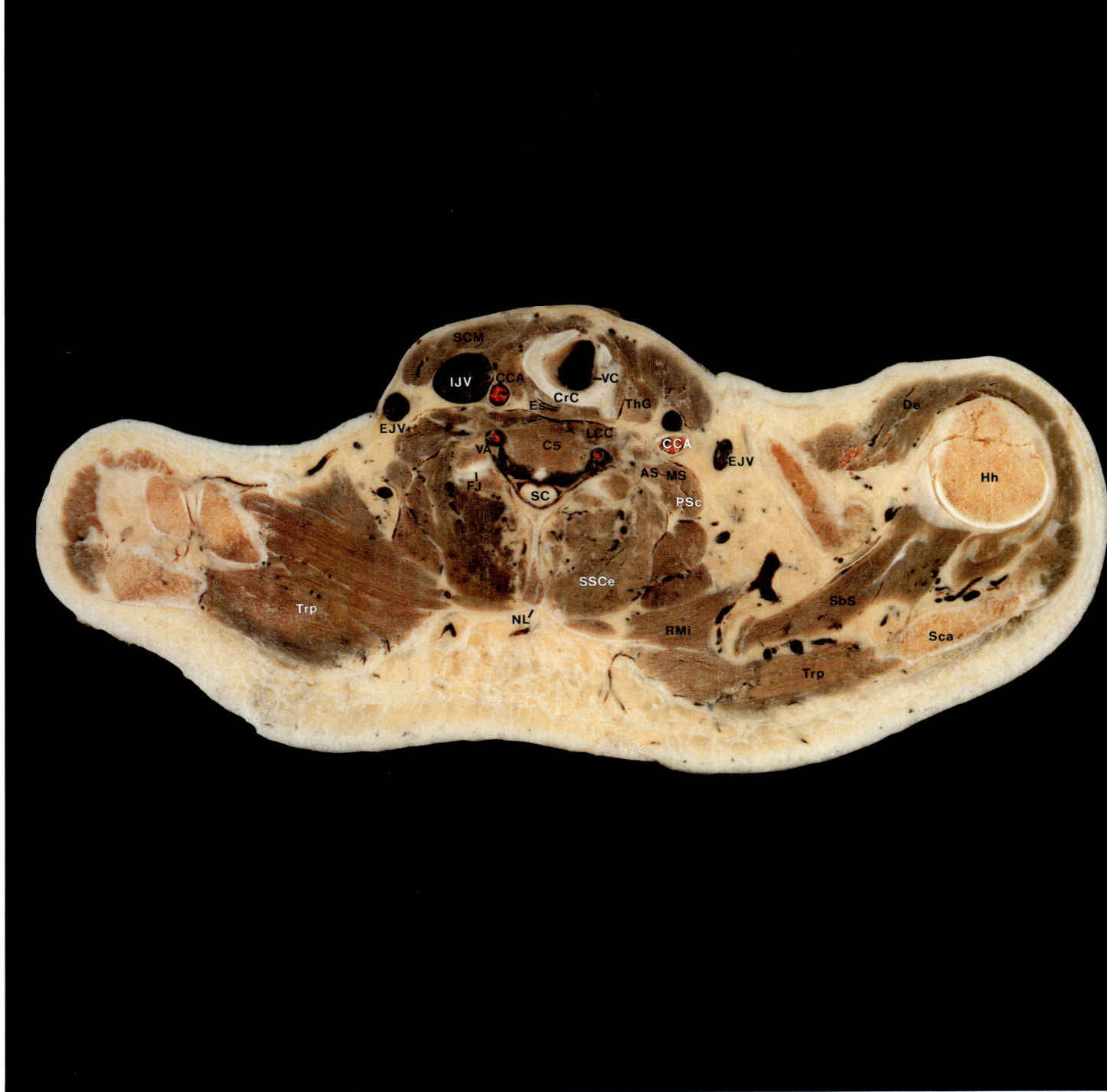

AS	Anterior scalene muscle	SSCe	Semispinalis cervicalis muscle
C5	C5 vertebral body	SbS	Subscapular muscle
CCA	Common carotid artery	Sca	Scapula
CrC	Cricoid cartilage	ThG	Thyroid gland
De	Deltoid muscle	Tr	Trachea
EJV	External jugular vein	TrF	Transverse foramen
Es	Esophagus	Trp	Trapezius muscle
FJ	Facet joint of cervical spine	VA	Vertebral artery
Hh	Humerus, head	VC	Vocal cord
IJV	Internal jugular vein		
LCC	Longus capitis & colli muscle		
MS	Middle scalene muscle		
NL	Nuchal ligament		
PSc	Posterior scalane muscle		
RMi	Rhomboideus minor muscle		
SC	Spinal cord		
SCM	Sternocleidomastoid muscle		
SCe	Spinalis cervicalis muscle		

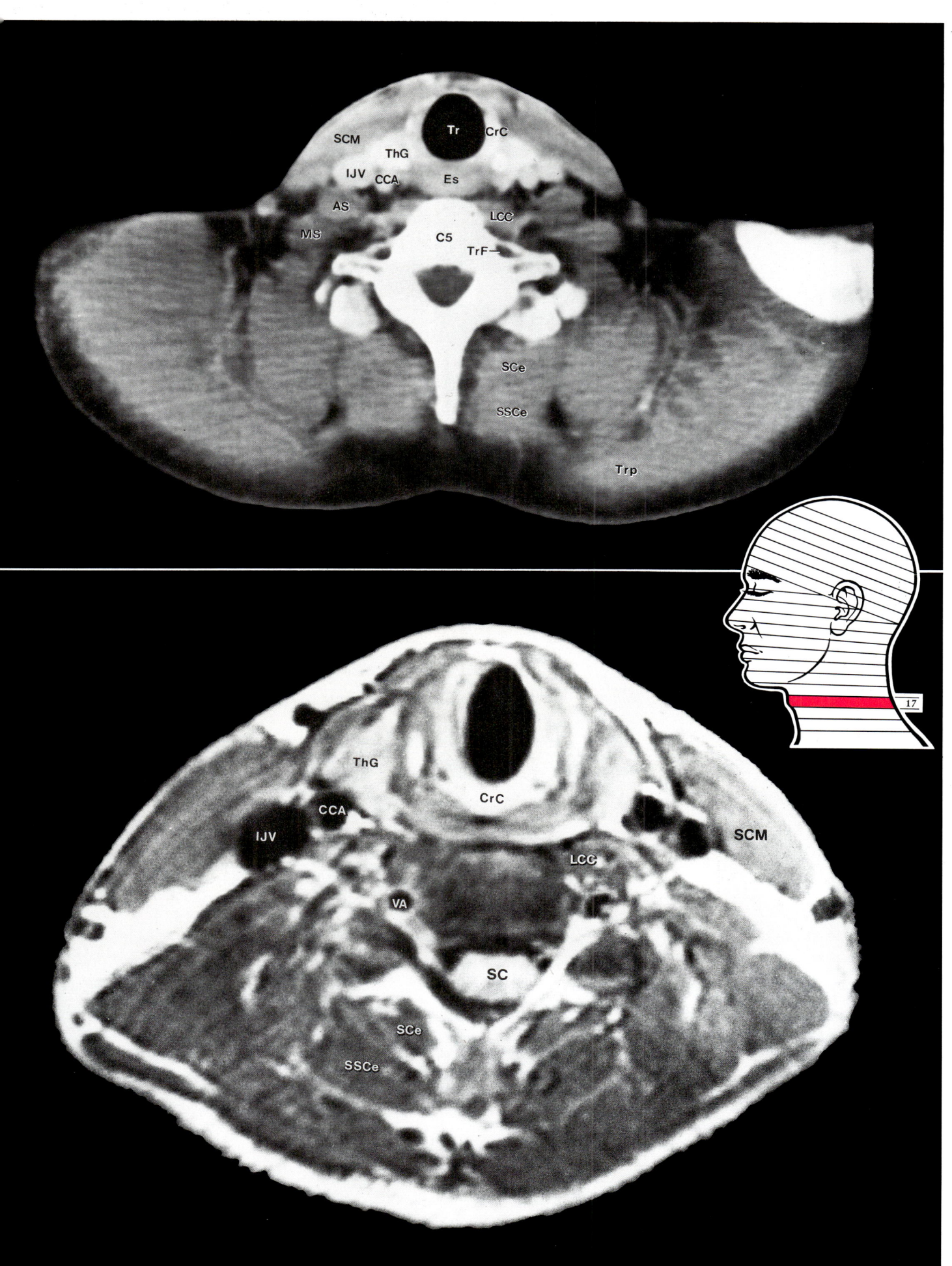

Plate 18. Transverse HEAD and NECK

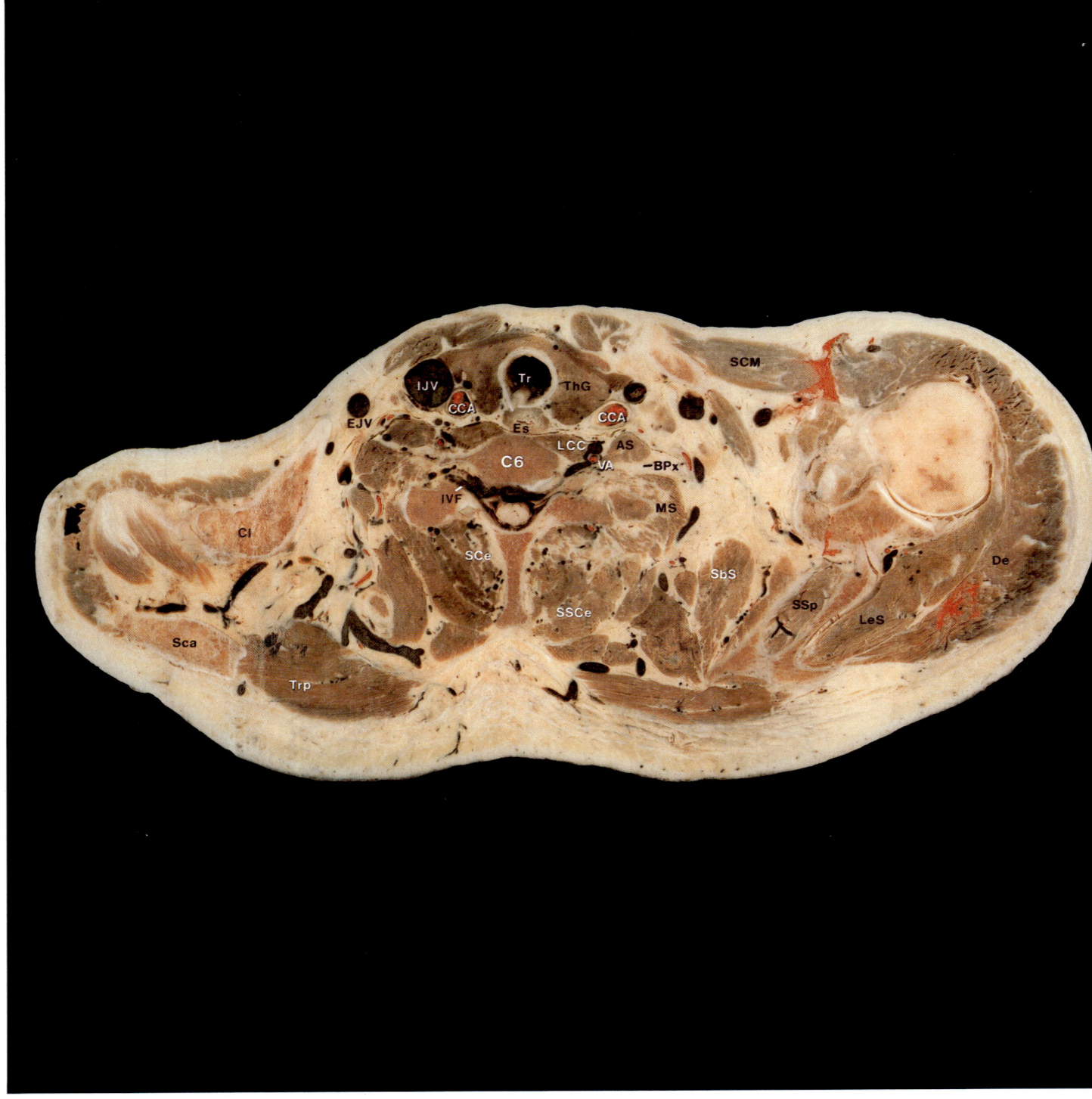

AS	Anterior scalene muscle	SbS	Subscapular muscle
BPx	Brachial plexus	Sca	Scapula
C6	C6 vertebral body	ThG	Thyroid gland
CCA	Common carotid artery	Tr	Trachea
Cl	Clavicle	Trp	Trapezius muscle
De	Deltoid muscle	VA	Vertebral artery
EJV	External jugular vein		
Es	Esophagus		
IJV	Internal jugular vein		
IVF	Intervertebral foramen		
LCC	Longus capitis & colli muscle		
LeS	Levator scapularis muscle		
MS	Middle scalene muscle		
SC	Spinal cord		
SCM	Sternocleidomastoid muscle		
SCe	Spinalis cervicalis muscle		
SSCe	Semispinalis cervicalis muscle		
SSp	Supraspinatus muscle		

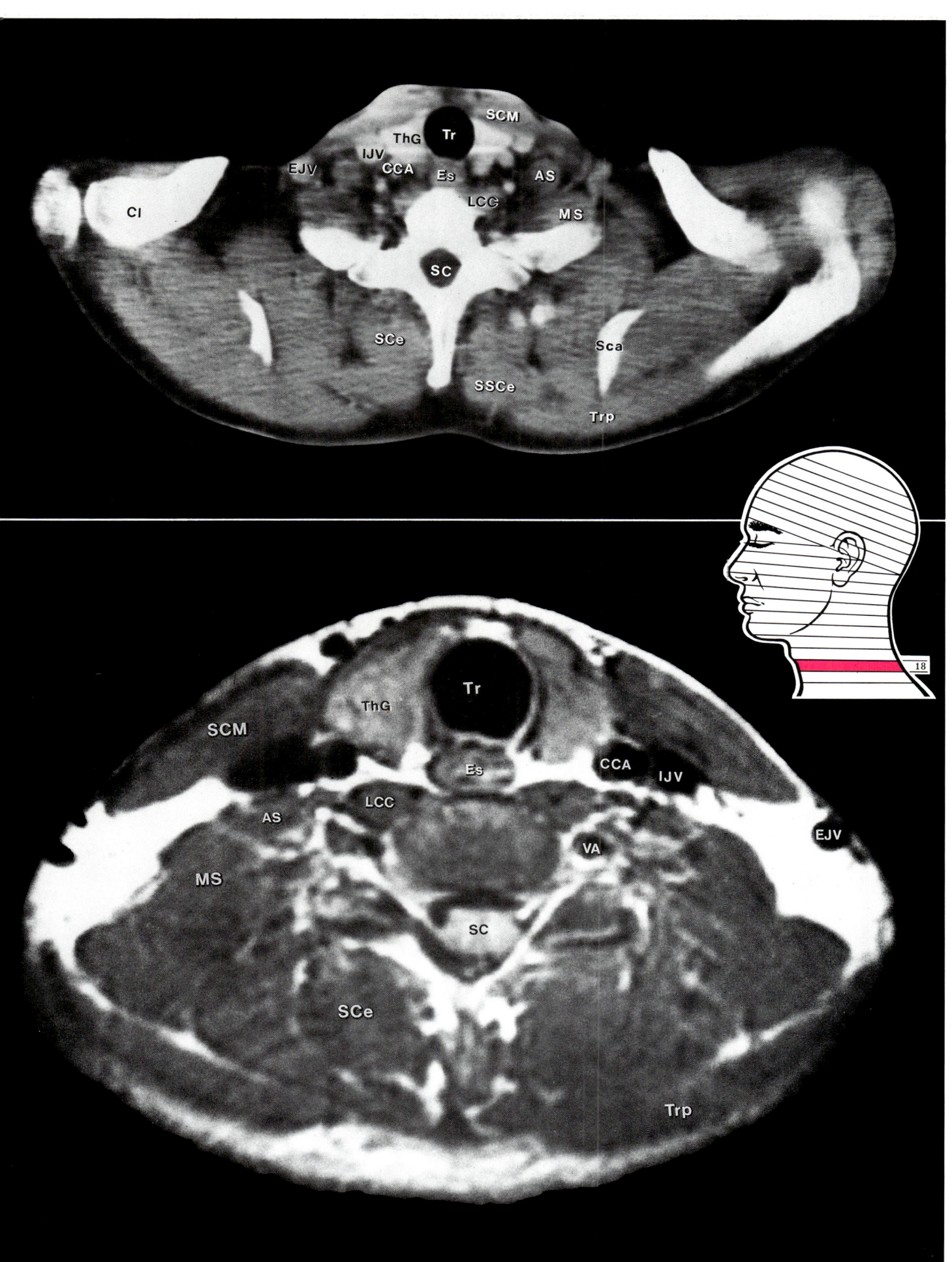

Plate 19. Transverse HEAD and NECK

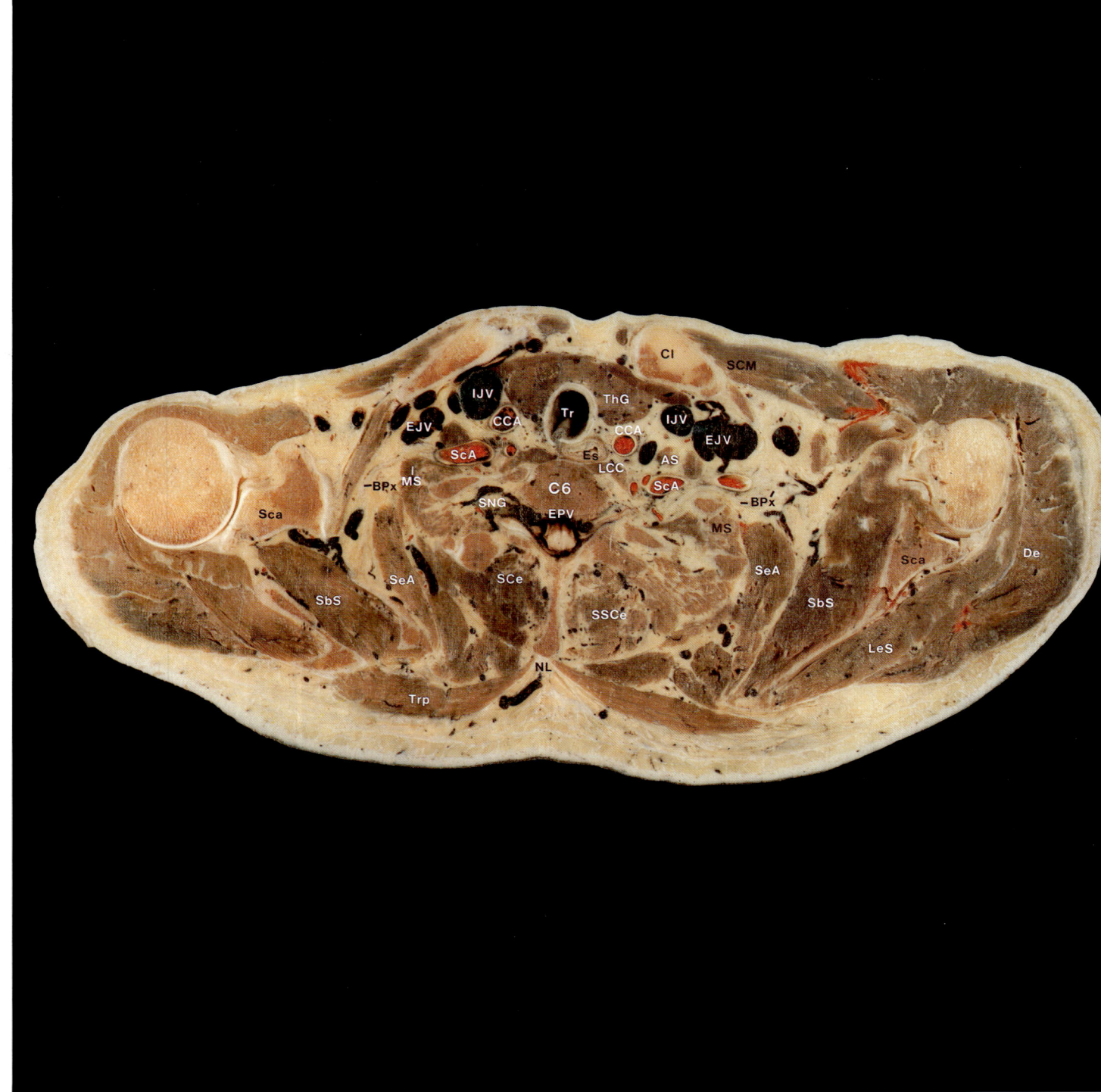

AS	Anterior scalene muscle	SSCe	Semispinalis cervicalis muscle
BPx	Brachial plexus	SbS	Subscapular muscle
C6	C6 vertebral body	ScA	Subclavian artery
CCA	Common carotid artery	Sca	Scapula
Cl	Clavicle	SeA	Serratus anterior muscle
De	Deltoid muscle	ThG	Thyroid gland
EJV	External jugular vein	Tr	trachea
EPV	Epidural venous plexus	Trp	Trapezius muscle
Es	Esophagus	VA	Vertebral artery
IJV	Internal jugular vein		
LCC	Longus capitis & colli muscle		
LeS	Levator scapularis muscle		
MS	Middle scalene muscle		
NL	Nuchal ligament		
SC	Spinal cord		
SCM	Sternocleidomastoid muscle		
SCe	Spinals cervicalis muscle		
SNG	Spinal nerve ganglion		

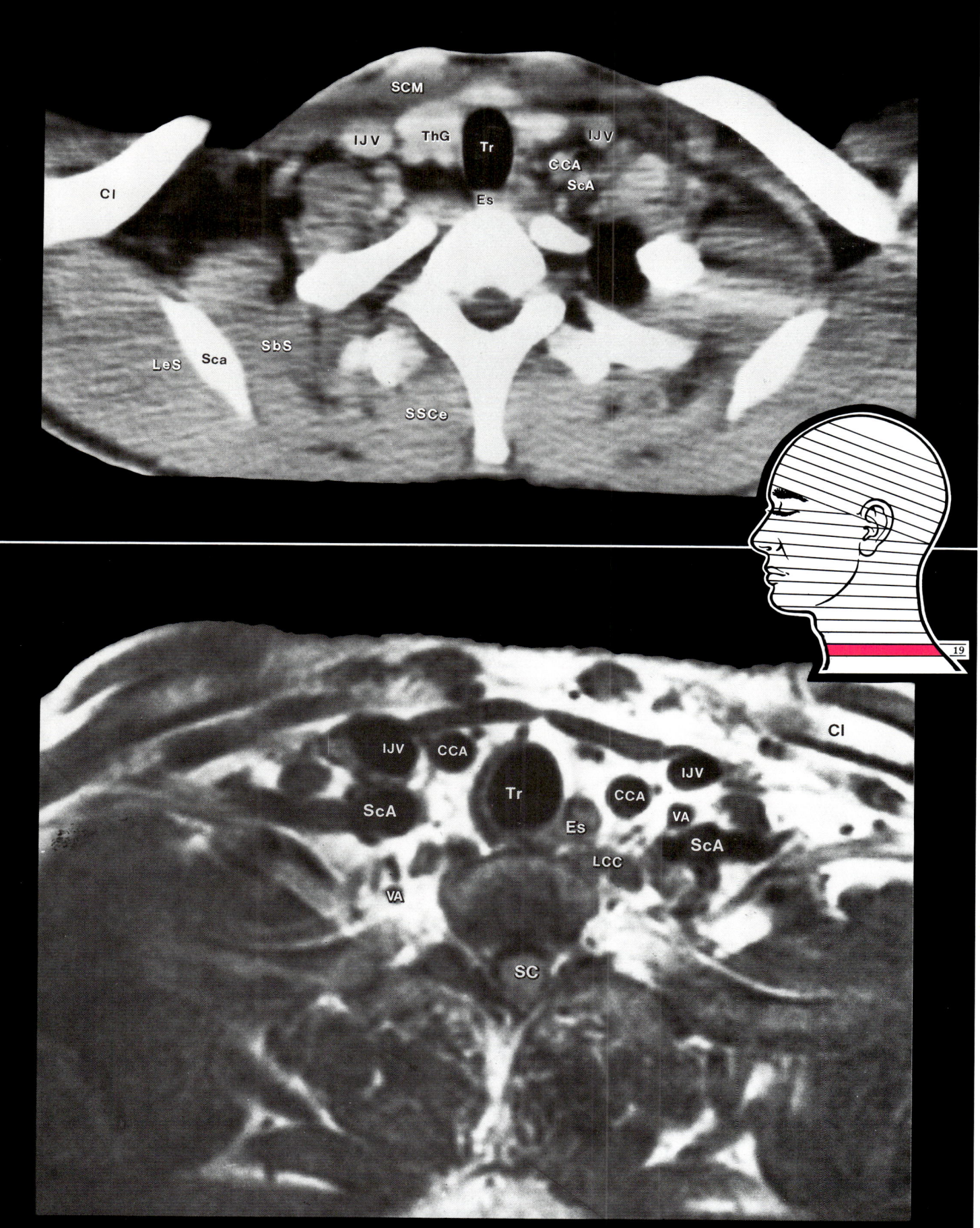

Coronal Section (Cadaver, CT & MRI) Plate 20-28

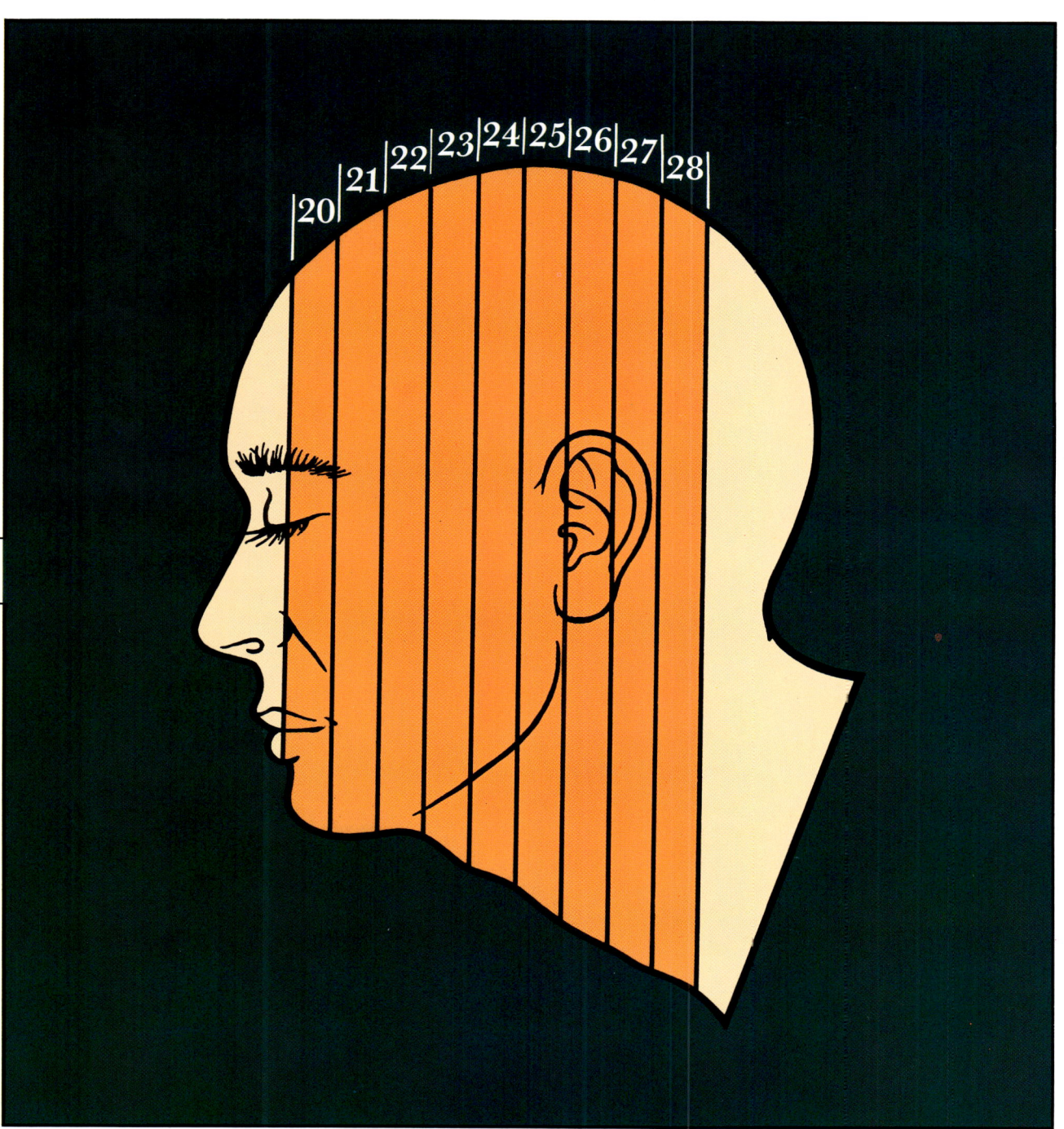

Plate 20. Coronal Brain, Head and Neck

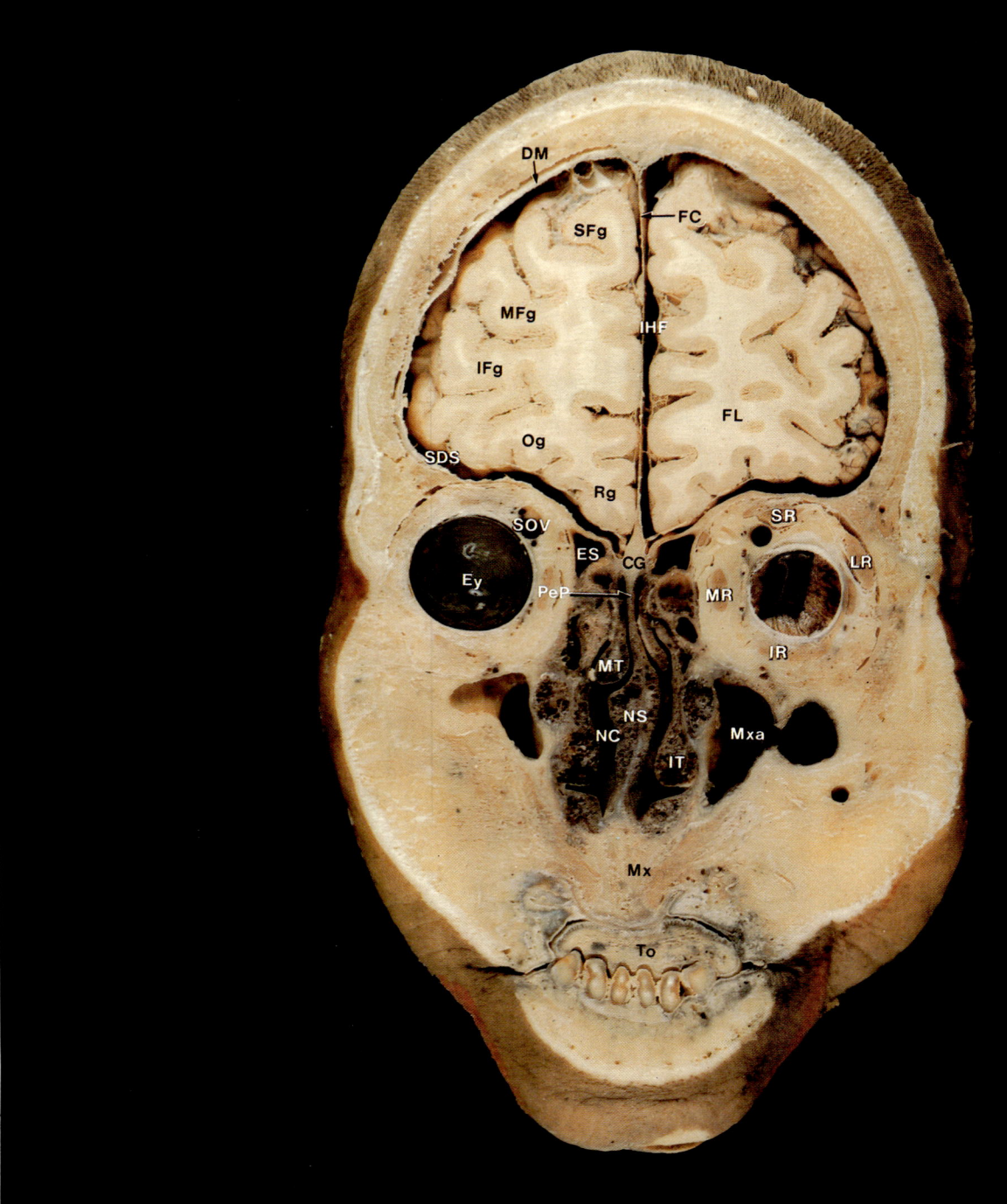

CG	Crista galli	NS	Nasal septum
DM	Dura mater	Og	Orbital gyrus
ES	Ethmoid sinus	PeP	Perpendicular plate
Ey	Eyeball	Rg	Rectal gyrus
FC	Falx cerebri	SDS	Subdural space
FL	Frontal lobe	SFg	Superior frontal gyrus
IFg	Inferior frontal gyrus	SOV	Superior ophthalmic vein, dilated
IHF	Interhemispheric fissure	SR	Superior rectus muscle
IR	Inferior rectus muscle	To	Tongue
IT	Inferior turbinate		
LR	Lateral rectus muscle		
LmP	Lamina papiracea		
MFg	Middle frontal gyrus		
MR	Medial rectus muscle		
MT	Middle turbinate		
Mx	Maxilla		
Mxa	Maxillary sinus, antrum		
NC	Nasal cavity		

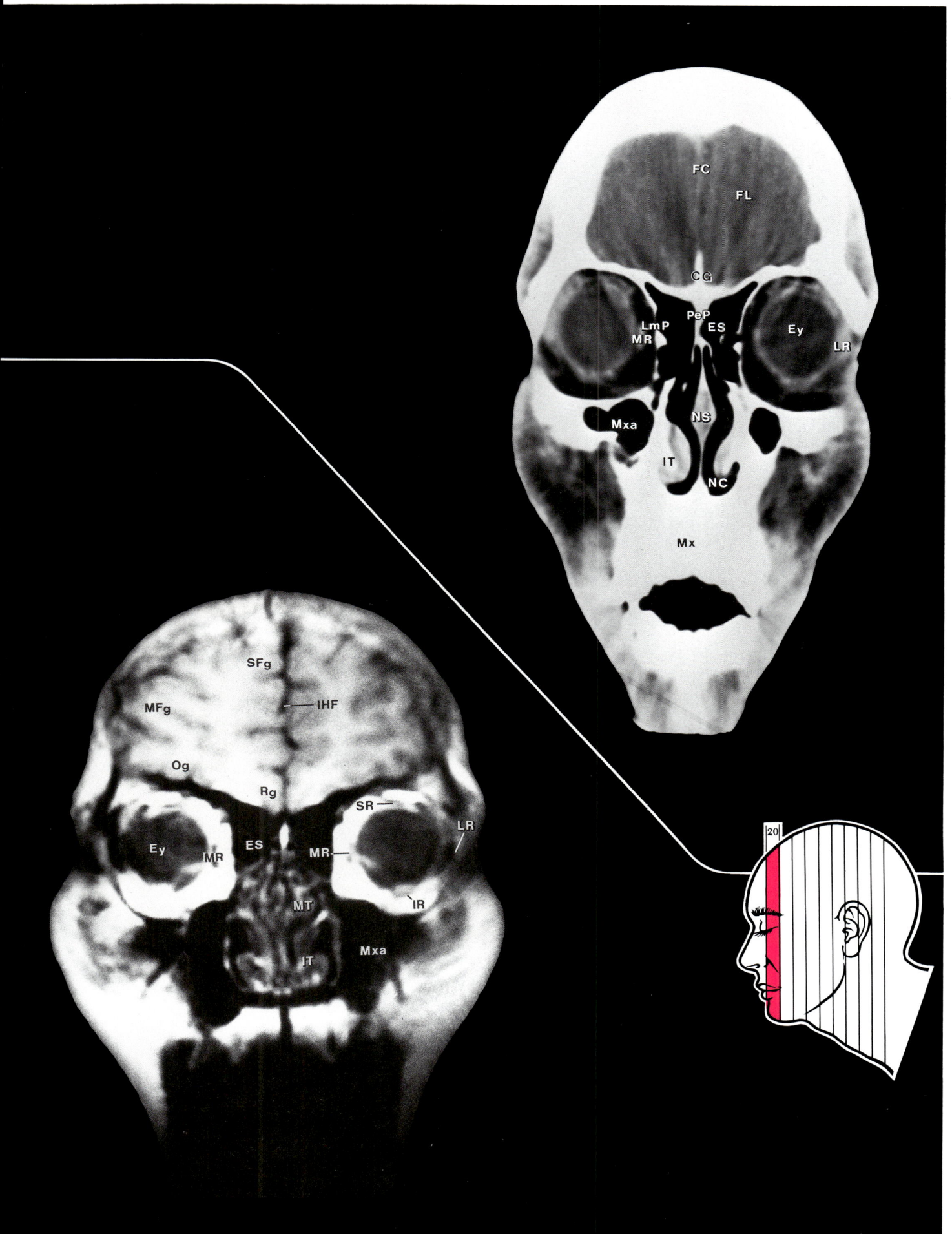

— 45 —

Plate 21. Coronal Brain, Head and Neck

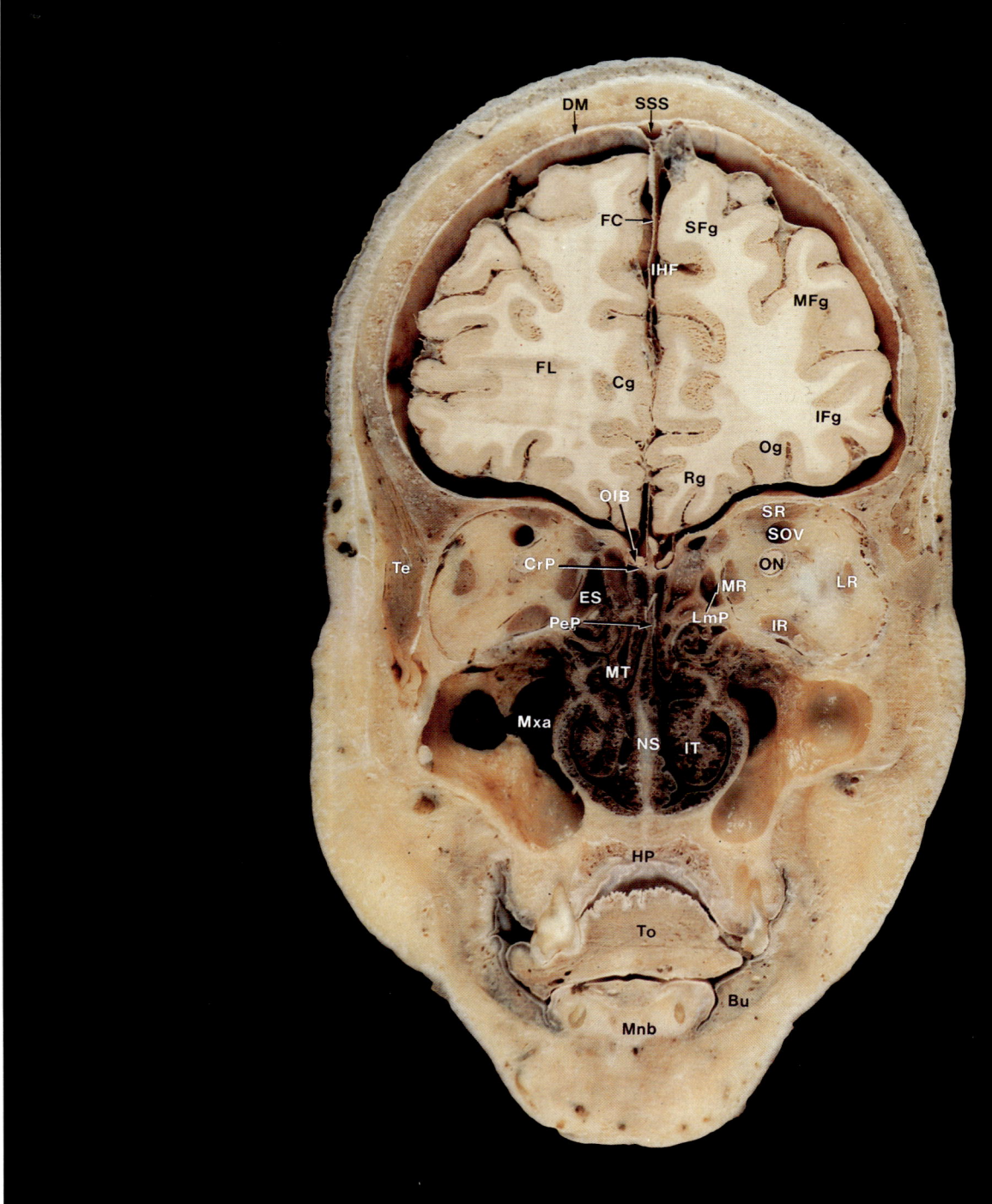

Bu	Buccinator muscle	Mnb	Mandible, body
CG	Crista galli	Mx	Maxilla
Cg	Cingulate gyrus	Mxa	Maxillary sinus, antrum
CrP	Cribriform plate	NS	Nasal septum
DM	Dura mater	ON	Optic nerve
ES	Ethmoid sinus	Og	Orbital gyrus
FC	Falx cerebri	OlB	Olfactory bulb
FL	Frontal lobe	PeP	Perpendicular plate
HP	Hard palate	Rg	Rectal gyrus
IFg	Inferior frontal gyrus	SFg	Superior frontal gyrus
IHF	Interhemispheric fissure	SOV	Superior ophthalmic vein, dilated
IR	Inferior rectus muscle	SR	Superior rectus muscle
IT	Inferior turbinate	SSS	Superior sagittal sinus
LR	Lateral rectus muscle	Te	Temporalis muscle
LmP	Lamina papiracea	To	Tongue
MFg	Middle frontal gyrus		
MR	Medial rectus muscle		
MT	Middle turbinate		

— 46 —

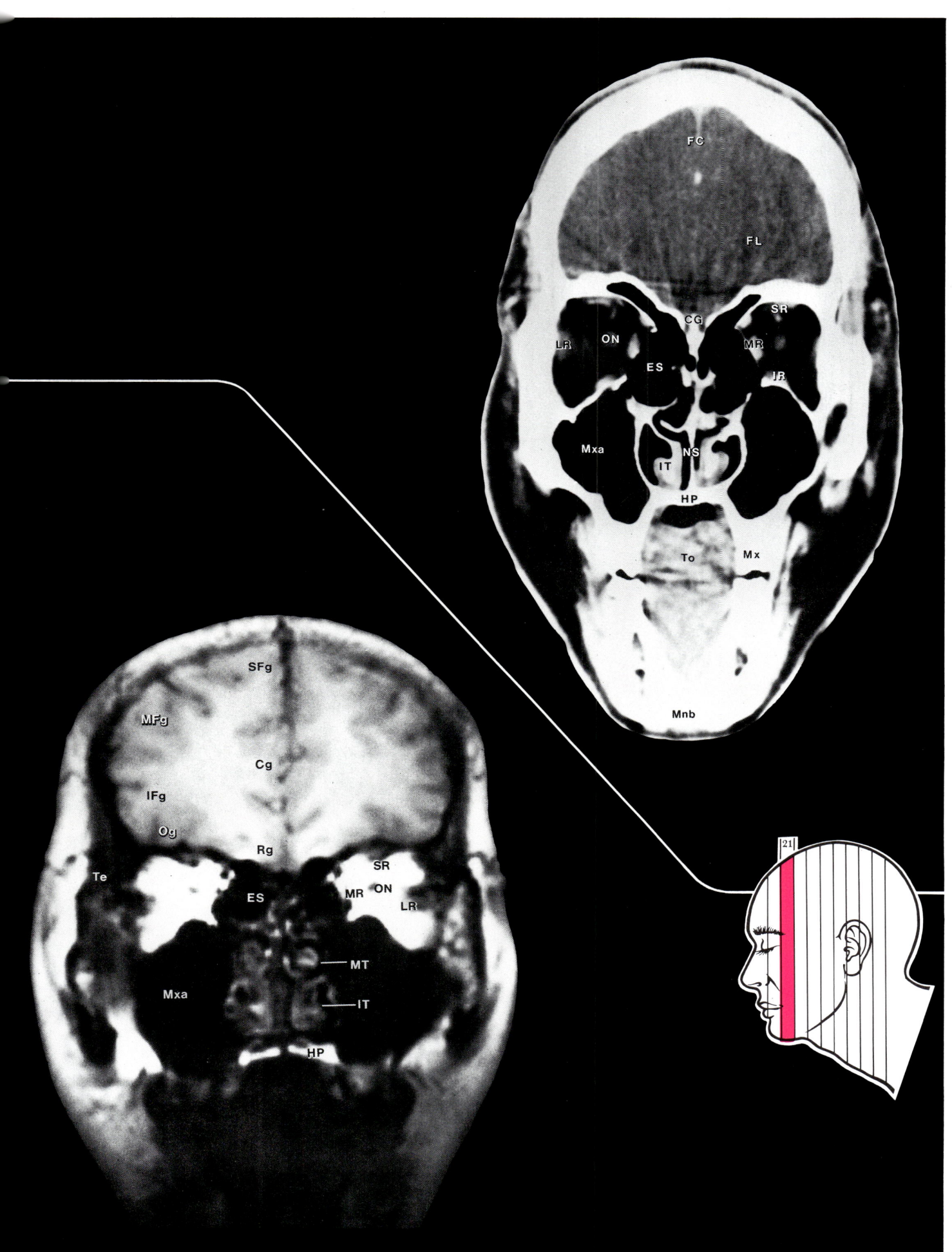

Plate 22. CORONAL BRAIN, HEAD AND NECK

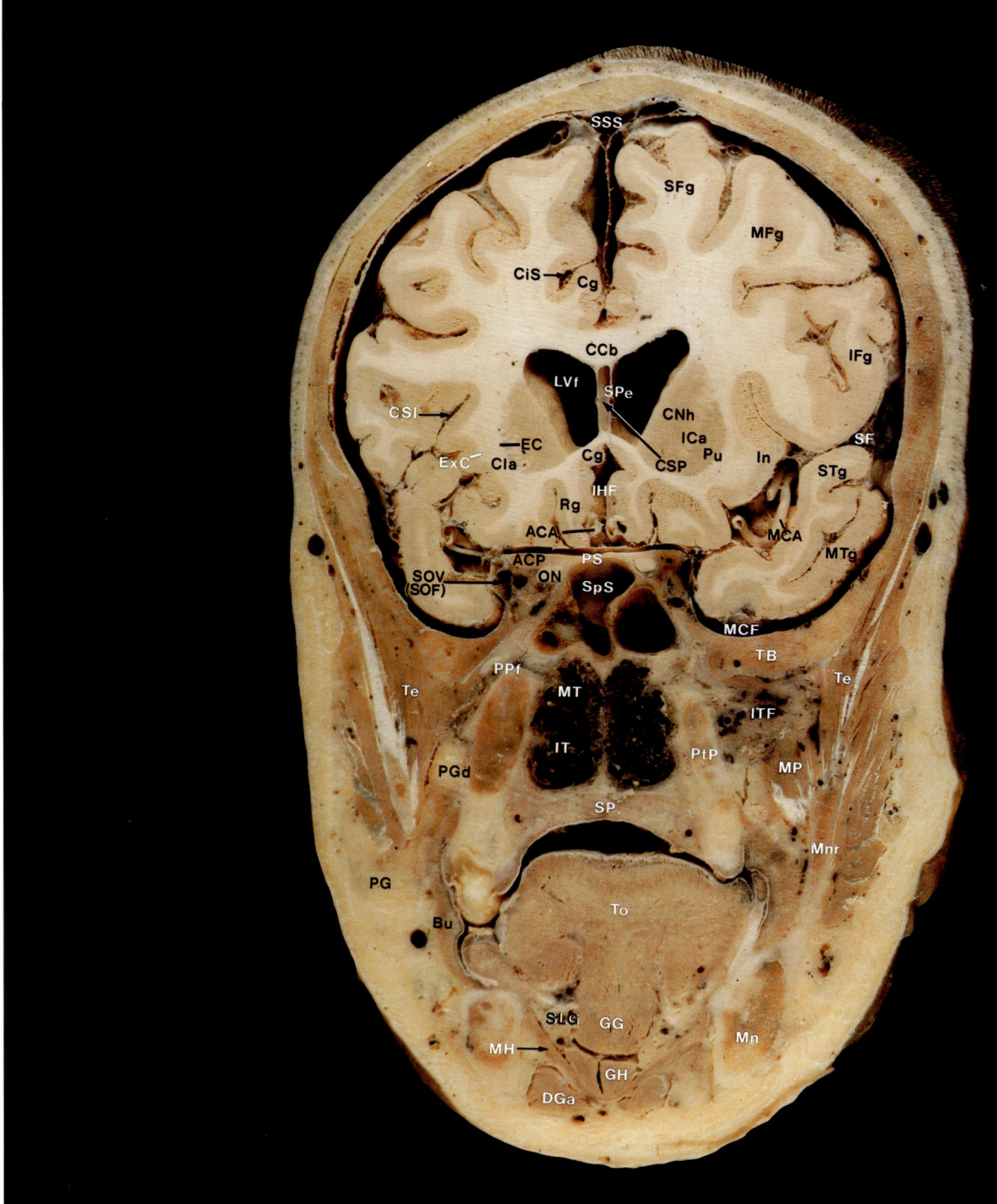

ACA	Anterior cerebral artery	IFg	Inferior frontal gyrus	PGd	Parotid gland, deep lobe
ACP	Anterior clinoid process	IHF	Interhemispheric fissure	PPf	Pterygopalatine fossa
Bu	Buccinator muscle	IT	Inferior turbinate	PS	Planum sphenoidale
CCb	Corpus callosum, body	ITF	Infratemporal fossa	PtP	Pterygoid plate
CNh	Caudate nucleus, head	In	Insula	Pu	Putamen
CSI	Circular sulcus of insula	LVf	Lateral ventricle, frontal horn	Rg	Rectal gyrus
CSP	Cavum septum pellucidum	MCA	Middle cerebral artery	SF	Sylvian fissure
Cg	Cingulate gyrus	MCF	Middle cranial fossa	SFg	Superior frontal gyrus
CiS	Cingulate sulcus	MFg	Middle frontal gyrus	SLG	Sublingual gland
Cla	Claustrum	MH	Mylohyoid muscle	SOF	Superior orbital fissure
DGa	Digastric muscle, anterior belly	MP	Medial pterygoid muscle	SOV	Superior ophthalmic vein, dilated
EC	External capsule	MT	Middle turbinate	SP	Soft palate
ExC	Extreme capsule	MTg	Middle temporal gyrus	SPe	Septum pellucidum
FC	Falx cerebri	Mn	Mandible	STg	Superior temporal gyrus
FL	Frontal lobe	Mnr	Mandible, ramus	SpS	Sphenoidal sinus
GG	Genioglossus muscle	NPh	Nasopharynx	TL	Temporal lobe
GH	Geniohyoid muscle	ON	Optic nerve	TS	Tuberculum sellae
ICa	Internal capsule, anterior limb	PG	Parotid gland	Te	Temporalis muscle

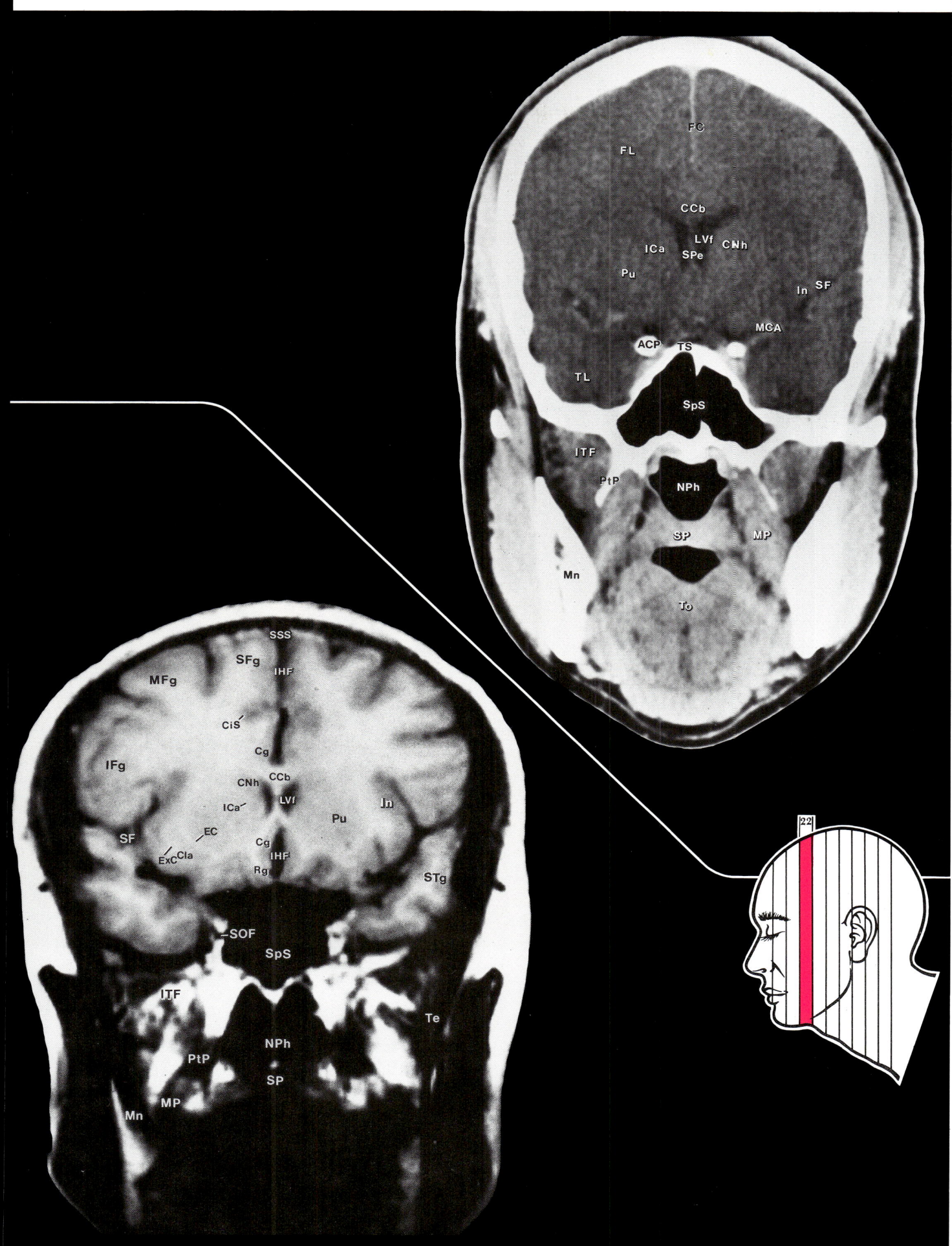

Plate 23. Coronal BRAIN, HEAD AND NECK

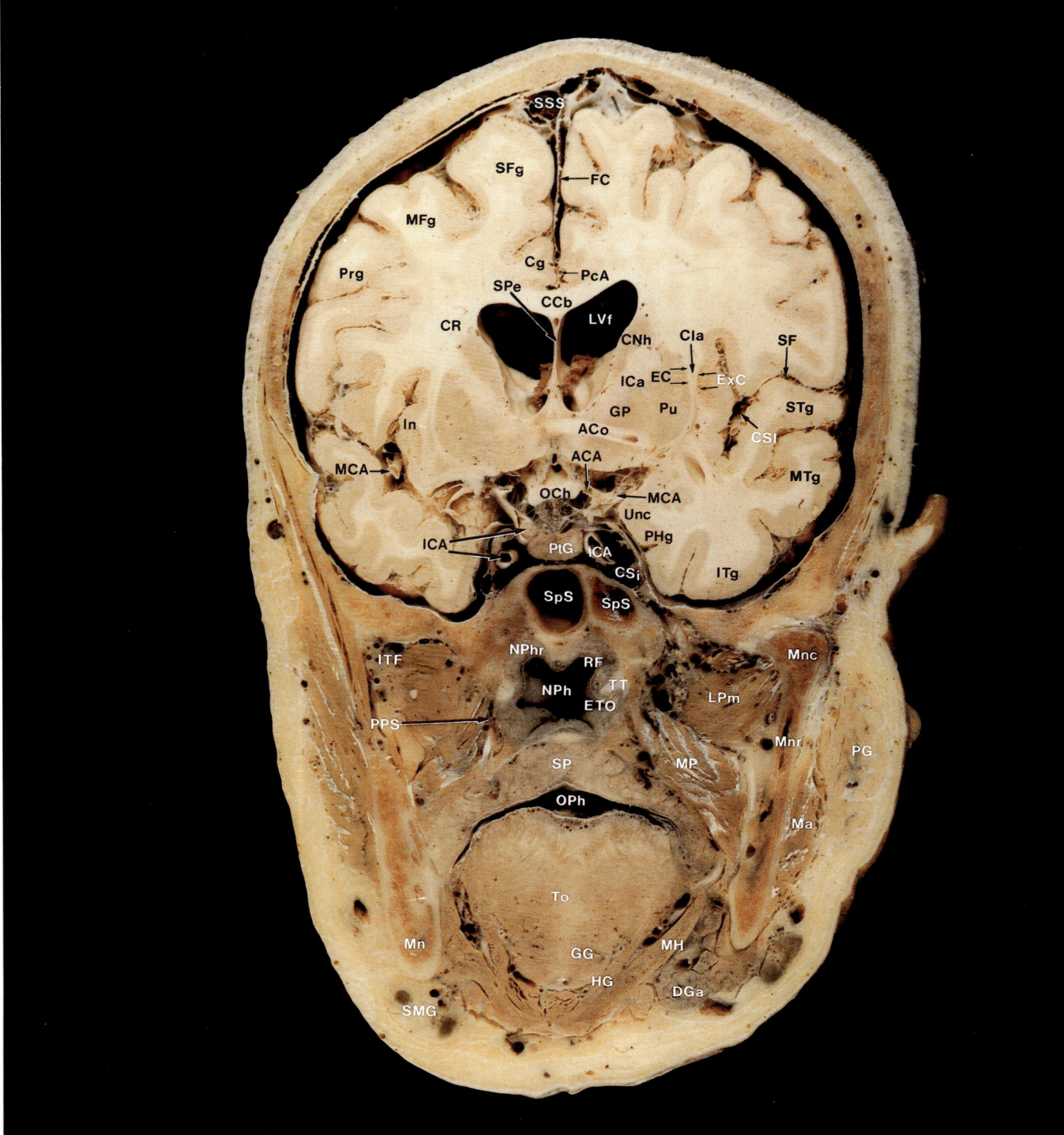

ACA	Anterior cerebral artery	ICA	Internal carotid artery	PHg	Parahippocampal gyrus
ACo	Anterior commissure	ICa	Internal capsule, anterior limb	PPS	Parapharyngeal space
BoF	Body of fornix	ITg	Inferior temporal gyrus	Prg	Precentral gyrus
CCb	Corpus callosum, body	In	Insula	PtG	Pituitary gland
CN	Caudate nucleus	LOTg	Lateral occipitotemporal gyrus	PtS	Pituitary stalk
CNh	Caudate nucleus, head	LPm	Lateral pterygoid muscle	Pu	Putamen
CR	Corona radiata	MFg	Middle frontal gyrus	RF	Rosenmuller fossa
CSI	Circular sulcus of insula	MH	Mylohyoid muscle	SFg	Superior frontal gyrus
CSi	Cavernous sinus	MP	Medial pterygoid muscle	SMG	Submandibular gland
Cg	Cingulate gyrus	MTg	Middle temporal gyrus	SP	Soft palate
Cla	Claustrum	Ma	Masseter muscle	SPe	Septum pellucidum
DGa	Digastric muscle, anterior belly	Mnc	Mandible, condylar process	SSS	Superior sagittal sinus
EC	External capsule	NPh	Nasopharynx	STg	Superior temporal gyrus
ETO	Eustachian tube orifice	NPhr	Nasopharynx, roof	SpS	Sphenoidal sinus
ExC	Extreme capsule	OCh	Optic chiasm	TT	Torus tubarius
GG	Genioglossus muscle	OPh	Oropharynx	Unc	Uncus
GP	Globus pallidus	PcA	Pericallosal artery		
HG	Hyoglossus muscle	PG	Parotid gland		

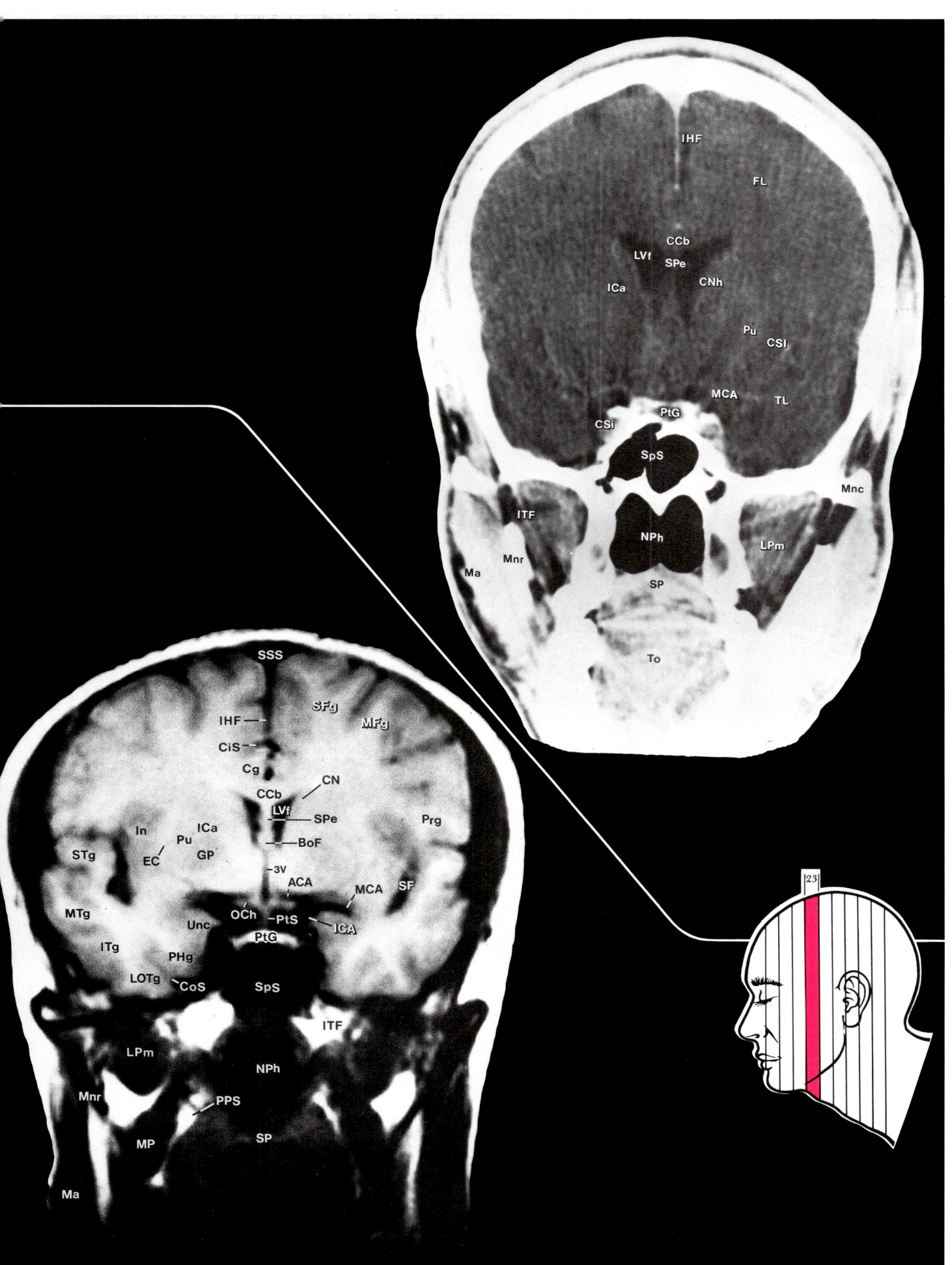

Plate 24. CORONAL BRAIN, HEAD AND NECK

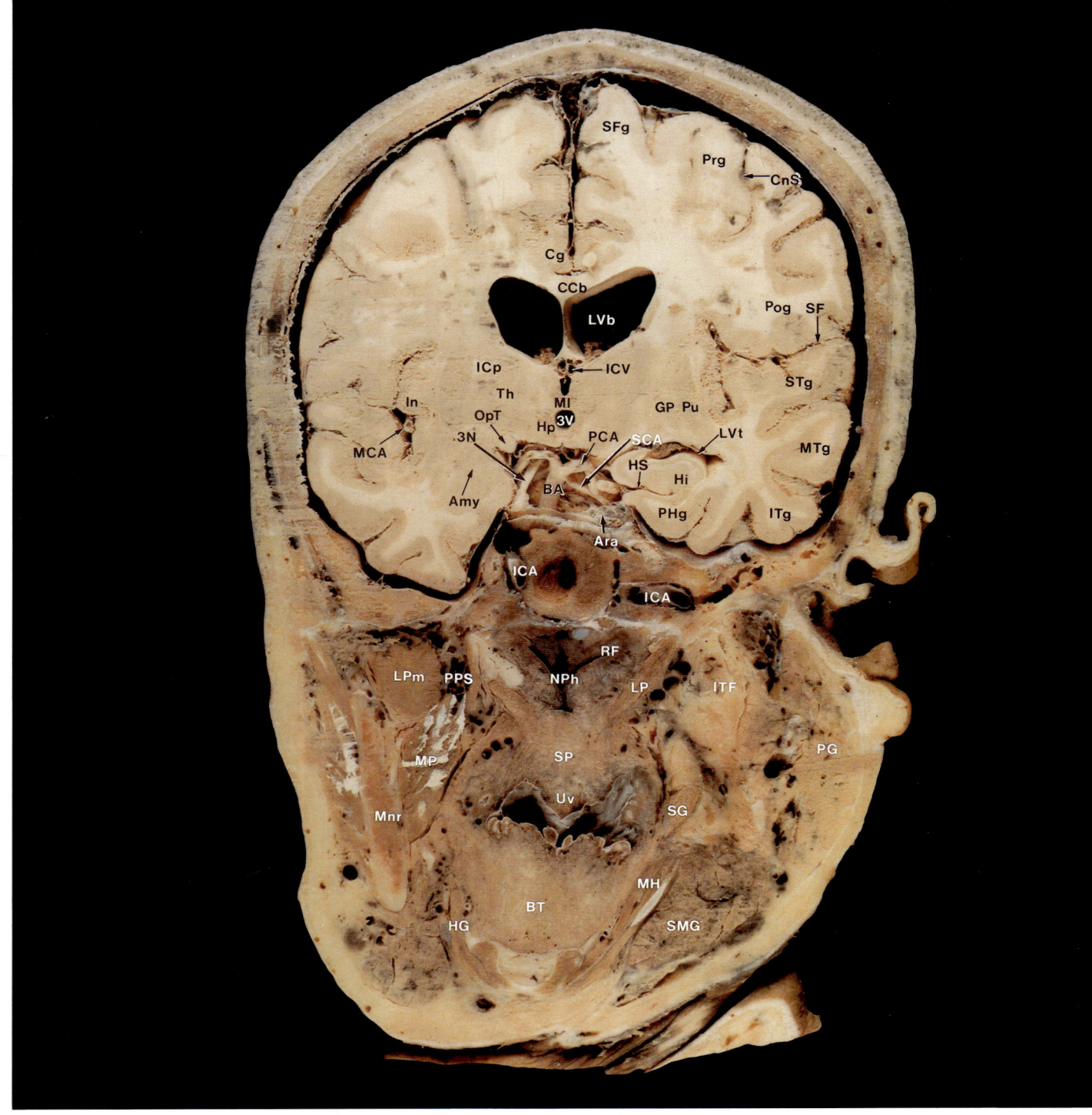

3N	3rd cranial nerve	ICp	Internal capsule, posterior limb	PCA	Posterior cerebral artery
Amy	Amygdala	ITF	Infratemporal fossa	PHg	Parahippocampal gyrus
Ara	Arachnoidal membrane	ITg	Inferior temporal gyrus	PL	Parietal lobe
BA	Basilar artery	In	Insula	Ph	Pharyngeal muscles
BT	Base of tongue	LOTg	Lateral occipitotemporal gyrus	Pog	Postcentral gyrus
CCb	Corpus callosum, body	LP	Levator palati muscle	Prg	Precentral gyrus
CNh	Caudate nucleus, head	LPm	Lateral pterygoid muscle	Pu	Putamen
Cg	Cingulate gyrus	LVb	Lateral ventricle, body	RF	Rosenmuller fossa
CiS	Cingulate sulcus	LVt	Lateral ventricle, temporal horn	SCA	Superior cerebellar artery
CnS	Central sulcus	MH	Mylohyoid muscle	SF	Sylvian fissure
EC	External capsule	MI	Massa intermedia	SFg	Superior frontal gyrus
GP	Globuls pallidus	MP	Medial pterygoid muscle	SG	Styloglossus muscle
HG	Hyoglossus muscle	MTg	Middle temporal gyrus	SMG	Submandibular gland
HS	Hippocampal sulcus	Ma	Masseter muscle	SP	Soft palate
Hi	Hippocampus	Mnr	Mandible, ramus	SPe	Septum pellucidum
Hp	Hypothalamus	NPh	Nasopharynx	STg	Superior temporal gyrus
ICA	Internal carotid artery	NPhr	Nasopharynx, roof	Th	Thalamus
ICV	Internal cerebral vein	OpT	Optic tract	Uv	Uvula

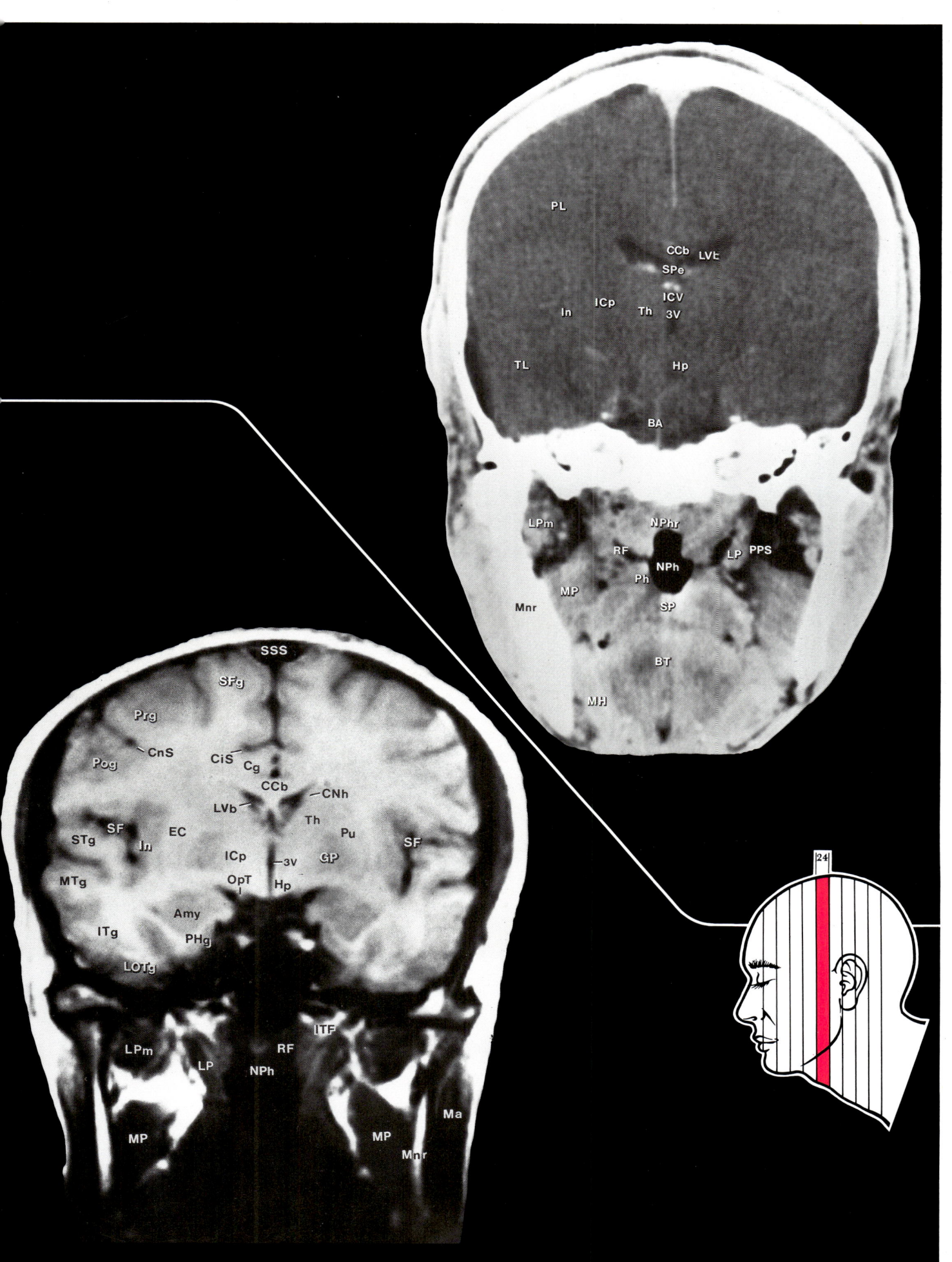

Plate 25. Coronal Brain, Head and Neck

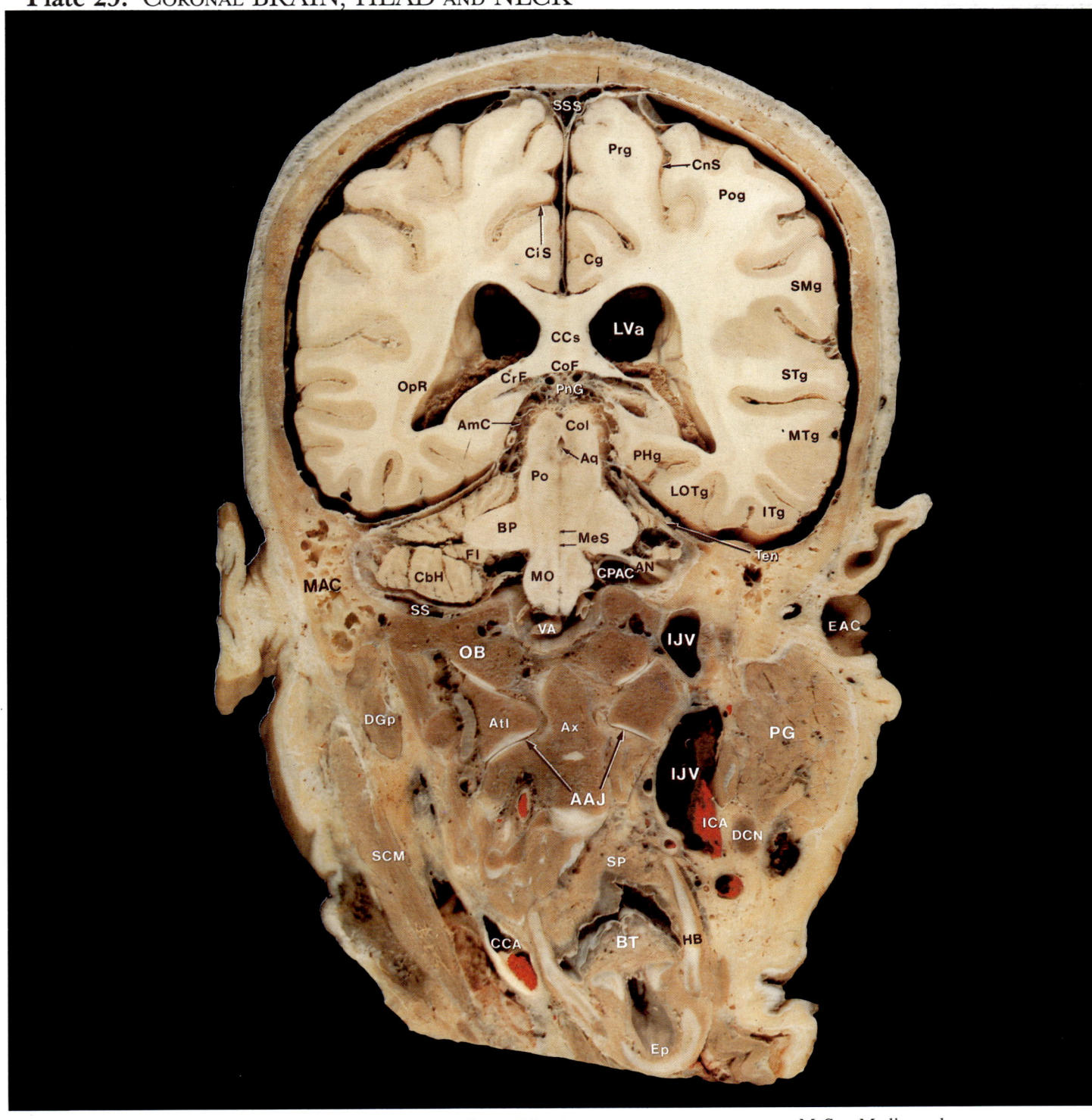

AAJ	Atlanto-axial joint	CrF	Crus of fornix
AN	Acoustic nerve	DCN	Deep cervical lymph node
AmC	Ambient cistern	DGp	Digastric muscle, posterior belly
Aq	Cerebral aqueduct	EAC	External auditory canal
Atl	Atlas	Ep	Epiglottis
Ax	Axis	Fl	Flocculus
BP	Brachium pontis	HB	Hyoid bone
BT	Base of tongue	ICA	Internal carotid artery
CCA	Common carotid artery	ICV	Internal cerebral vein
CCs	Corpus callosum, splenium	IJV	Internal jugular vein
CPAC	Cerebellopontine angle cistern	IPLo	Inferior parietal lobule
CbH	Cerebellar hemisphere	ITg	Inferior temporal gyrus
Cg	Cingulate gyrus	JF	Jugular foramen
ChP	Choroid plexus	LOTg	Lateral occipitotemporal gyrus
CiS	Cingulate sulcus	LVa	Lateral ventricle, antrum
CnS	Central sulcus	MAC	Mastoid air cells
CoF	Commissure of fornix	MO	Medulla oblongata
Col	Colliculi	MTg	Middle temporal gyrus
MeS	Median sulcus		
Mi	Midbrain		
OB	Occipital bone		
OpR	Optic radiation		
PG	Parotid gland		
PHg	Para-hippocampal gyrus		
Pal	Paracentral lobule		
PnG	Pineal gland		
Po	Pons		
Pog	Postcentral gyrus		
Prg	Precentral gyrus		
SCM	Sternocleidomastoid muscle		
SMg	Supramarginal gyrus		
SS	Sigmoid sinus		
STg	Superior temporal gyrus		
Ten	Tentorium cerebelli		
Th	Thalamus		
VA	Vertebral artery		

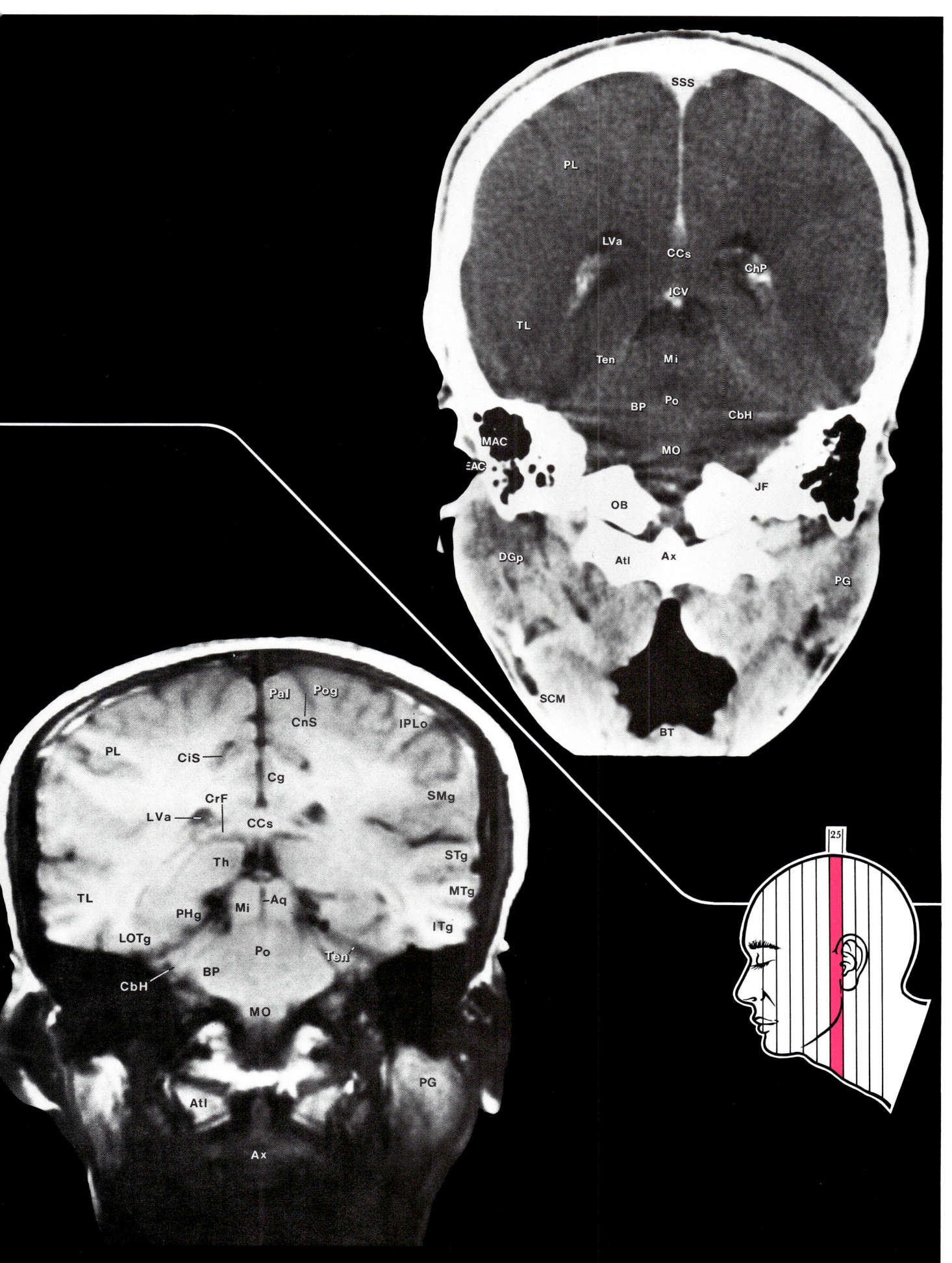

Plate 26. CORONAL BRAIN, HEAD AND NECK

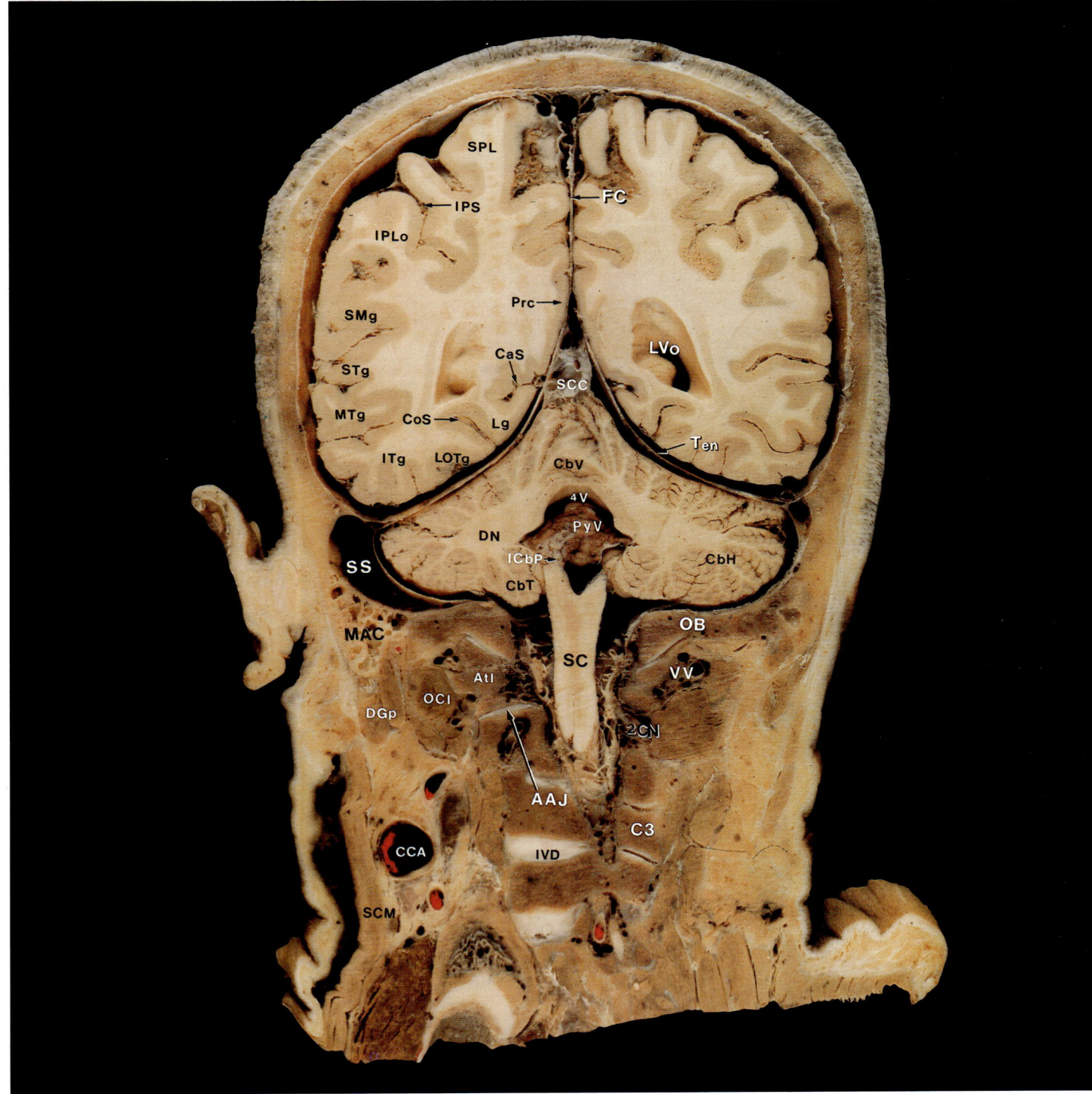

2CN	Second cervical nerve	IPS	Intraparietal sulcus	SCM	Sternocleidomastoid muscle
4V	4th ventricle	ITg	Inferior temporal gyrus	SF	Sylvian fissure
AAJ	Atlanto-axial joint	IVD	Intervertebral disc	SMg	Supramarginal gyrus
Atl	Atlas	LOTg	Lateral occipitotemporal gyrus	SPL	Superior parietal lobule
C3	C3 vertebral body	LVo	Lateral ventricle, occipital horn	SS	Sigmoid sinus
CCA	Common carotid artery	Lg	Lingual gyrus	STg	Superior temporal gyrus
CaS	Calcarine sulcus	MAC	Mastoid air cells	TL	Temporal lobe
CbH	Cerebellar hemisphere	MO	Medulla oblongata	Ten	Tentorium cerebelli
CbT	Cerebellar tonsil	MTg	Middle temporal gyrus	VG	Vein of Galen
CbV	Cerebellar vermis	OB	Occipital bone	VV	Vertebral vein
Cg	Cingulate gyrus	OCI	Obliquus capitis inferior muscle		
ChP	Choroid plexus	OpR	Optic radiation		
CoS	Collateral sulcus	PL	Parietal lobe		
DGp	Digastric muscle, posterior belly	Pal	Paracentral lobule		
DN	Dentate nucleus	Prc	Precuneus		
FC	Falx cerebri	PyV	Pyramis vermis		
ICbP	Inferior cerebellar peduncle	SC	Spinal cord		
IPLo	Inferior parietal lobule	SCC	Superior cerebellar cistern		

— 56 —

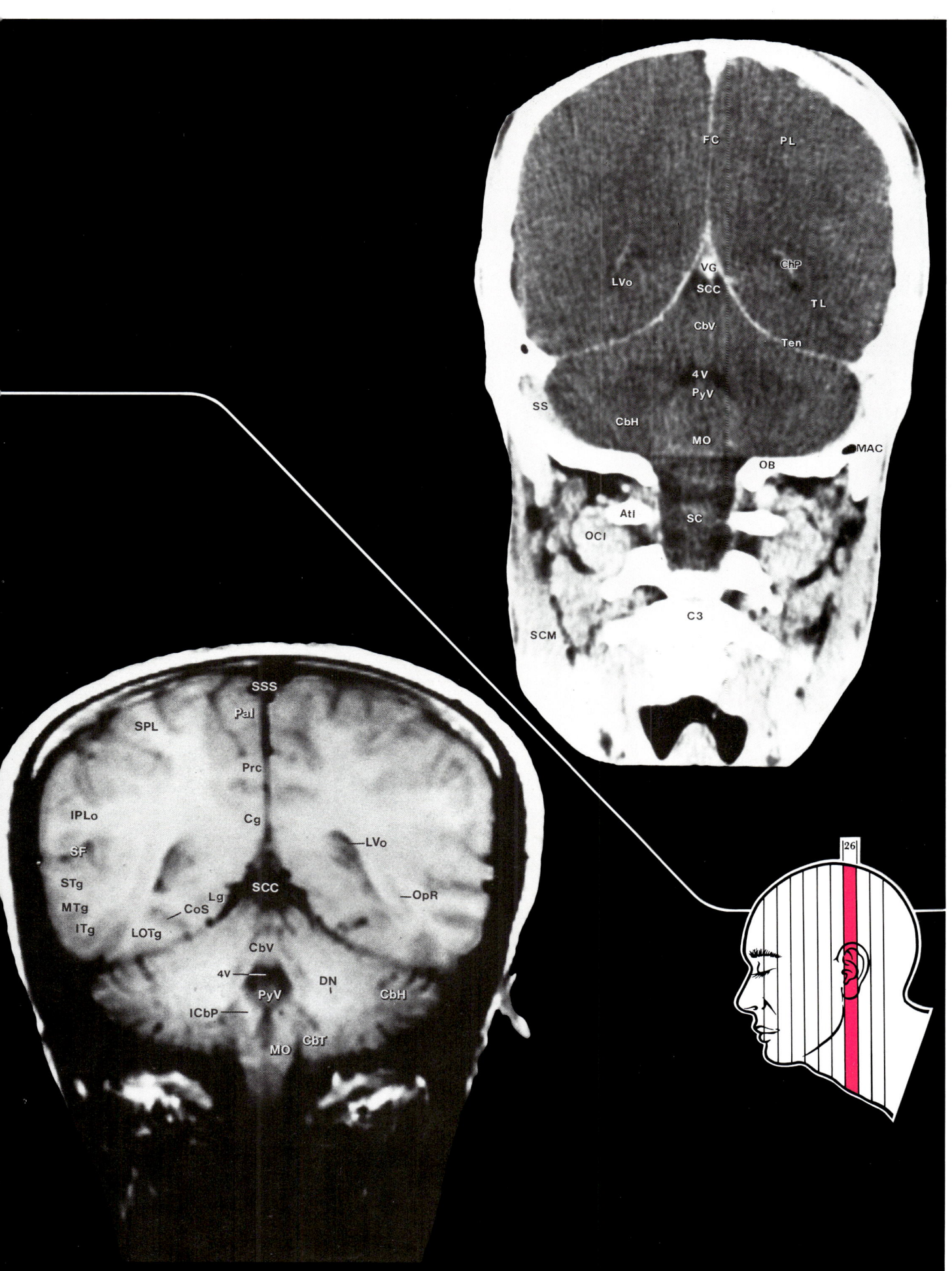

Plate 27. Coronal Brain, Head and Neck

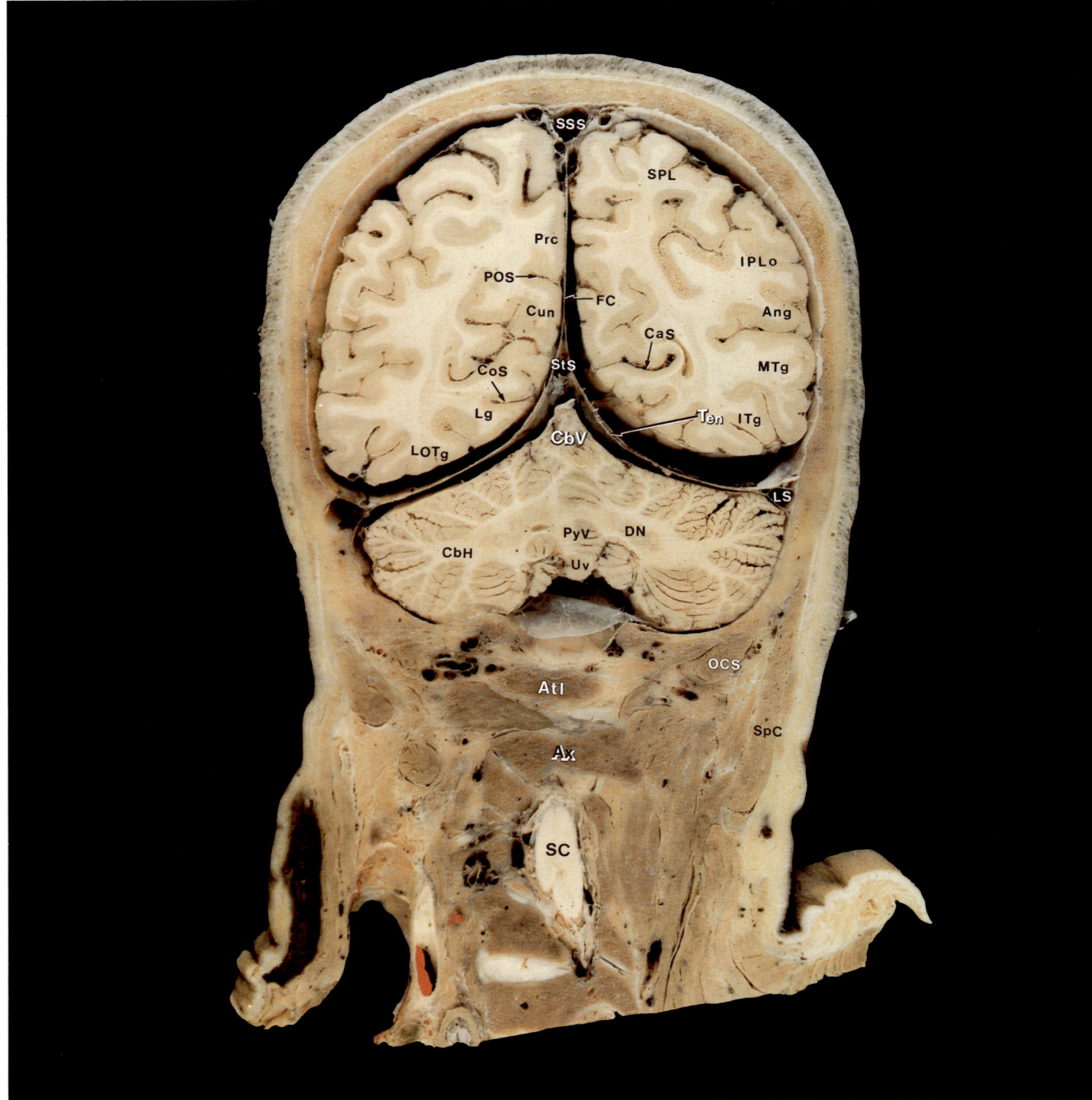

Ang	Angular gyrus	POS	Parietooccipital sulcus
Atl	Atlas	Prc	Precuneus
Ax	Axis	PyV	Pyramis vermis
CaS	Calcarine sulcus	SC	Spinal cord
CbH	Cerebellar hemisphere	SPL	Superior parietal lobule
CbV	Cerebellar vermis	SSS	Superior sagittal sinus
CoS	Collateral sulcus	SpC	Splenius capitis muscle
Cun	Cuneus	StS	Straight sinus
DN	Dentate nucleus	TL	Temporal lobe
FC	Falx cerebri	Ten	Tentorium cerebelli
IPLo	Inferior parietal lobule	Uv	Uvula
ITg	Inferior temporal gyrus		
LOTg	Lateral occipitotemporal gyrus		
LS	Lateral sinus		
Lg	Lingual gyrus		
MTg	Middle temporal gyrus		
OCS	Obliquus capitis superior muscle		
PL	Parietal lobe		

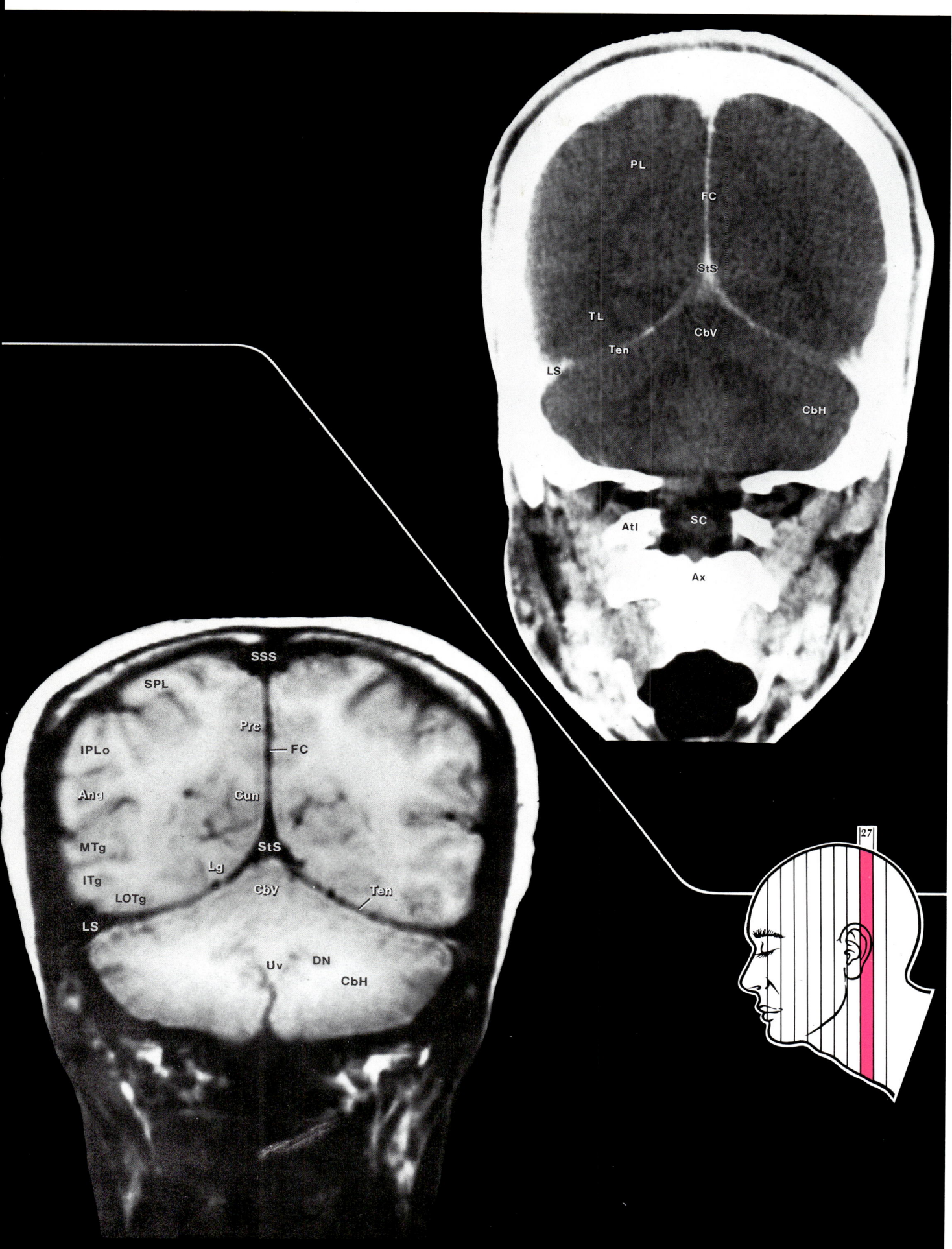

Plate 28. Coronal BRAIN, HEAD AND NECK

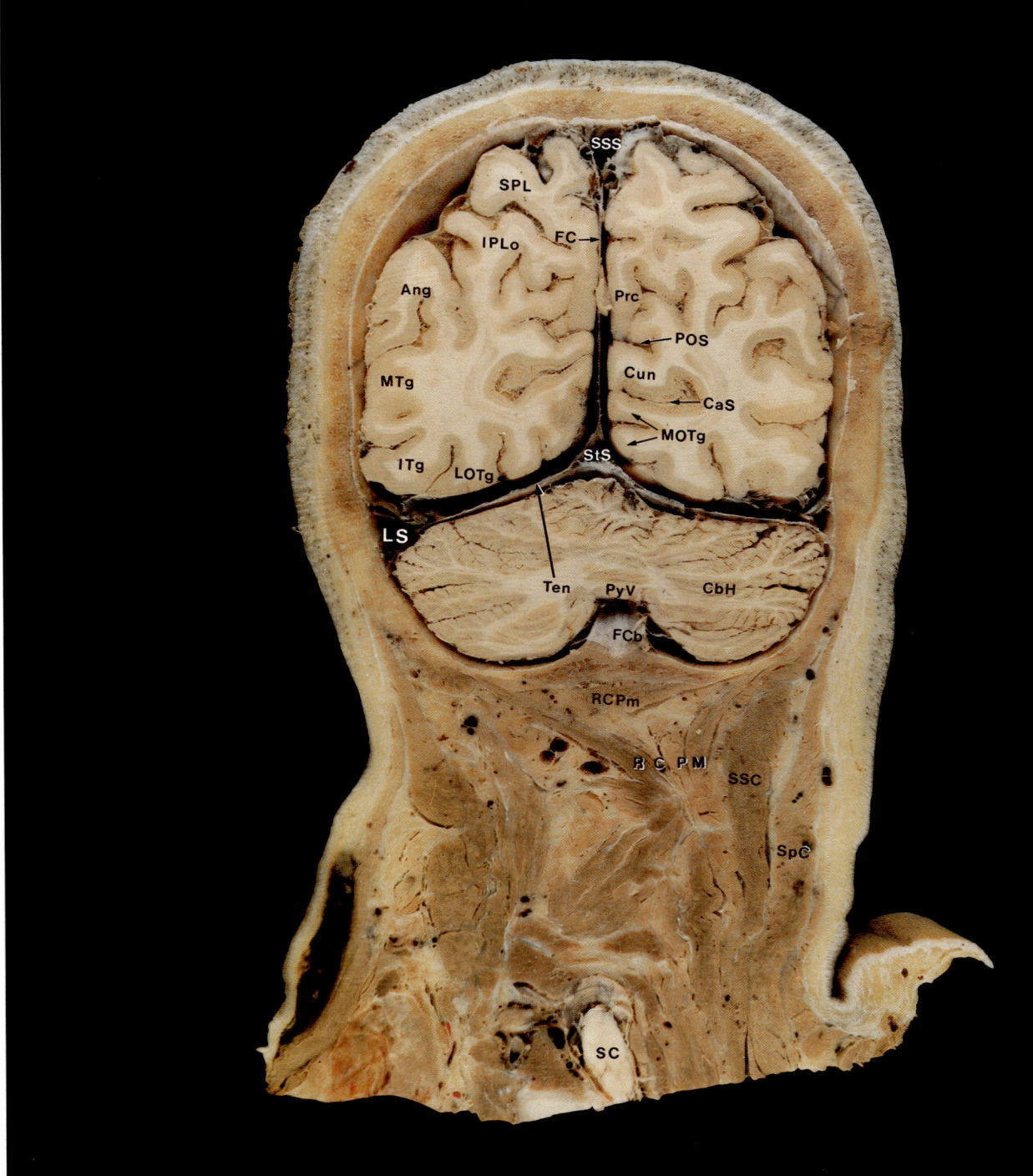

Ang	angular gyrus	
CaS	Calcarine sulcus	
CbH	Cerebellar hemisphere	
CbV	Cerebellar vermis	
Cun	Cuneus	
FC	Falx cerebri	
FCb	Falx cerebelli	
IPLo	Inferior parietal lobule	
ITg	Inferior temporal gyrus	
LOTg	Lateral occipitotemporal gyrus	
LS	Lateral sinus	
MOTg	Medial occipitotemporal gyrus	
MTg	Middle temporal gyrus	
OB	Occipital bone	
OL	Occipital lobe	
POS	Parietooccipital sulcus	
Prc	Precuneus	
PyV	Pyramis vermis	
RCPM	Rectus capitis posterior major muscle	
RCPm	Rectus capitis posterior minor muscle	
SC	Spinal cord	
SPL	Superior parietal lobule	
SSC	Semispinalis capitis muscle	
SSS	Superior sagittal sinus	
SpC	Splenius capitis muscle	
StS	Straight sinus	
Ten	Tentorium cerebelli	

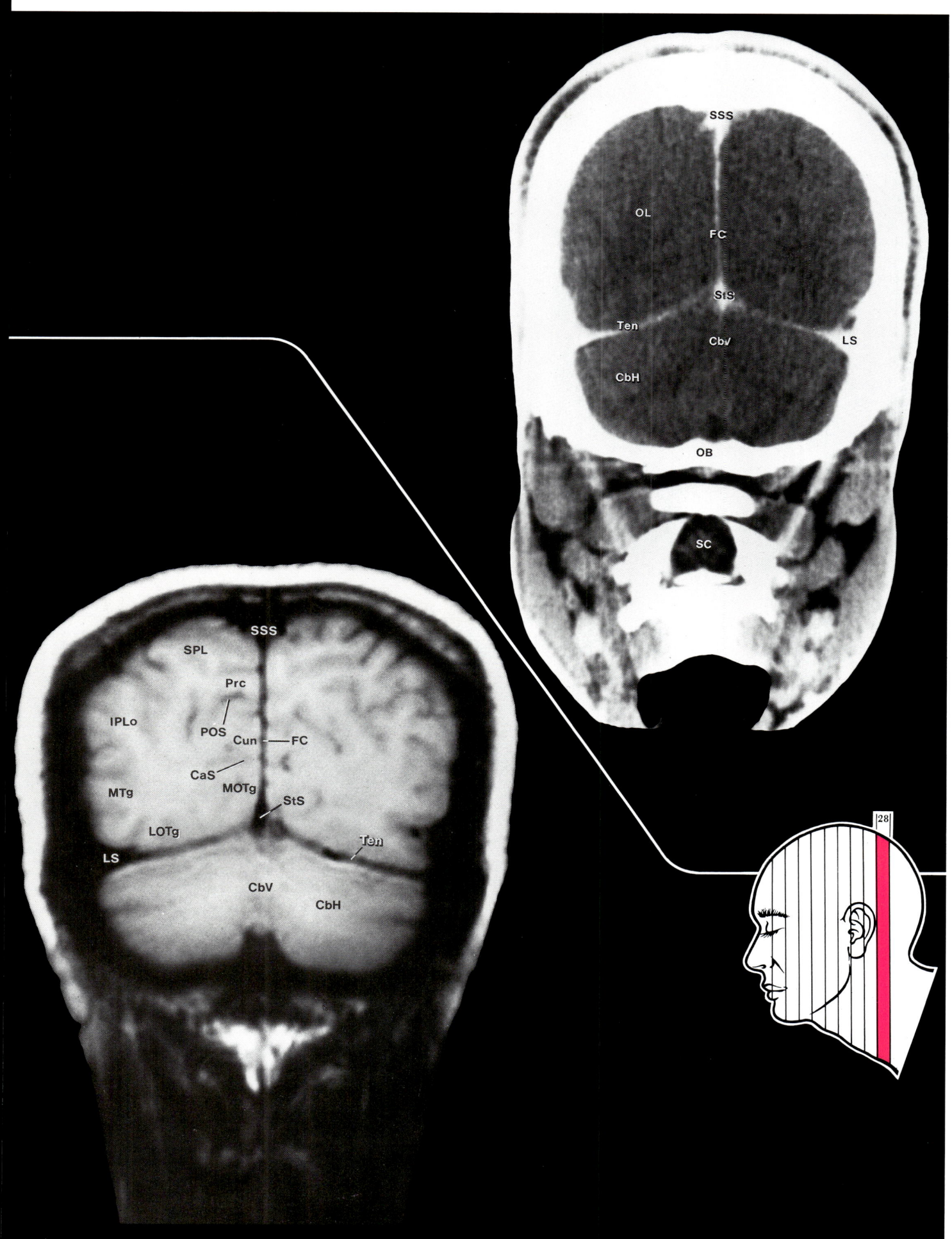

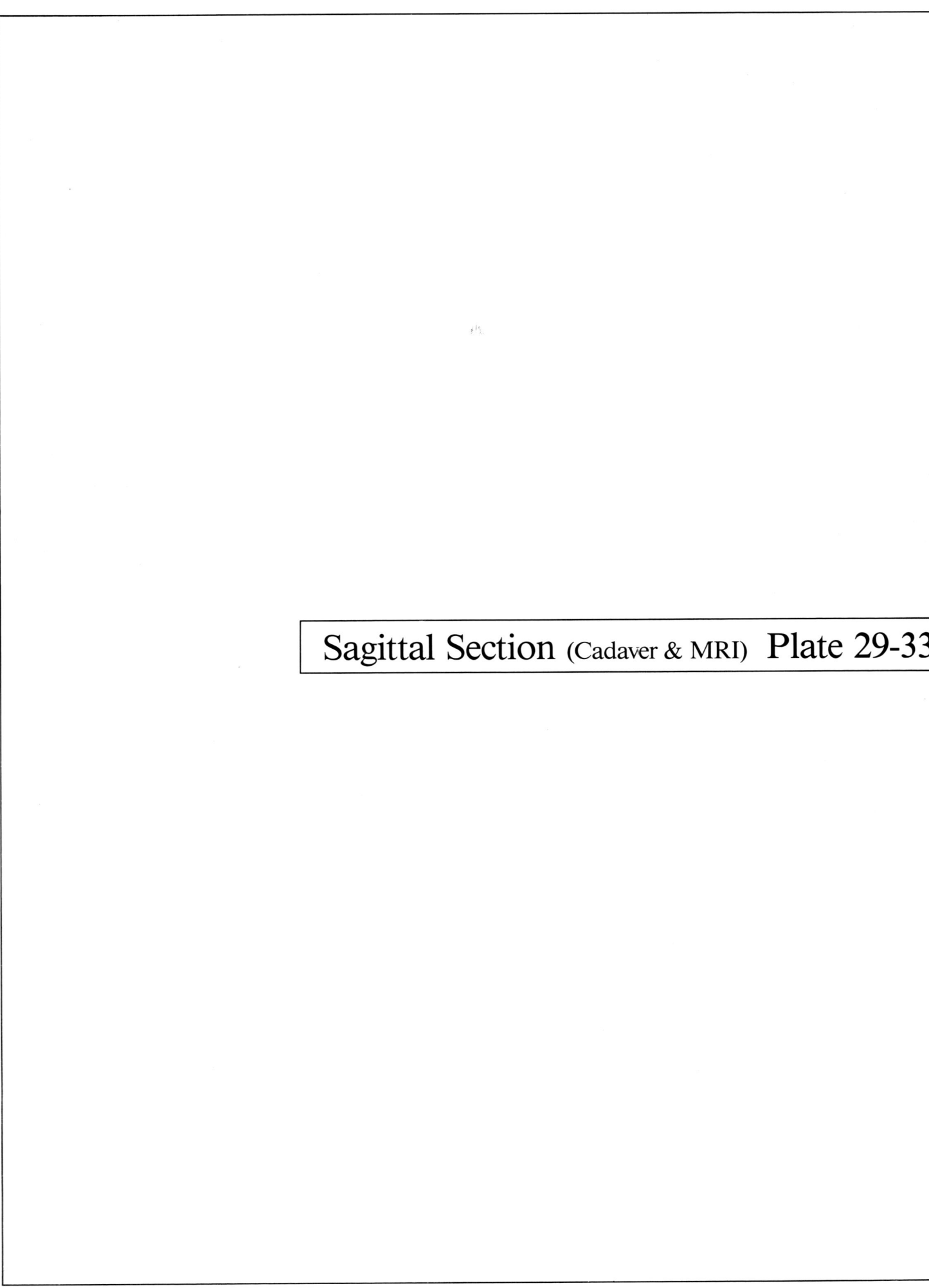

Sagittal Section (Cadaver & MRI) Plate 29-33

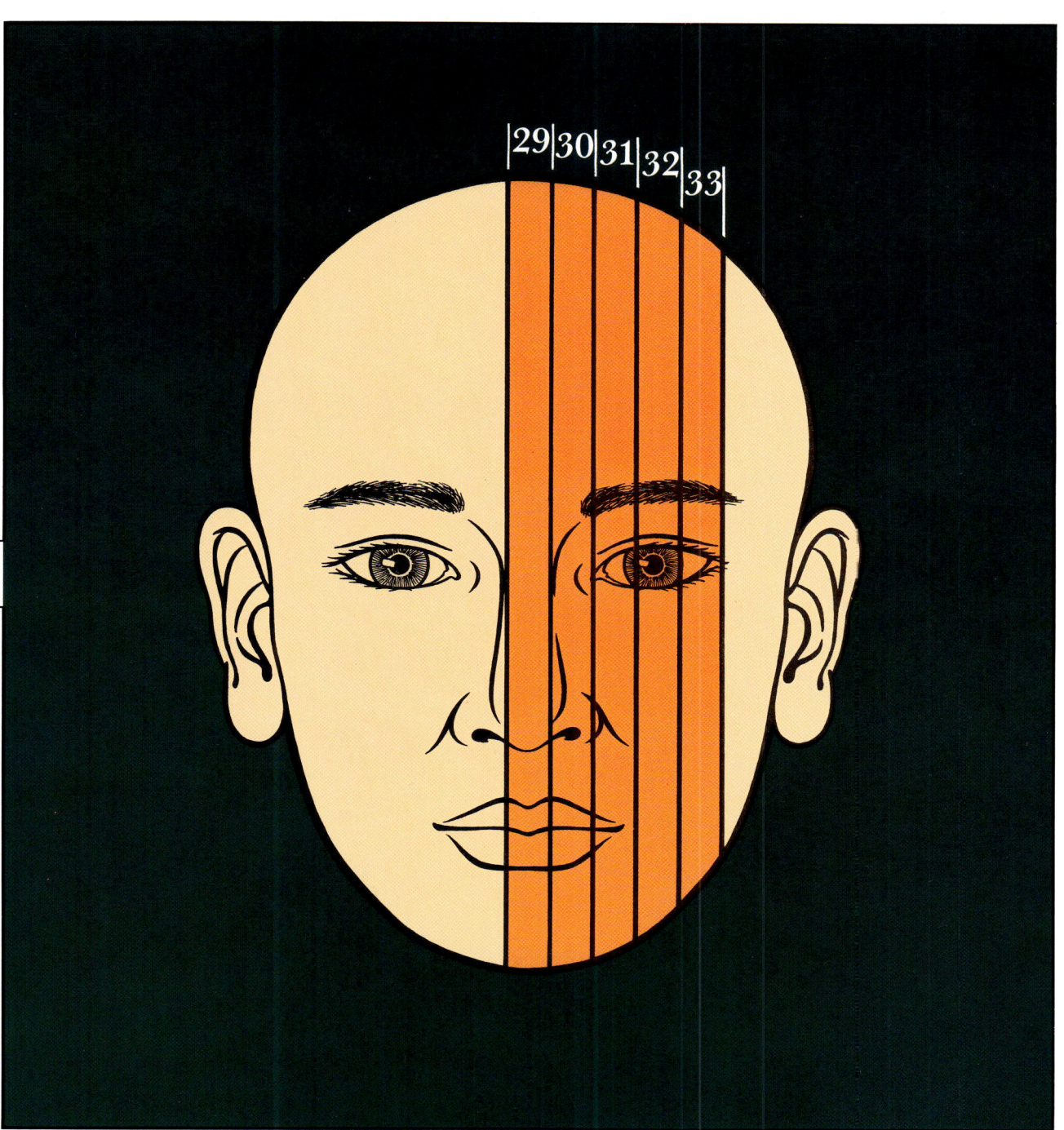

Plate 29. Sagittal BRAIN

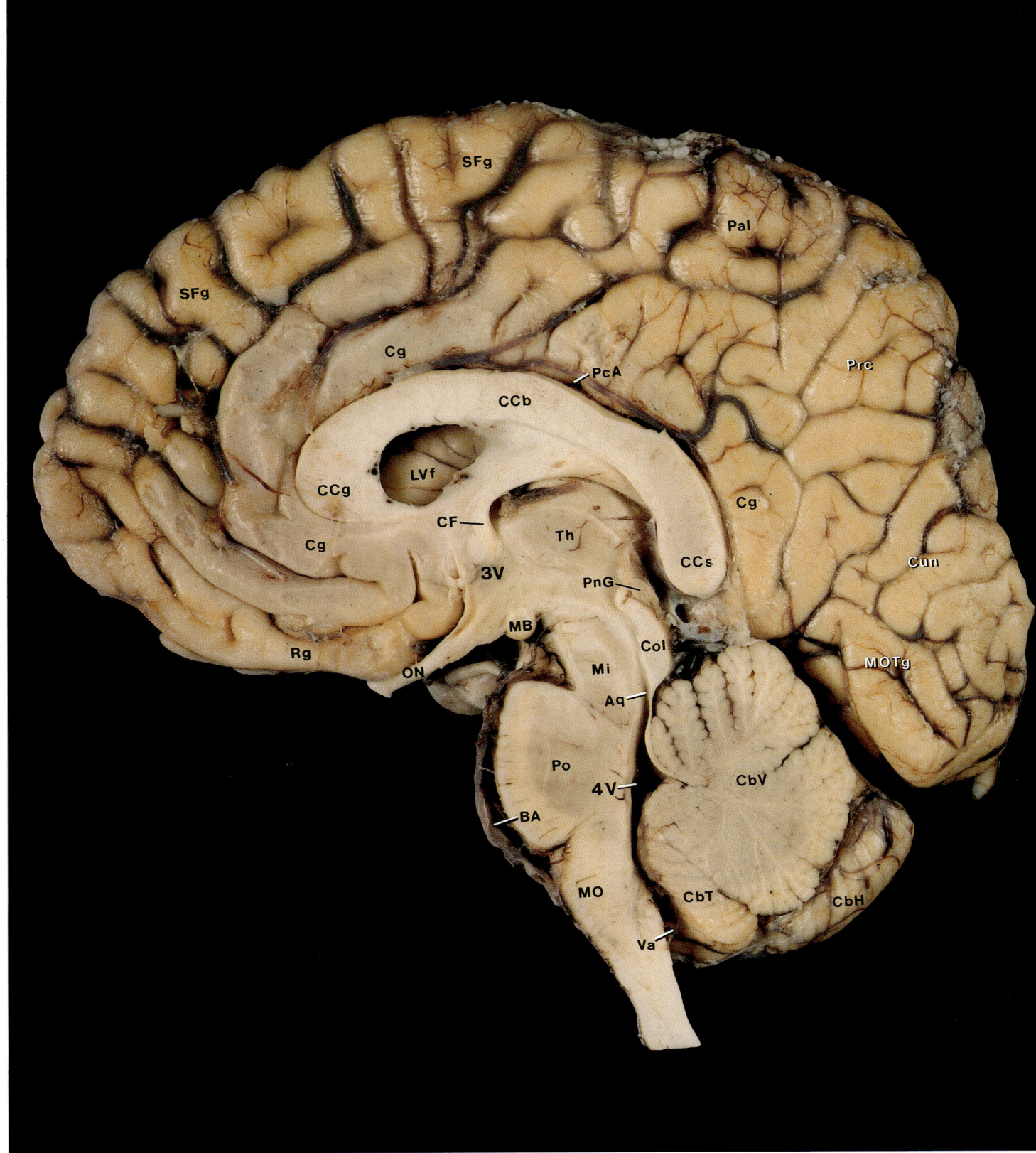

3V	3rd ventricle	Cg	Cingulate gyrus	PnG	Pineal gland
4V	4th ventricle	Col	Colliculus	Po	Pons
Aq	Aqueduct of sylvius	Cun	Cuneus	Prc	Precuneus
BA	Basilar artery	LVf	Lateral ventricle, frontal horn	Rg	Rectus gyrus
CCb	Corpus callosum body	MB	Mamillary body	SFg	Superior frontal gyrus
CCg	Corpus callosum genu	MO	Medulla oblongata	Th	Thalamus
CCs	Corpus callosum splenium	MOTg	Medial occiptotemporal gyrus	Va	Vallecula
CF	Column of fornix	Mi	Midbrain		
CbH	Cerebellar hemisphere	ON	Optic nerve		
CbT	Cerebellar tonsil	Pal	Paracentral lobule		
CbV	Cerebellar vermis	PcA	Pericallosal artery		

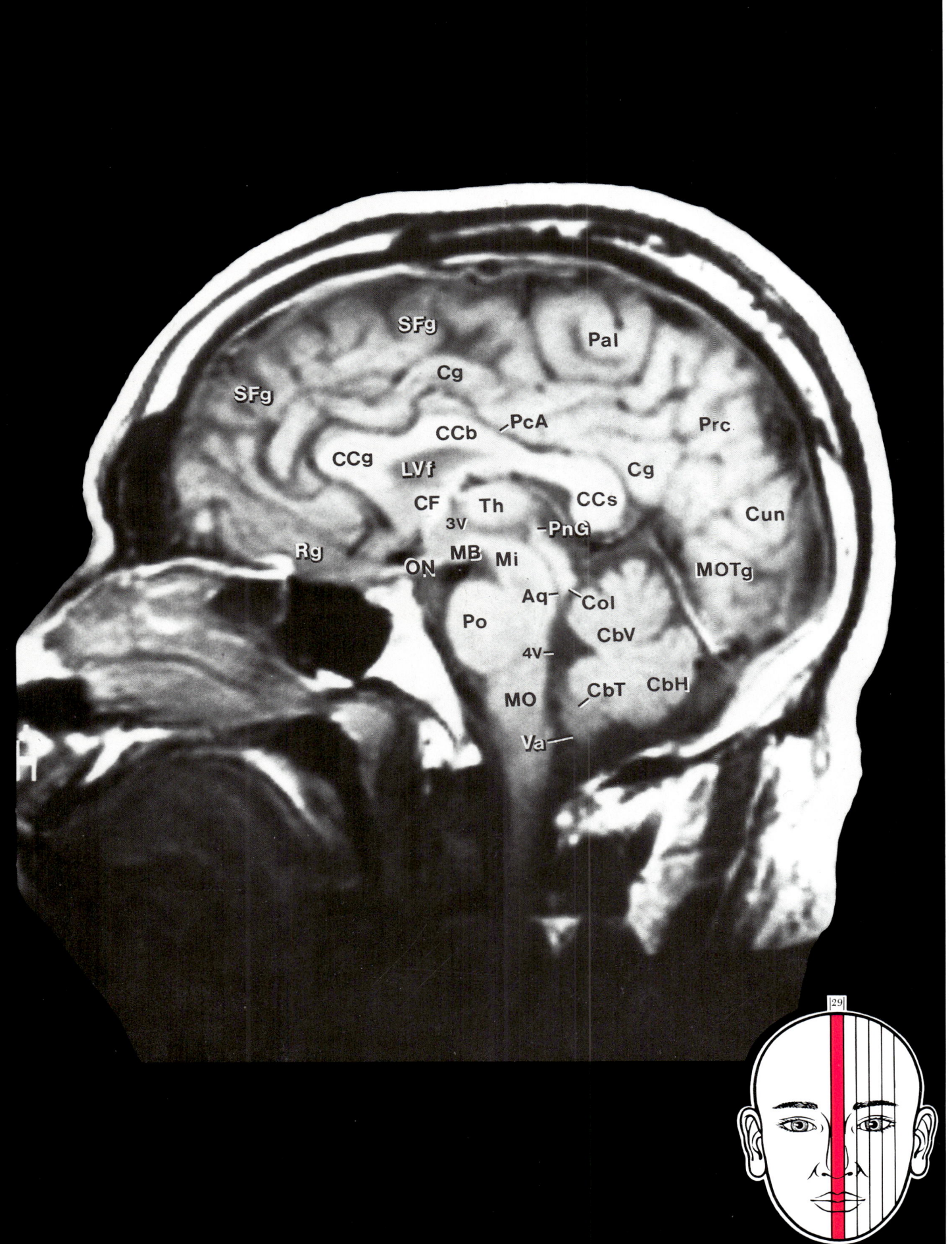

Plate 30. Sagittal BRAIN

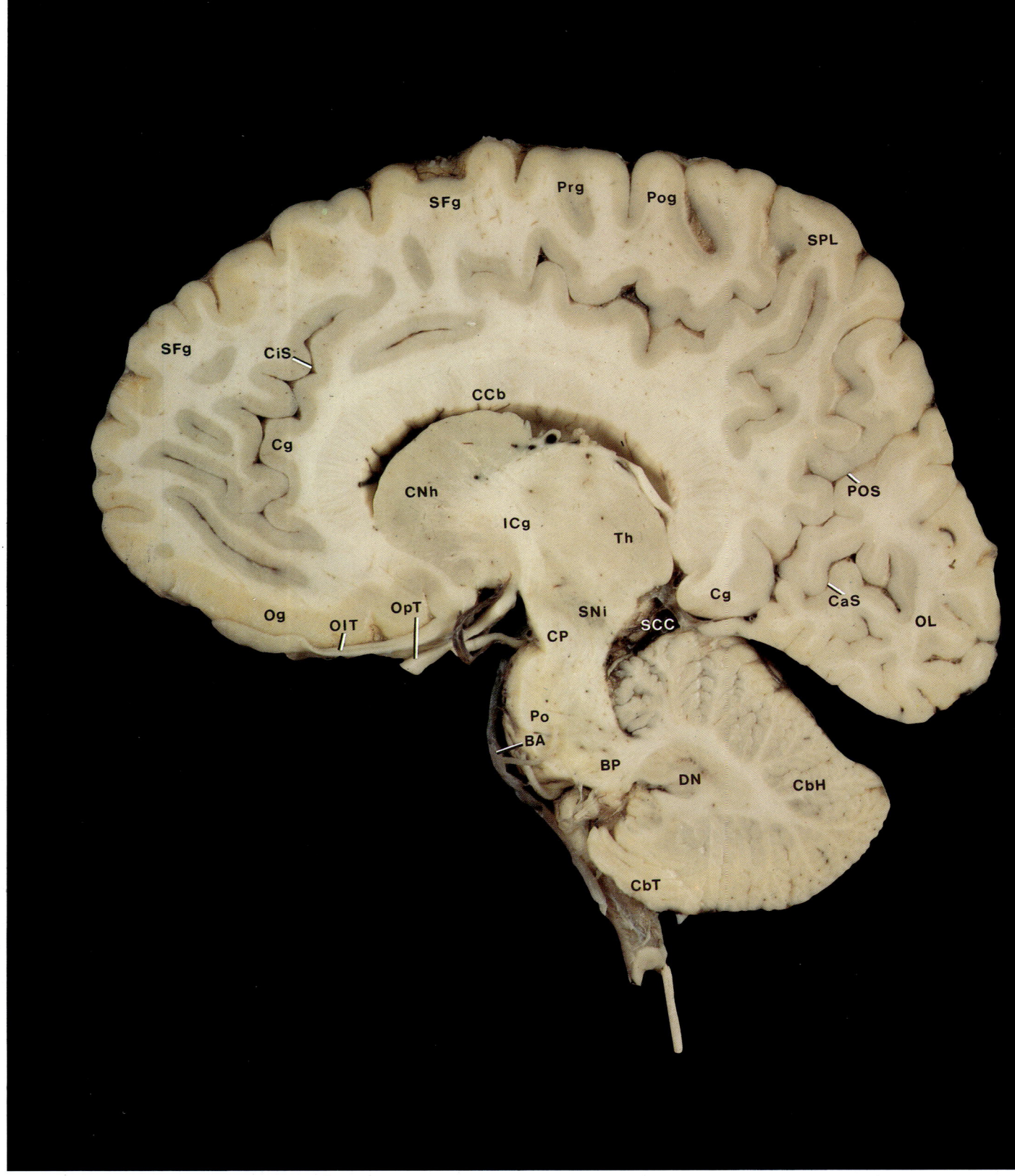

BA	Basilar artery	GP	Globus pallidus
BP	Brachium pontis	ICg	Internal capsule, genu
CCb	Corpus callosum, body	OL	Occipital lobe
CNh	Caudate nucleus, head	Og	Olfactory gyrus
CP	Cerebral peduncle	OlT	Olfactory tract
CaS	Calcarine sulcus	OpT	Optic tract
CbH	Cerebellar hemisphere	POS	Parietooccipital sulcus
CbT	Cerebellar tonsil	Po	Pons
Cg	Cirgulate gyrus	Pog	Postcentral gyrus
CiS	Cingalate sulcus	Prg	Precentral gyrus
DN	Dentate nucleus	SCC	Superior cerebellar cistern

SFg	Superior frontal gyrus
SNi	Subtantia nigra
SPL	Superior parietal lobule
Th	Thalamus

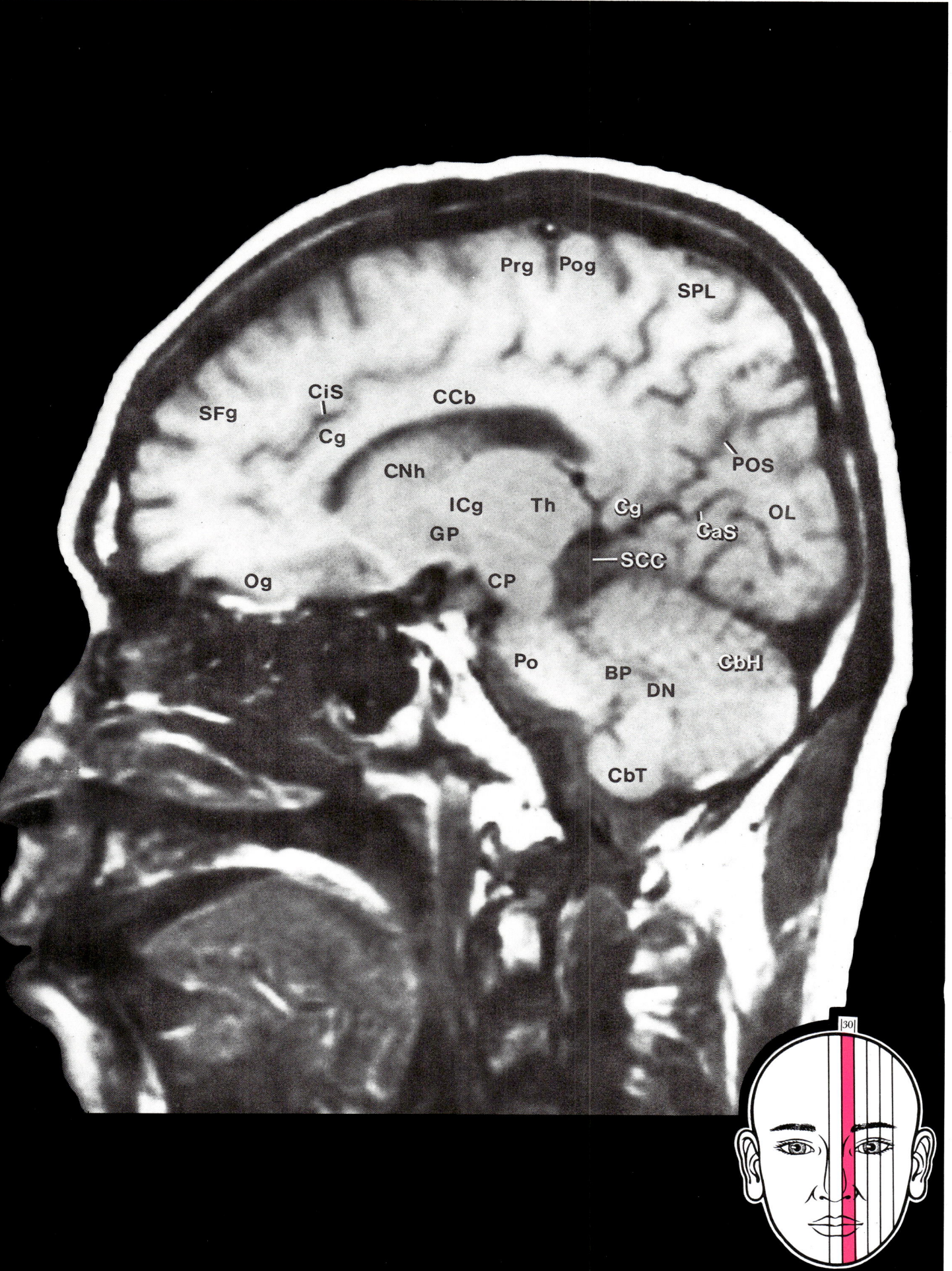

Plate 31. Sagittal BRAIN

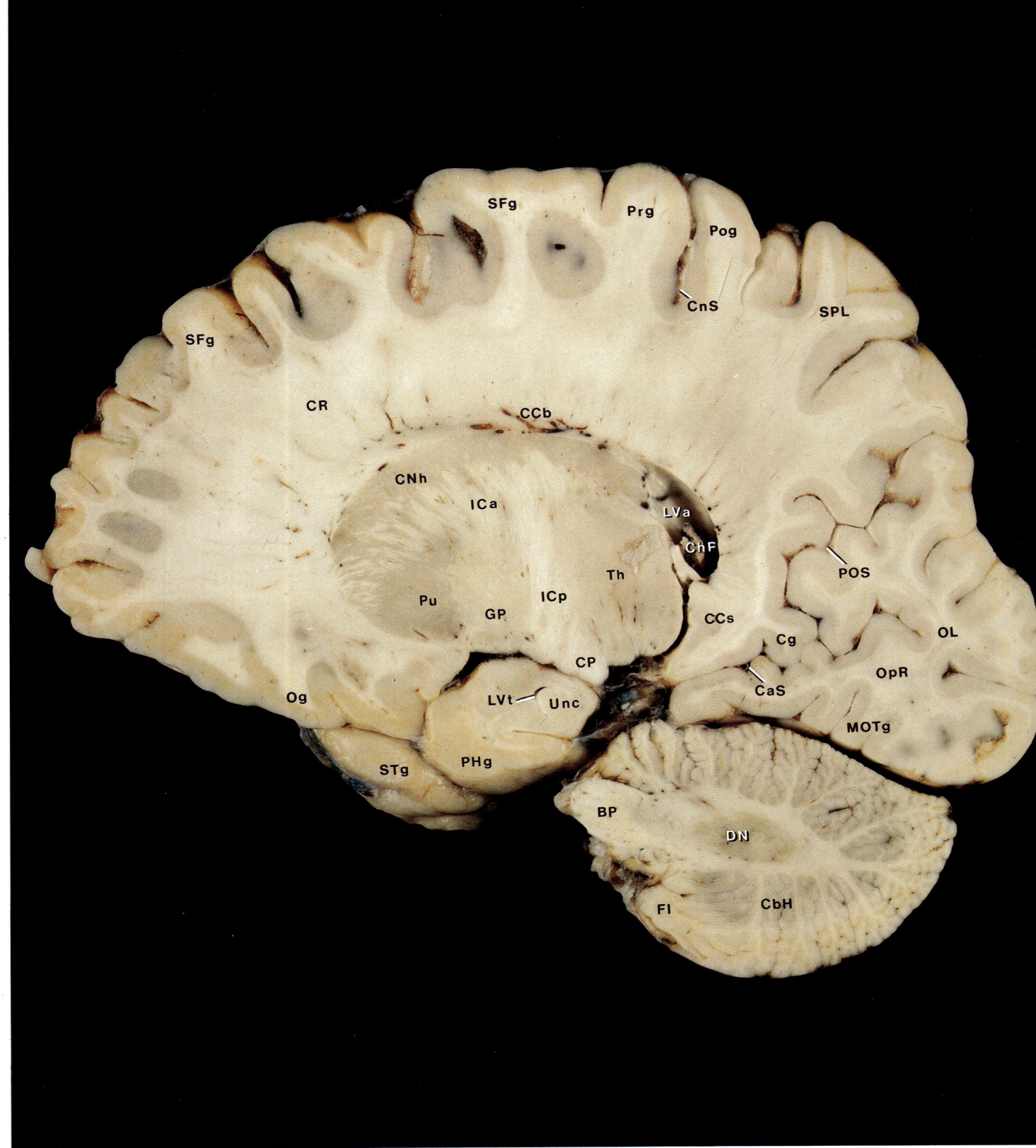

BP	Brachium pontis	DN	Dentate nucleus	PHg	Parahippocampal gyrus
CCb	Corpus callosum, body	Fl	Flocculus	POS	Parietooccipital sulcus
CCs	Corpus callosum, splenium	GP	Golbus pallidus	Pog	Postcentral gyrus
CNh	Caudate nucleus, head	ICa	Internal capsule, anterior limb	Prg	Precentral gyrus
CP	Cerebral peduncle	ICp	Internal capsule, posterior limb	Pu	Putamen
CR	Corona radiata	LVa	Lateral ventricle, atrium	SFg	Superior frontal gyrus
CaS	Calcarine sulcus	LVt	Lateral ventricle, temporal horn	SPL	Superior parietal lobule
CbH	Cerebellar hemisphere	MOTg	Medial occipitotemporal gyrus	STg	Superior temporal gyrus
Cg	Cingulate gyrus	OL	Occipital lobe	Th	Thalamus
ChP	Choroid plexus	Og	Olfactory gyrus	Unc	Uncus
CnS	Central sulcus	OpR	Optic radiation		

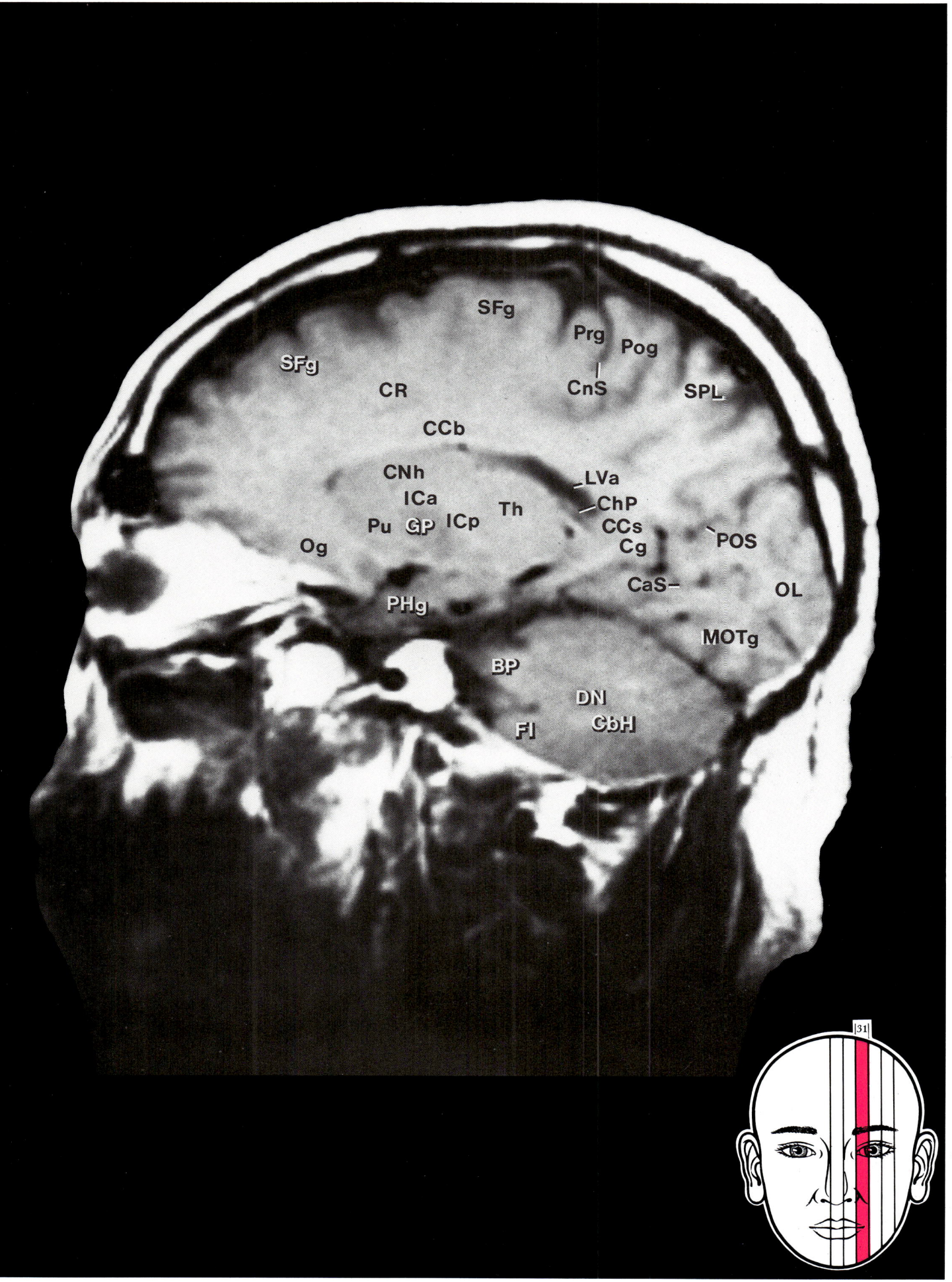

Plate 32. Sagittal BRAIN

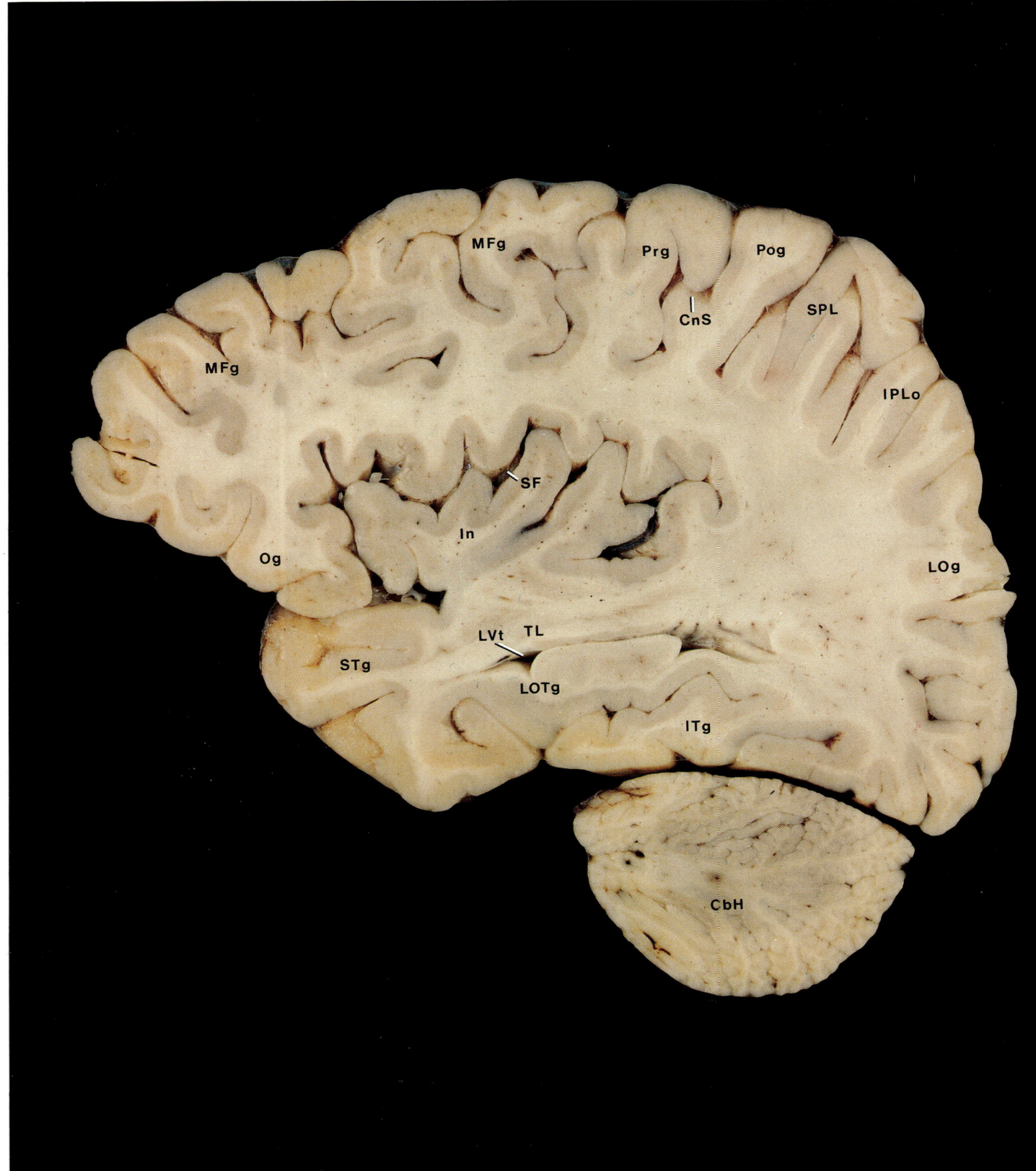

CbH	Cerebellar hemisphere	Prg	Precentral gyrus
CnS	Central sulcus	SF	Sylvian fissure
IPLo	Inferior parietal lobule	SPL	Superior parietal lobule
ITg	Inferior temporal gyrus	STg	Superior temporal gyrus
In	Incus	TL	Temporal lobe
LOTg	Lateral occipitotemporal gyrus		
LOg	Lateral occipital gyrus		
LVt	Lateral ventricle, temporal horn		
MFg	Middle frontal gyrus		
Og	Olfactory gyrus		
Pog	Postcentral gyrus		

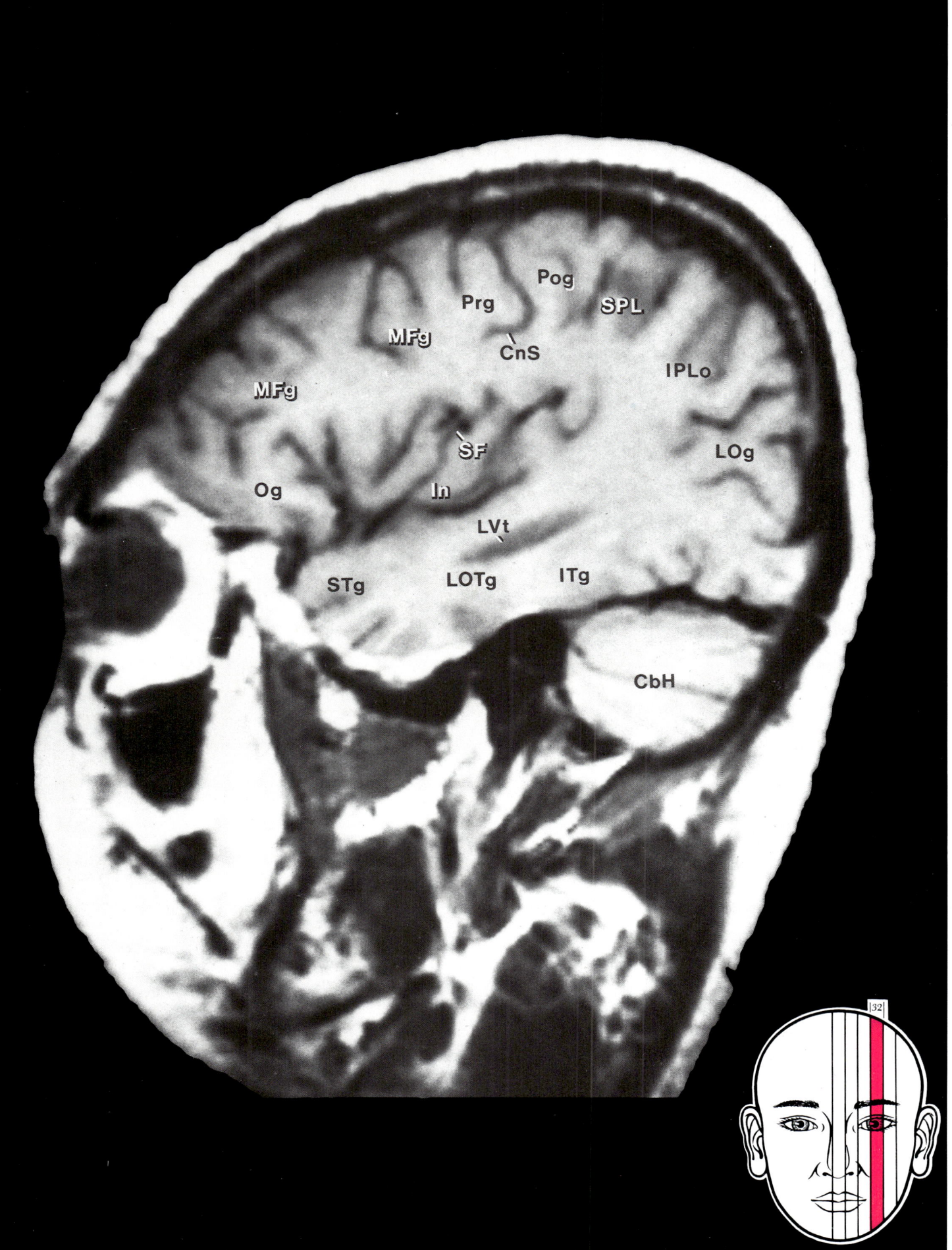

Plate 33. SAGITTAL BRAIN

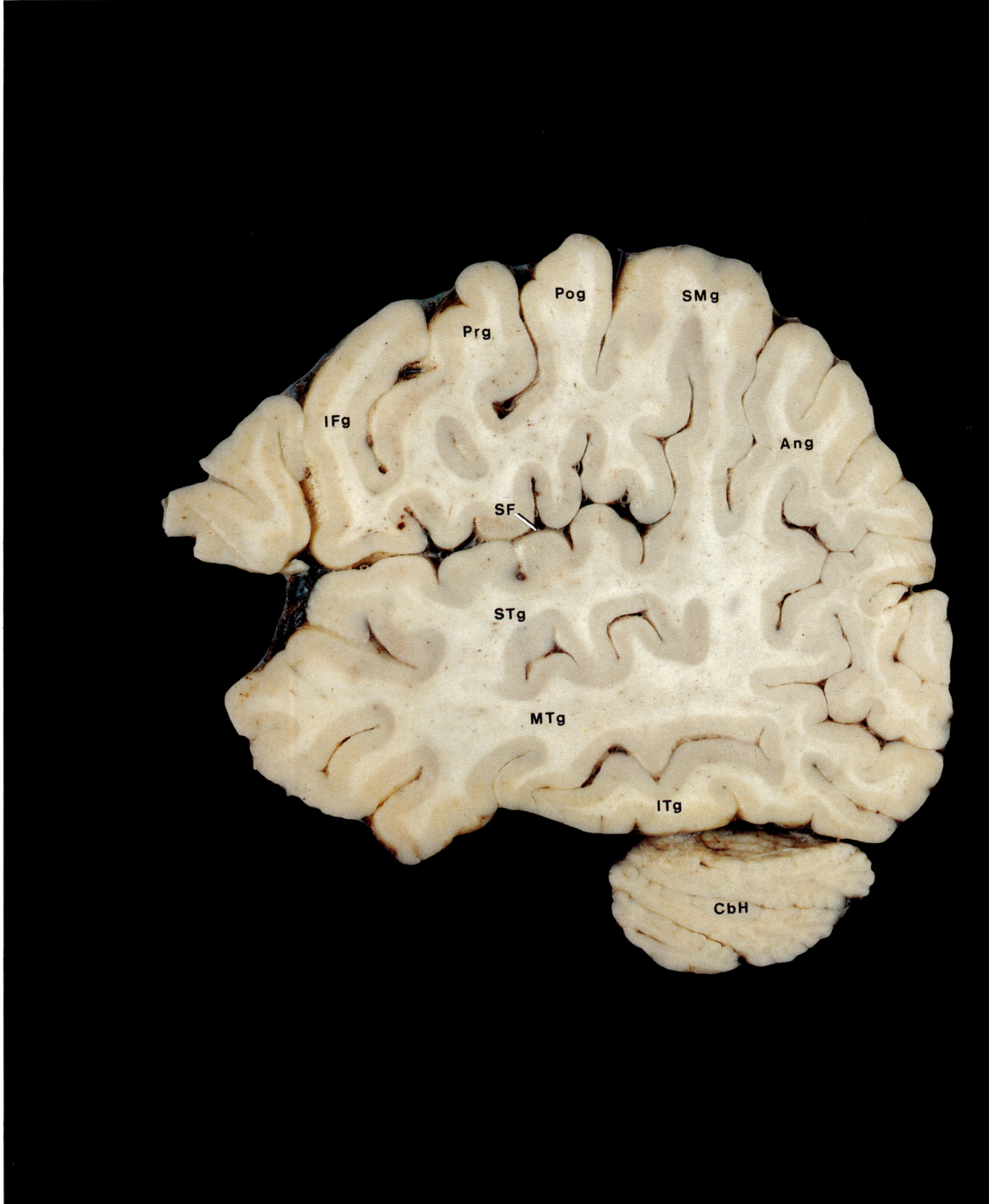

Ang	Angular gyrus
CbH	Cerebellar hemisphere
IFg	Inferior frontal gyrus
ITg	Inferior temporal gyrus
MTg	Middle temporal gyrus
Pog	Postcentral gyrus
Prg	Precentral gyrus
SF	Sylvian fissure
SMg	Supramarginal gyrus
STg	Superior temporal gyrus

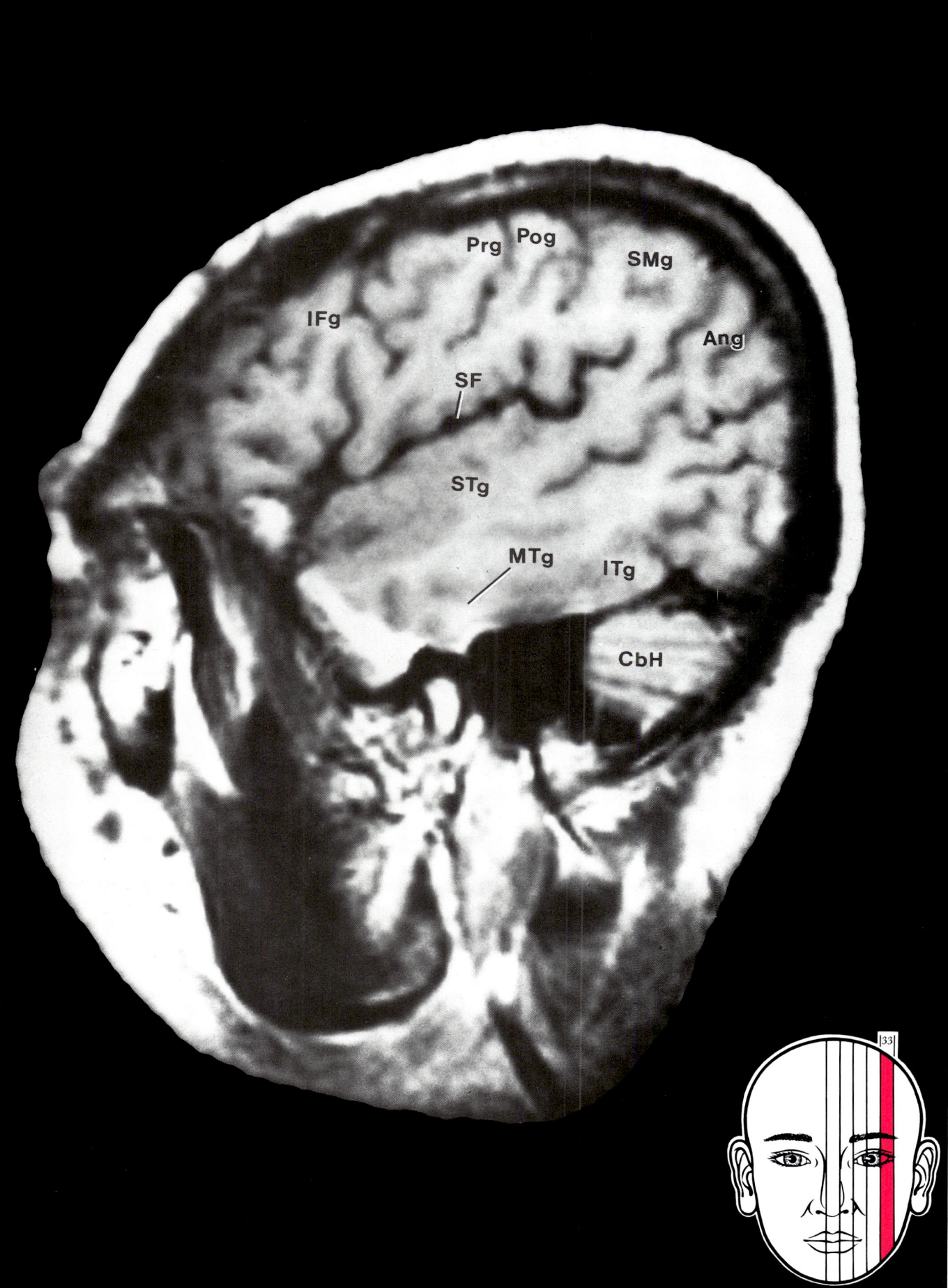

PART 2
CHEST

Transverse Section-male (Cadaver, CT & MRI) Plate 34-42

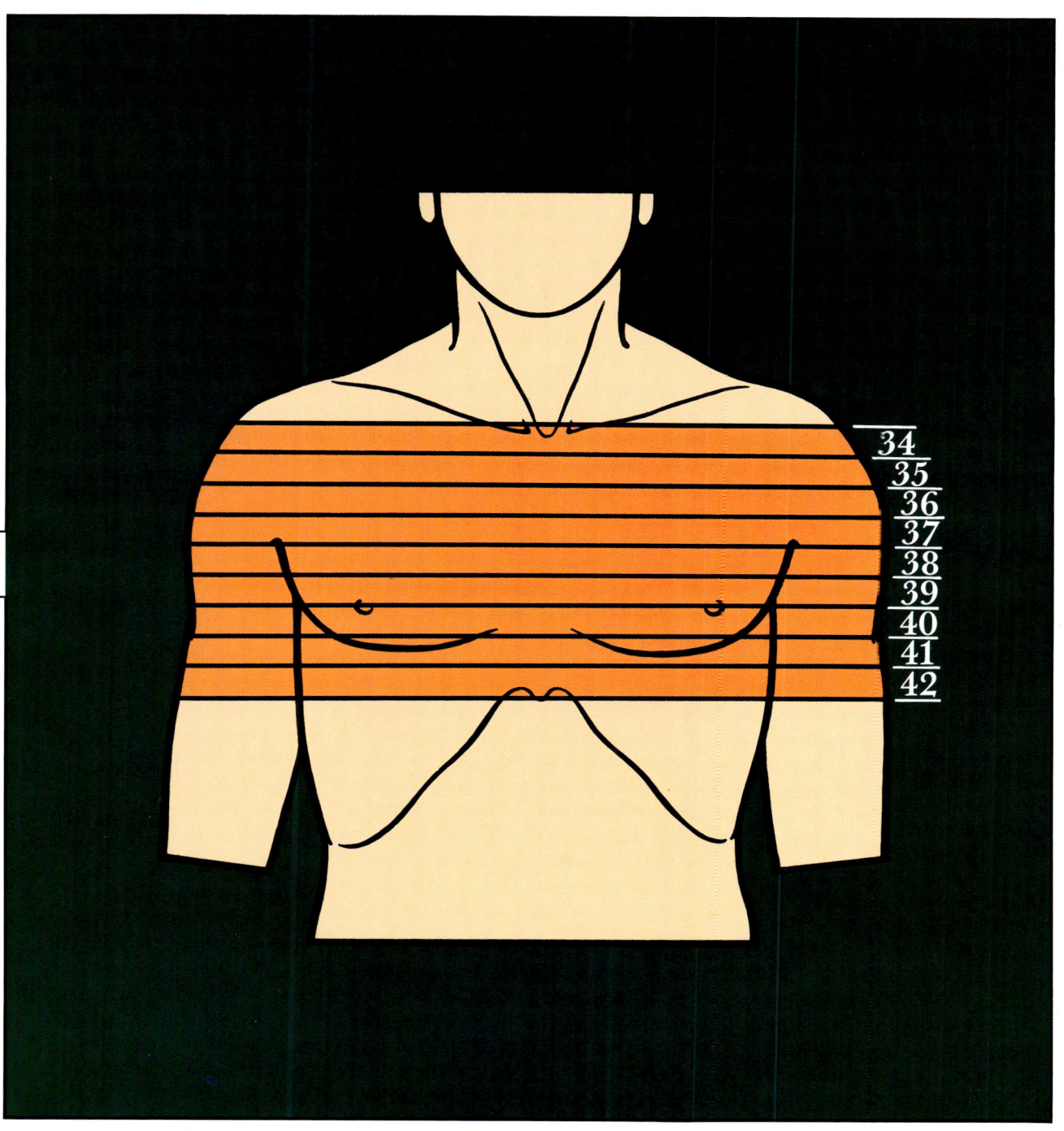

Plate 34. Transverse CHEST

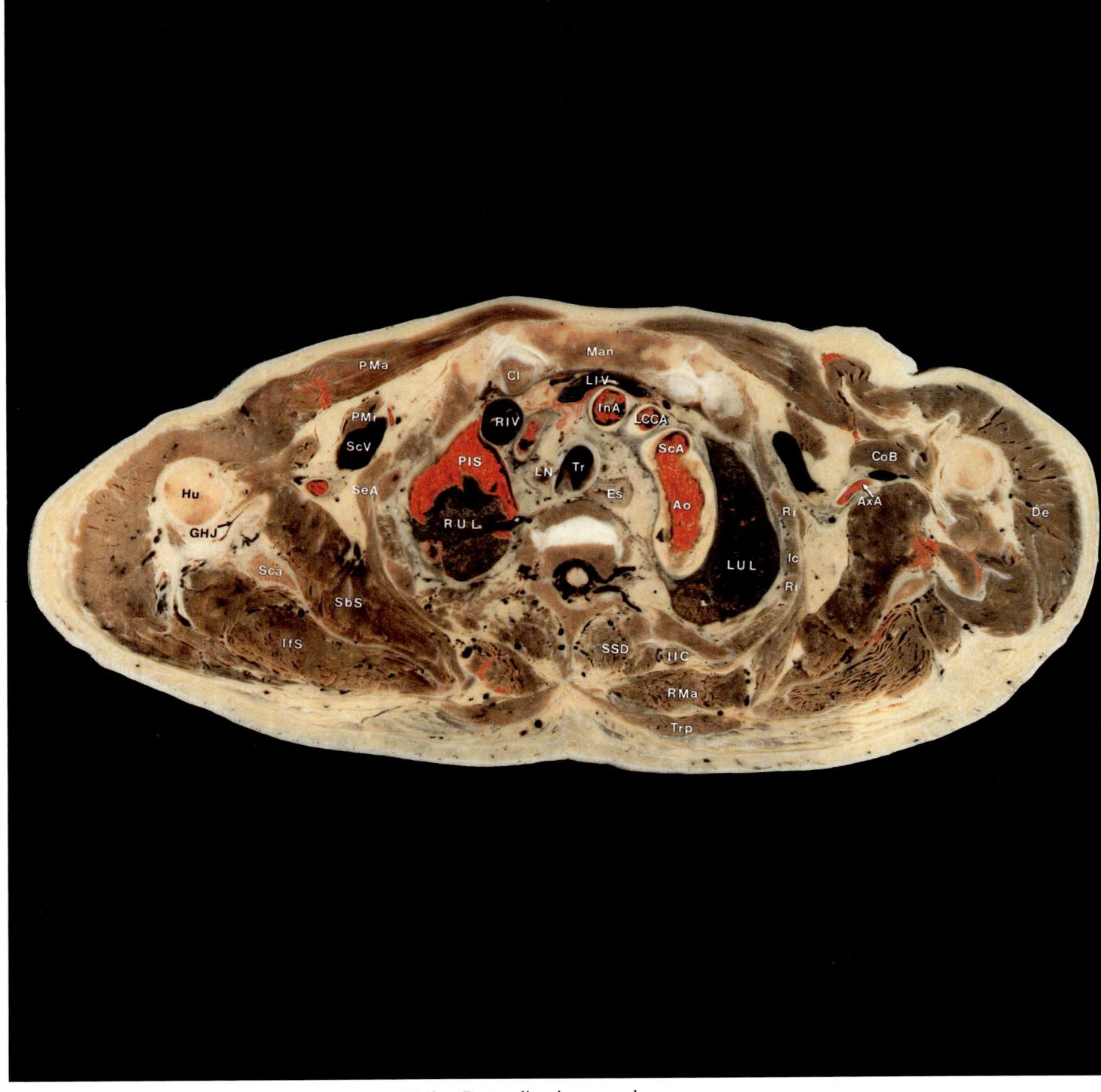

Ao	Aorta	PMi	Pectoralis minor muscle
AxA	Axillary artery	PlS	Pleural space
Cl	Clavicle	RIV	Right innominate vein
CoB	Coracobrachialis muscle	RMa	Rhomboideus major muscle
De	Deltoid muscle	RUL	Right upper lobe of lung
Es	Esophagus	Ri	Rib
GHJ	Glenohumeral joint	SSD	Semispinalis dorsi muscle
Hu	Humerus	SbS	Subscapularis muscle
Ic	Intercostal muscle	ScA	Subclavian artery
IfS	Infraspinatus muscle	ScV	Subclavian vein
IlC	Iliocostalis muscle	Sca	Scapula
InA	Innominate artery	SeA	Serratus anterior muscle
LCCA	Left common carotid artery	Tr	Trachea
LIV	Left innominate vein	Trp	Trapezius muscle
LN	Lymph node		
LUL	Left upper lobe of lung		
Man	Manubrium		
PMa	Pectoralis major muscle		

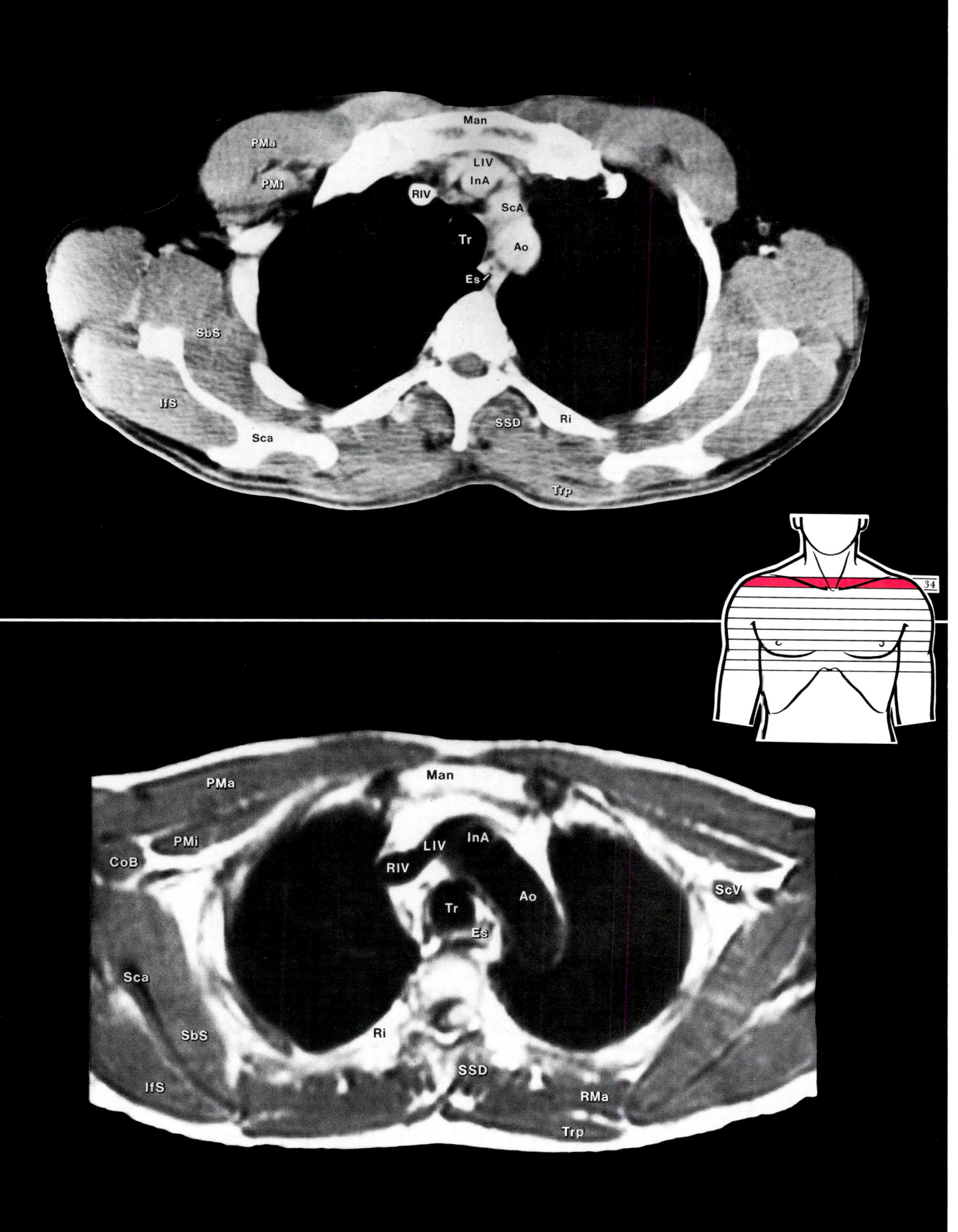

Plate 35. TRANSVERSE CHEST

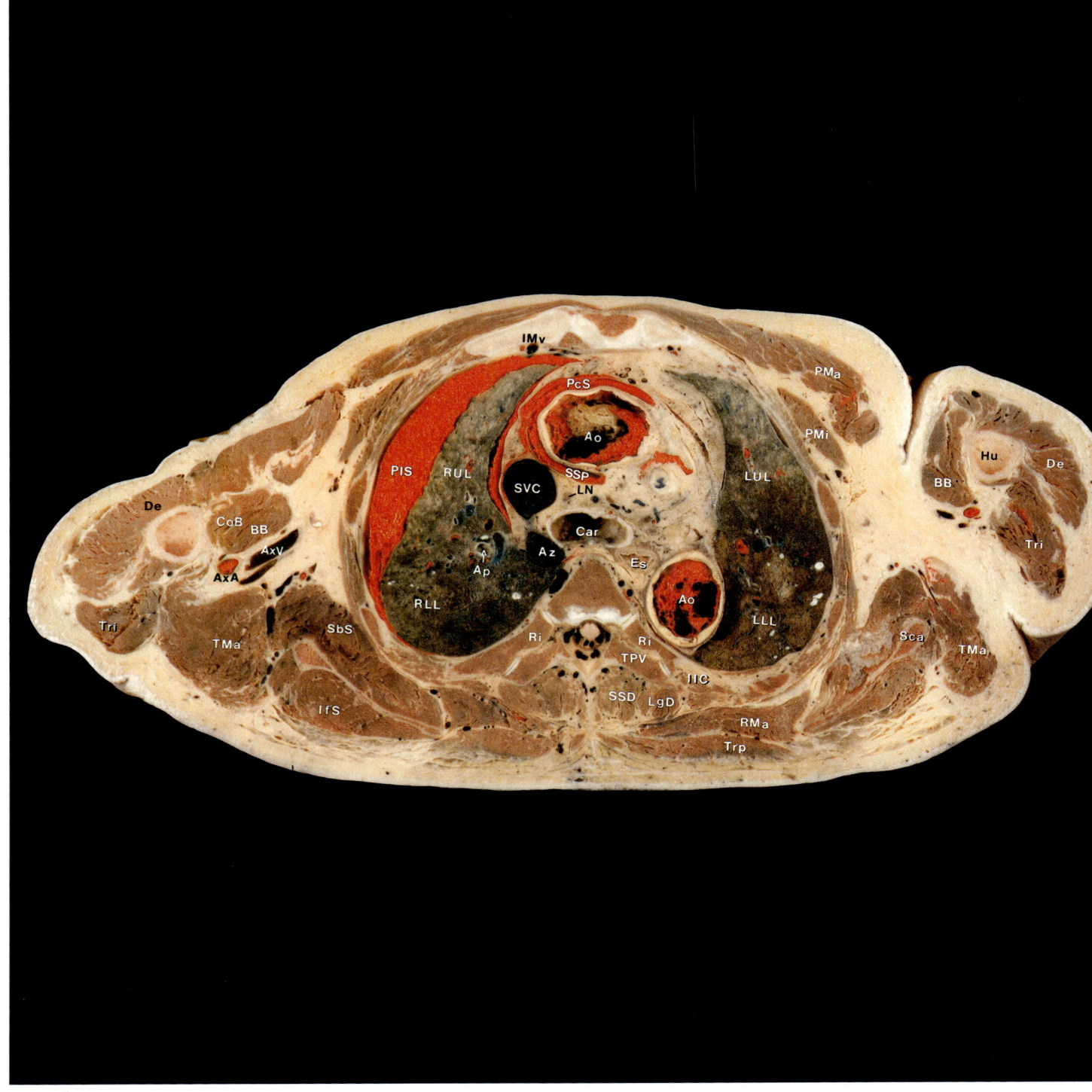

Ao	Aorta	LgD	Longissimus dorsi muscle	Trp	Trapezius muscle
Ap	Apical segment of right upper lobe bronchus	PMa	Pectoralis major muscle		
		PMi	Pectoralis minor muscle		
AxA	Axillary artery	PcS	Pericardial space		
AxV	Axillary vein	PlS	Pleural space		
Az	Azygos vein	RLL	Right lower lobe of lung		
BB	Biceps brachii muscle	RMa	Rhomboideus major muscle		
Car	Carina	RUL	Right upper lobe of lung		
CoB	Coracobrachialis muscle	Ri	Rib		
De	Deltoid muscle	SSD	Semispinalis dorsi muscle		
Es	Esophagus	SSP	Superior sinus of pericardium		
Hu	Humerus	SVC	Superior vena cava		
IMv	Internal mammary vessel	SbS	Subscapularis muscle		
IfS	Infraspinatus muscle	ScV	Subclavian vein		
IlC	Iliocostalis muscle	Sca	Scapula		
LLL	Left lower lobe of lung	TMa	Teres major muscle		
LN	Lymph node	TPV	Transverse process of vertebra		
LUL	Left upper lobe of lung	Tri	Triceps brachii muscle		

— 80 —

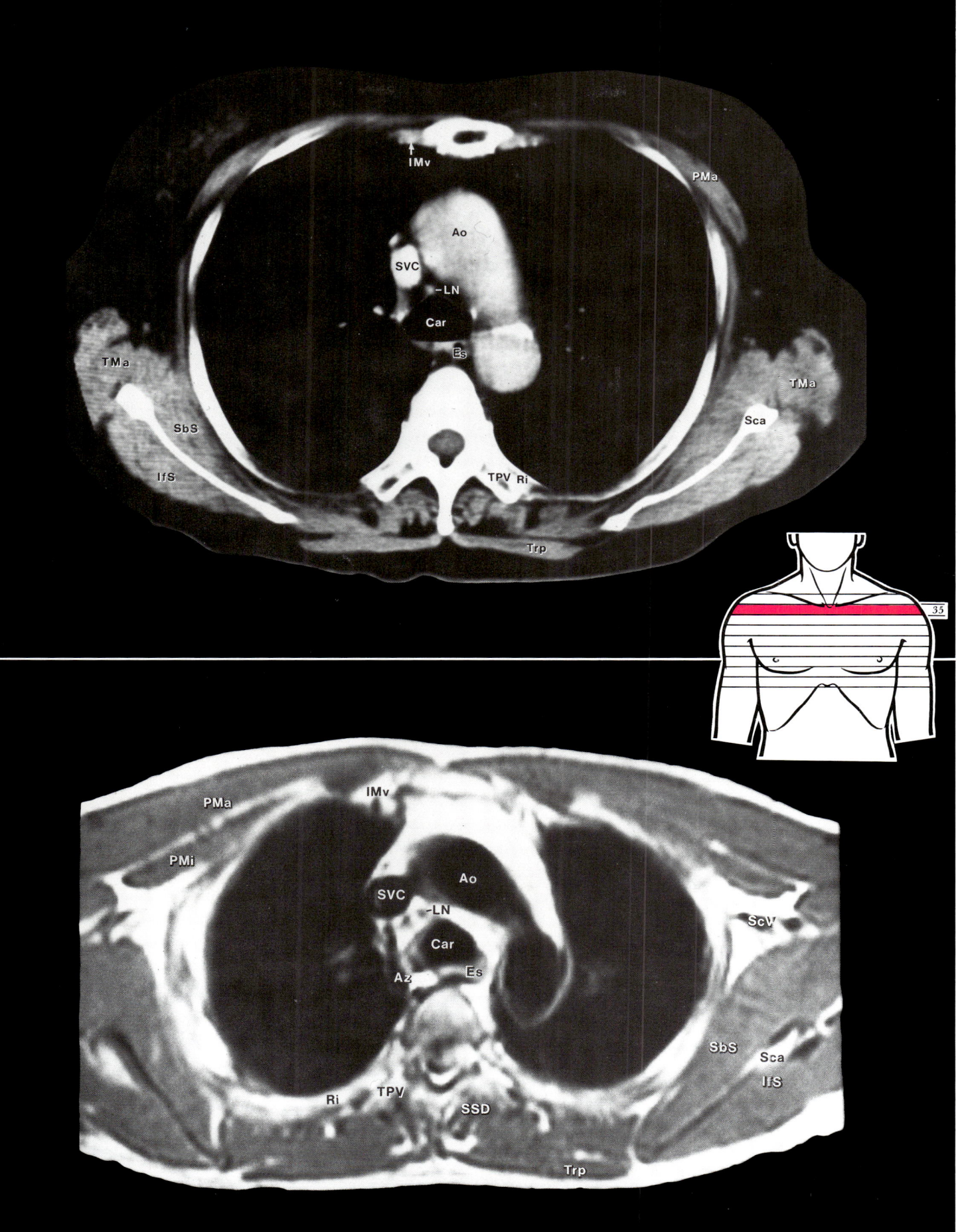

Plate 36. Transverse CHEST

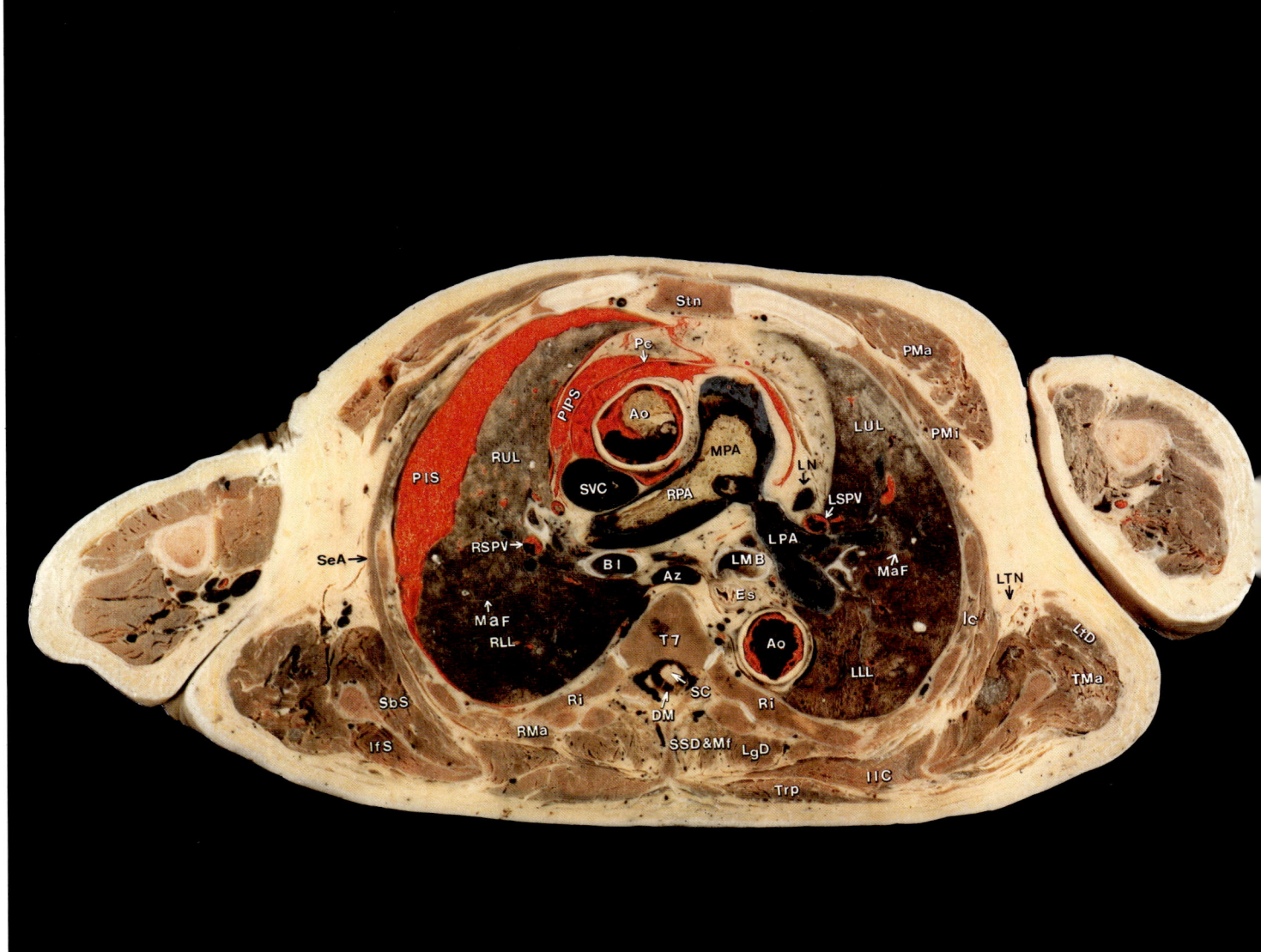

Ao	Aorta	MaF	Major fissure	SeA	Serratus anterior muscle
Az	Azygos vein	Mf	Multifidus muscle	Stn	Sternum
BI	Bronchus intermedius	PMa	Pectoralis major muscle	T7	T7 vertebral body
DM	Dura mater	PMi	Pectoralis minor muscle	TMa	Tres major muscle
Es	Esophagus	Pc	Pericardium	Trp	Trapezius muscle
Ic	Intercostal muscle	PlPS	Pleuropericardial space		
IfS	Infraspinatus muscle	PlS	Pleural space		
IlC	Iliocostalis muscle	RLL	Right lower lobe of lung		
LLL	Left lower lobe of lung	RMa	Rhomboideus major muscle		
LMB	Left main bronchus	RPA	Right pulmonary artery		
LN	Lymph node	RSPV	Right superior pulmonary vein		
LPA	Left pulmonary artery	RUL	Right upper lobe of lung		
LSPV	Left superior pulmonary vein	Ri	Rib		
LTN	Long thoracic nerve	SC	Spinal cord		
LUL	Left upper lobe of lung	SSD	Semispinalis dorsi muscle		
LgD	Longissimus dorsi muscle	SVC	Superior vena cava		
LtD	Latissimus dorsi muscle	SbS	Subscapularis muscle		
MPA	Main pulmonary artery	Sca	Scapula		

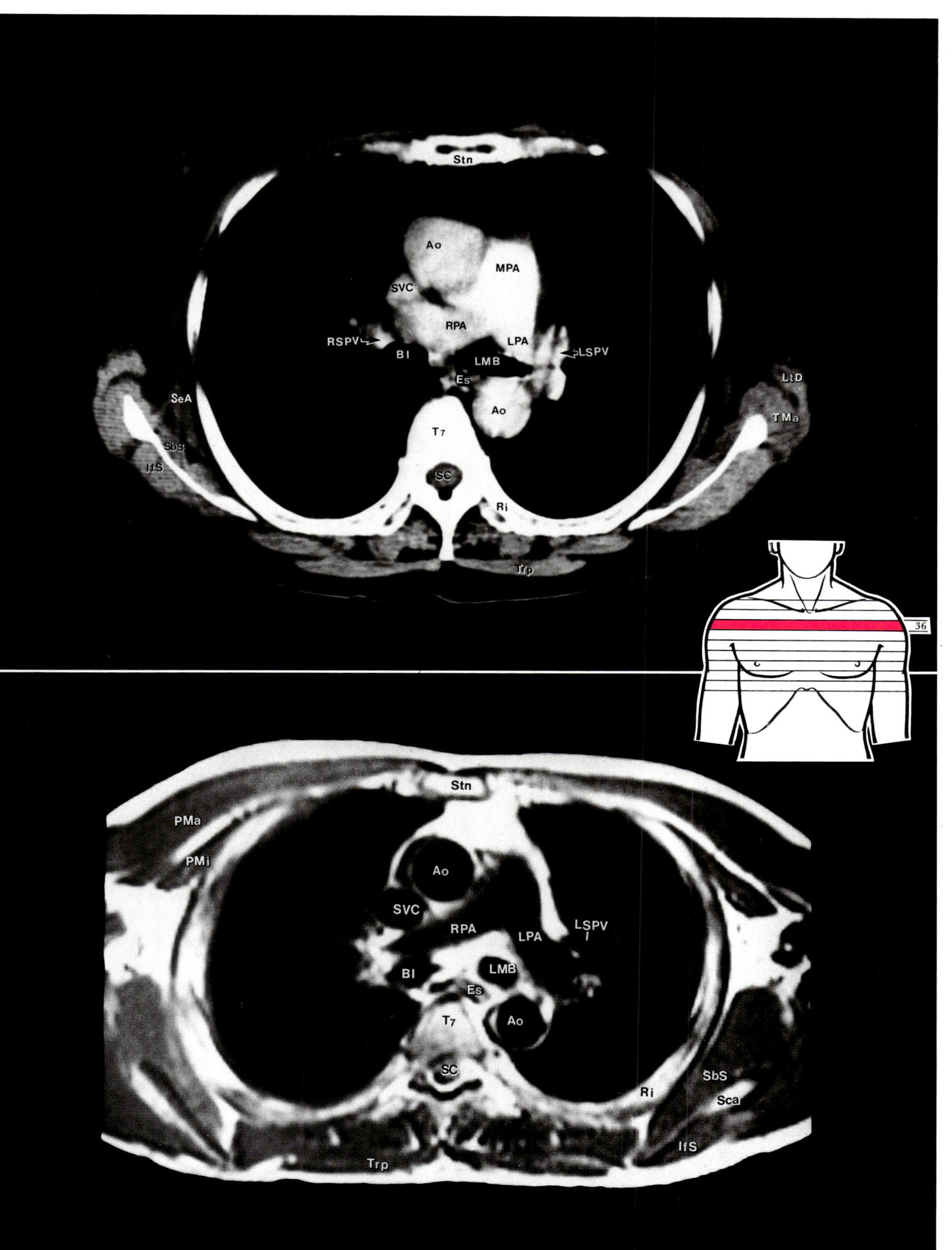

Plate 37. TRANSVERSE CHEST

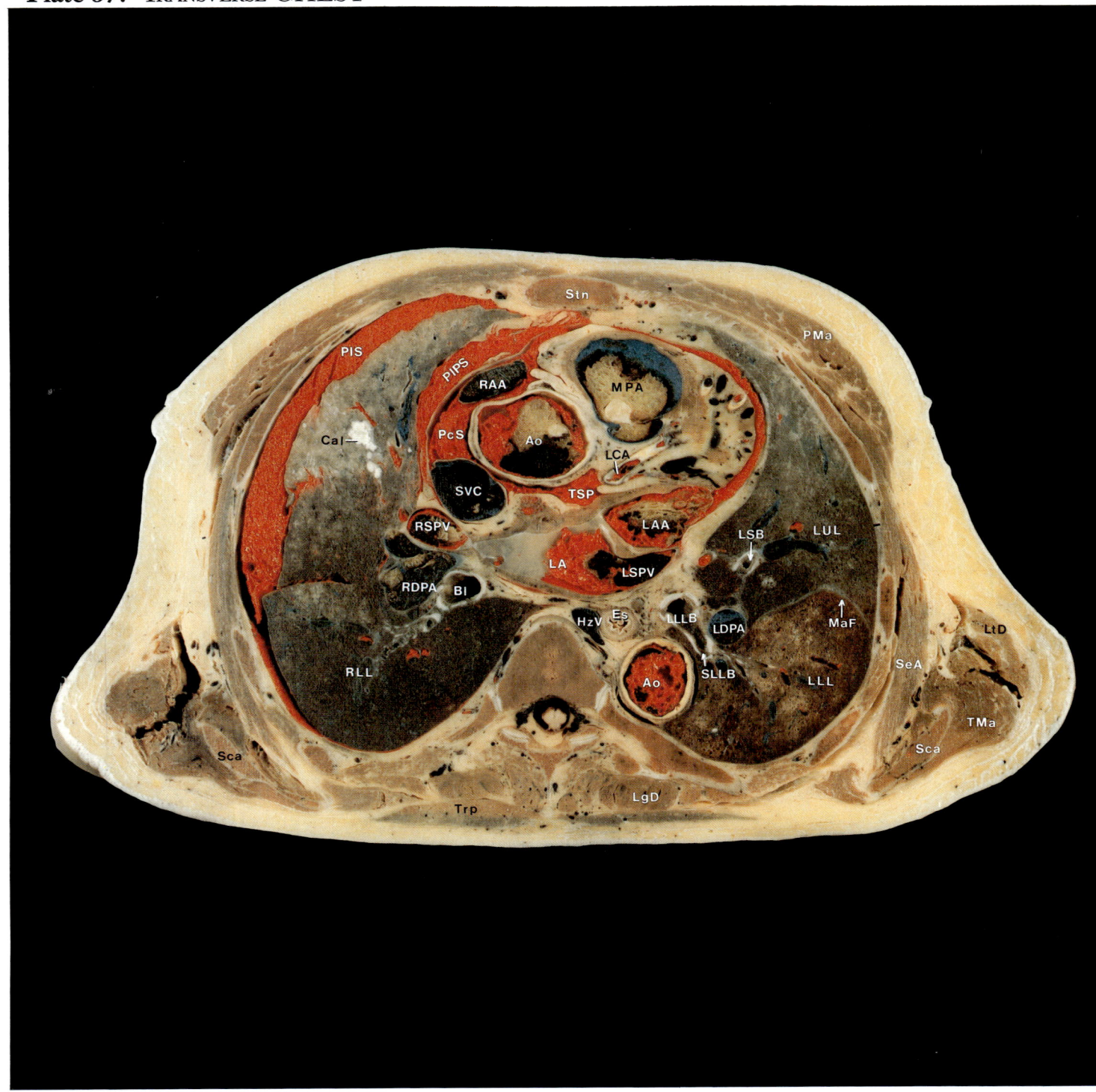

Ao	Aorta	MPA	Main pulmonary artery	TSP	Transverse sinus of pericardium
Az	Azygos vein	MaF	Major fissure	Trp	Trapezius muscle
BI	Bronchus intermedius	PMa	Pectoralis major muscle		
Cal	Calcification of lung	PcS	Pericardial space		
Es	Esophagus	PlPS	Pleuropericardial space		
HzV	Hemiazygos vein	PlS	Pleural space		
IcV	Intercostal vein	RAA	Right atrial appendage of heart		
LA	Left atrium of heart	RDPA	Right descending pulmonary artery		
LAA	Left atrial appendage of heart	RLL	Right lower lobe of lung		
LCA	Left coronary artery	RLLB	Right lower lobe bronchus		
LDPA	Left descending pulmonary artery	RSPV	Right superior pulmonary vein		
LLL	Left lower lobe of lung	SLLB	Superior segment of left lower lobe bronchus		
LLLB	Left lower lobe bronchus	SVC	Superior vena cava		
LSB	Lingular segmental bronchus	Sca	Scapula		
LSPV	Left superior pulmonary vein	SeA	Serratus anterior muscle		
LUL	Left upper lobe of lung	Stn	Sternum		
LgD	Longissimus dorsi muscle	TMa	Teres major muscle		
LtD	Latissimus dorsi muscle				

— 84 —

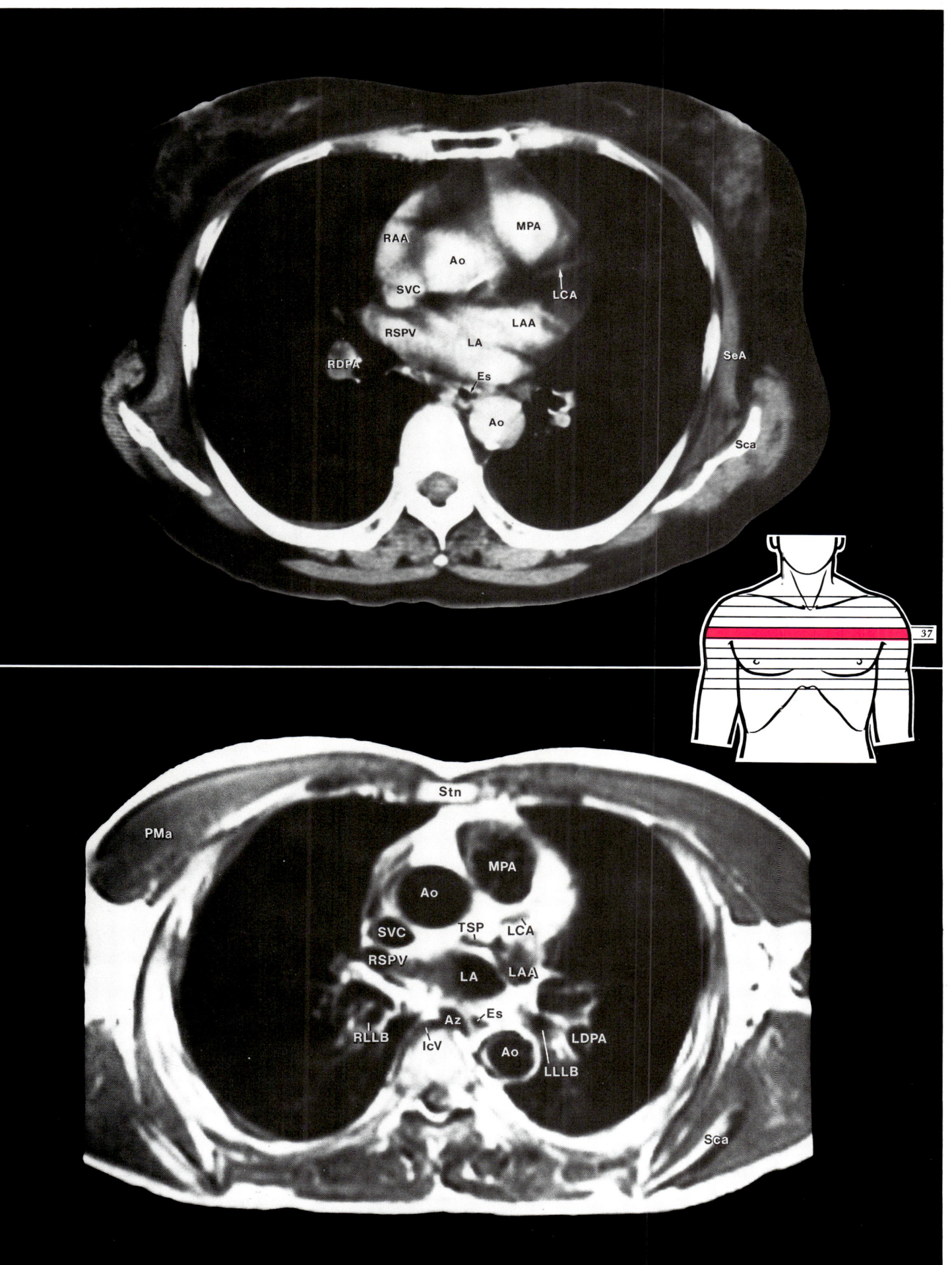

Plate 38. Transverse CHEST

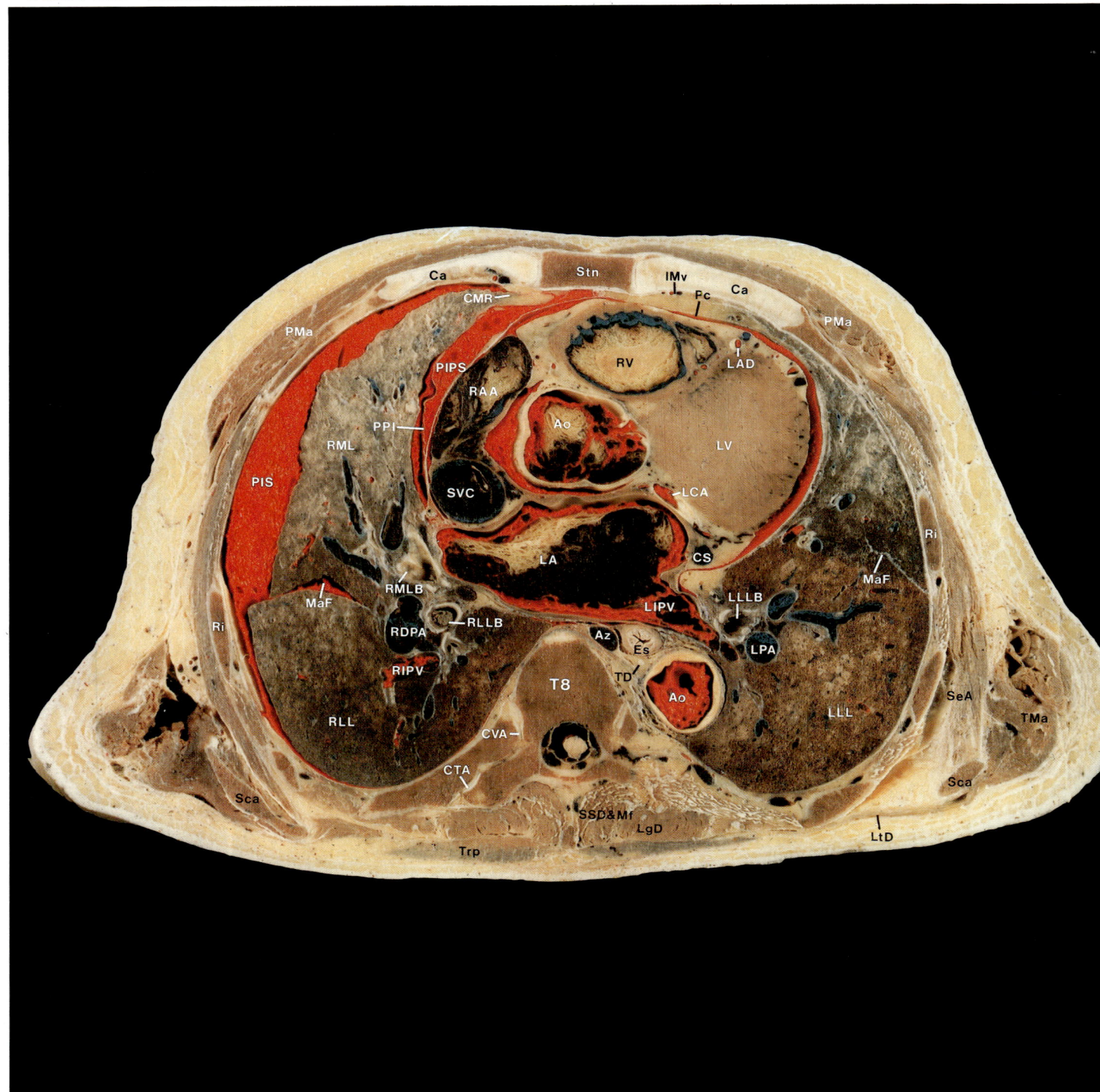

Ao	Aorta	LgD	Longissimus dorsi muscle
Az	Azygos vein	LtD	Latissimus dorsi muscle
CMR	Costomediastinal recess	MaF	Major fissure
CS	Coronary sinus	Mf	Multifidus muscle
CTA	Costotransverse articulation	PMa	Pectoralis major muscle
CVA	Costovertebral articulation	PPl	Parietal pleura
Ca	Cartilage	Pc	Pericardium
Es	Esophagus	PlPS	Pleuropericardial space
IMv	Internal mammary vessel	PlS	Pleural space
LA	Left atrium of heart	RAA	Right atrial appendage of heart
LAD	Left anterior descending branch of left coronary artery	RDPA	Right descending pulmonary artery
		RIPV	Right inferior pulmonary vein
LCA	Left coronary artery	RLL	Right lower lobe of lung
LIPV	Left inferior pulmonary vein	RLLB	Right lower lobe bronchus
LLL	Left lower lobe of lung	RML	Right middle lobe of lung
LLLB	Left lower lobe bronchus	RMLB	Right middle lobe bronchus
LPA	Left pulmonary artery	RV	Right ventricle of heart
LV	Left ventricle of heart	Ri	Rib

SSD	Semispinalis dorsi muscle
SVC	Superior vena cava
Sca	Scapula
SeA	Serratus anterior muscle
Stn	Sternum
T8	T8 vertebral body
TD	Thoracic duct
TMa	Teres major muscle
Trp	Trapezius muscale

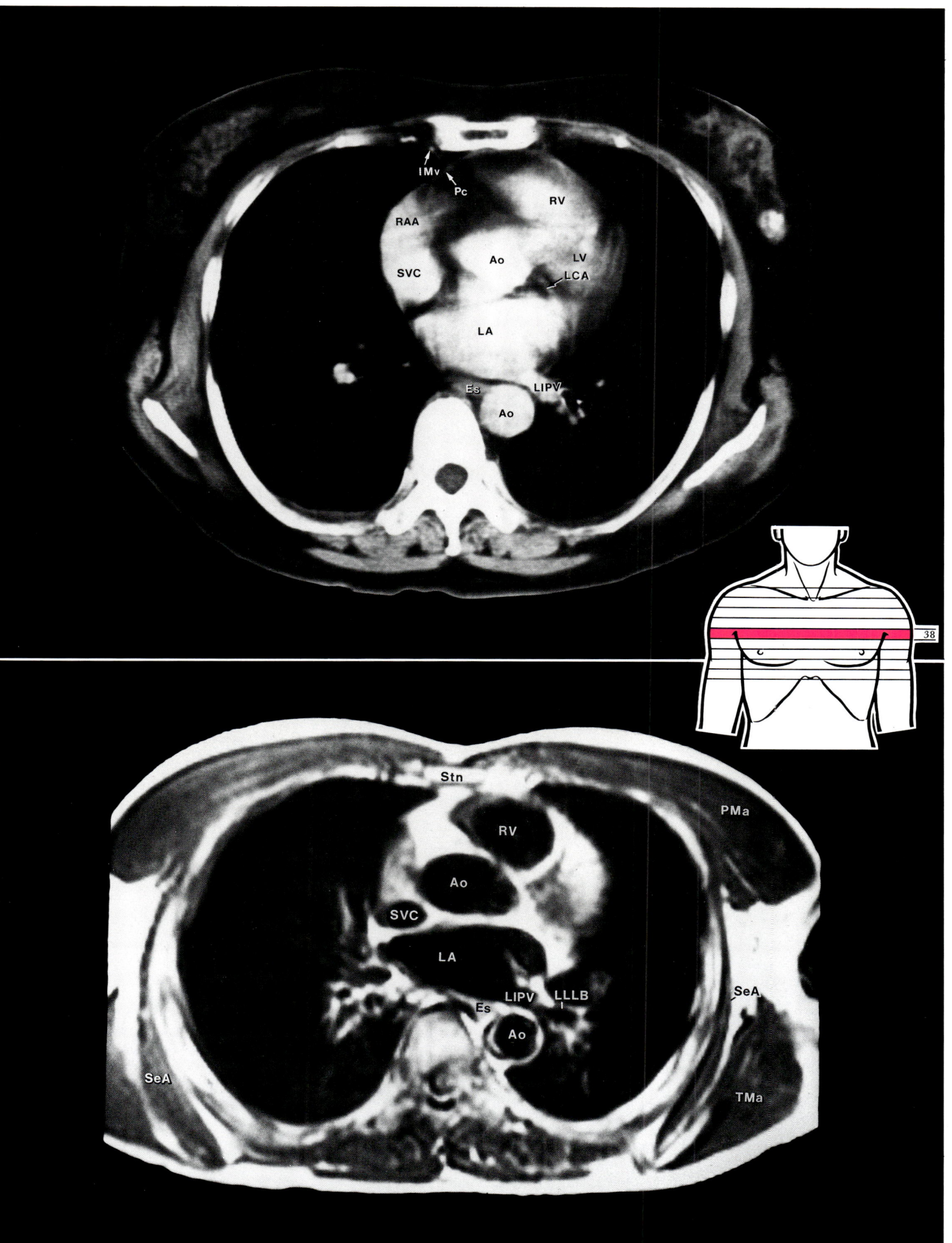

Plate 39. Transverse CHEST

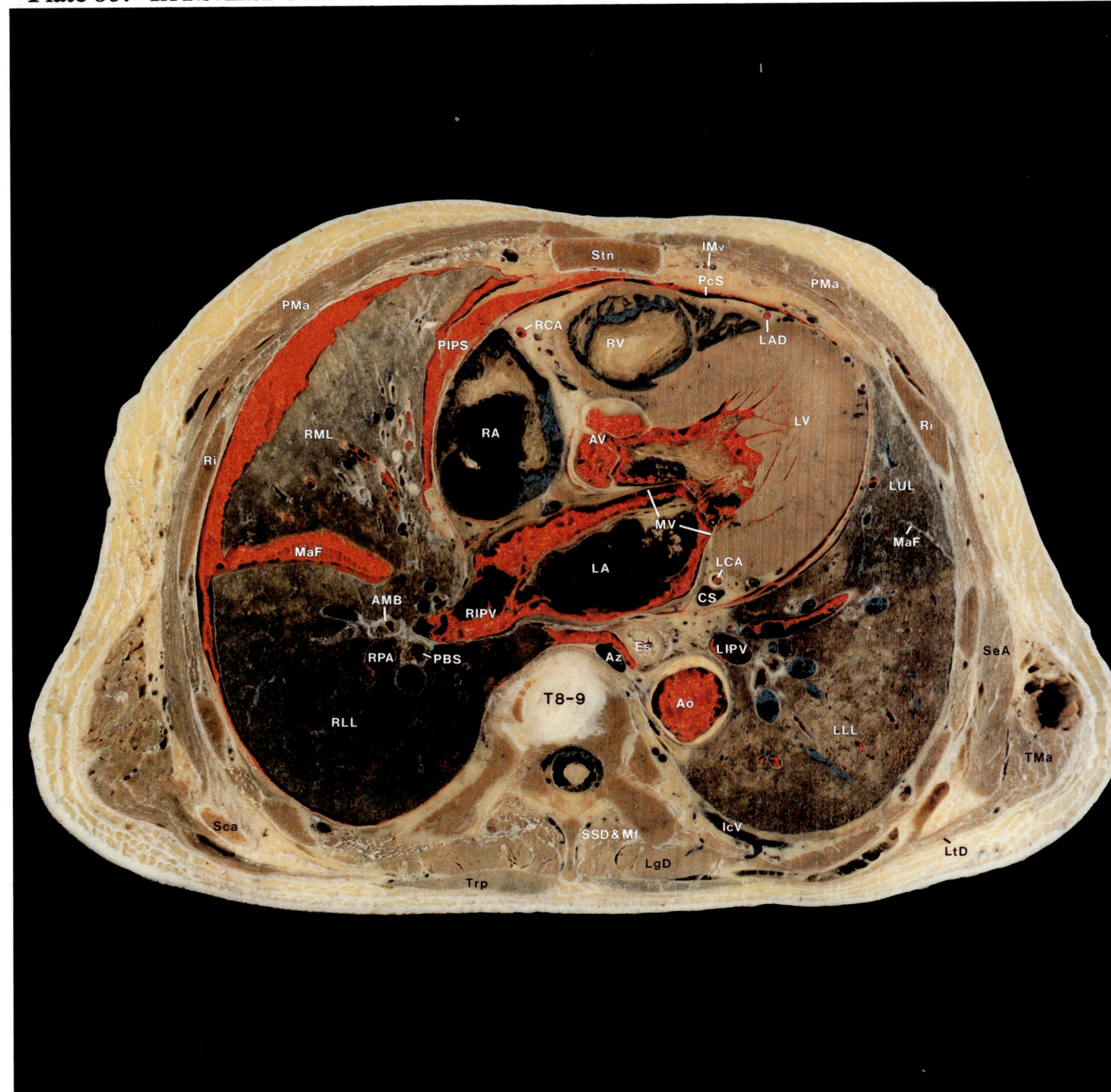

AMB	Anteromedial basal segment of lung	MV	Mitral valve	Sca	Scapula
AV	Aortic valve	MaF	Major fissure	SeA	Serratus anterior muscle
Ao	Aorta	Mf	Multifidus muscle	Stn	Sternum
Az	Azygos vein	PBS	Posterolateral basal segment of lung	T8-9	T8-9 intervertebral disc
CS	Coronary sinus	PMa	Pectoralis major muscle	TMa	Teres major muscle
Es	Esophagus	PcS	Pericardial space	Trp	Trapezius muscle
IMv	Internal mammary vessel	PlPS	Pleuropericardial space		
IcV	Intercostal vein	RA	Right atrium of heart		
LA	Left atrium of heart	RAA	Right atrial appendage of heart		
LAD	Left anterior descending branch of left coronary artery	RCA	Right coronary artery		
		RIPV	Right inferior pulmonary vein		
LCA	Left coronary artery	RLL	Right lower lobe of lung		
LIPV	Left inferior pulmonary vein	RML	Right middle lobe of lung		
LLL	Left lower lobe of lung	RPA	Right pulmonary artery		
LUL	Left upper lobe of lung	RV	Right ventricle of heart		
LV	Left ventricle of heart	Ri	Rib		
LgD	Longissimus dorsi muscle	SSD	Semispinalis dorsi muscle		
LtD	Latissimus dorsi muscle	SVC	Superior vena cava		

— 88 —

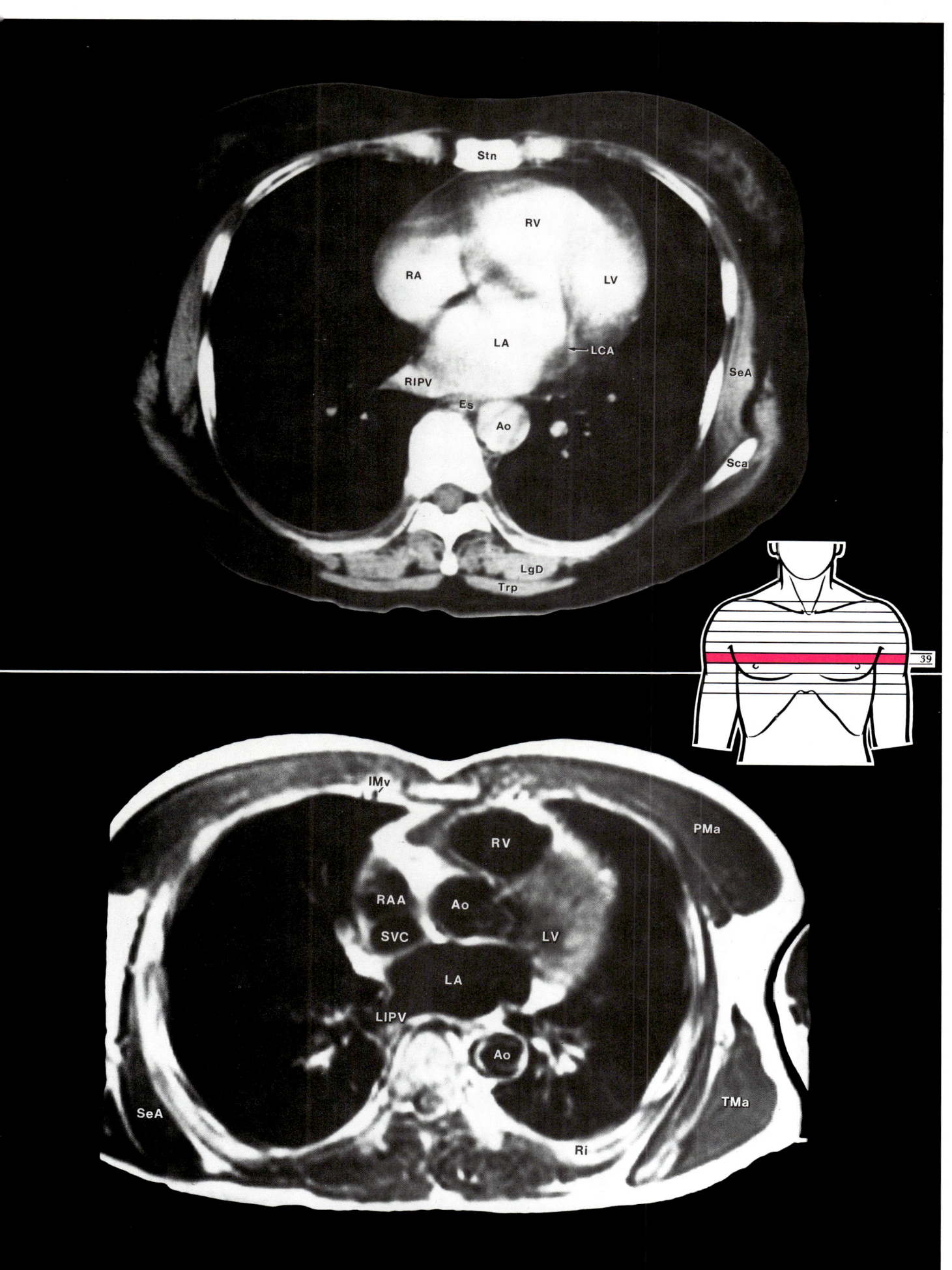

Plate 40. Transverse CHEST

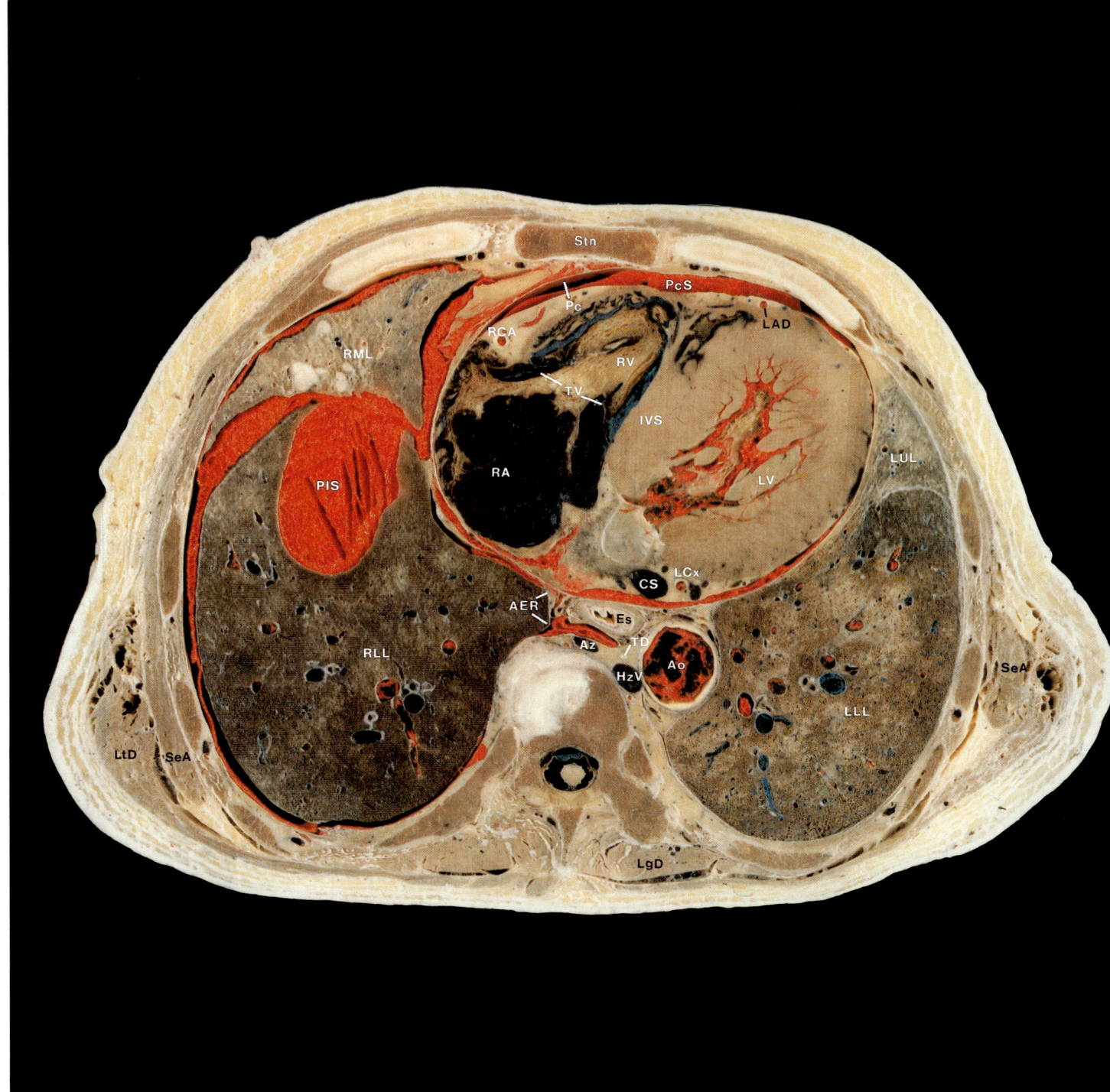

AER	Azygoesophageal recess	Pc	Pericardium
Ao	Aorta	PcS	Pericardial space
Az	Azygos vein	PlS	Pleural space
CS	Coronary sinus	RA	Right atrium of heart
Es	Esophagus	RCA	Right coronary artery
HzV	Hemiazygos vein	RLL	Right lower lobe of lung
IVS	Interventricular septum	RML	Right middle lobe of lung
LA	Left atrium of heart	RV	Right ventricle of heart
LAD	Left anterior descending branch of left coronary artery	SC	Spinal cord
		SeA	Serratus anterior muscle
LCx	Left circumflex artery	Stn	Sternum
LLL	Left lower lobe of lung	TD	Thoracic duct
LUL	Left upper lobe of lung	TV	Tricuspid valve
LV	Left ventricle of heart		
LgD	Longissimus dorsi muscle		
LtD	Latissimus dorsi muscle		
MV	Mitral valve		
PMa	Pectoralis major muscle		

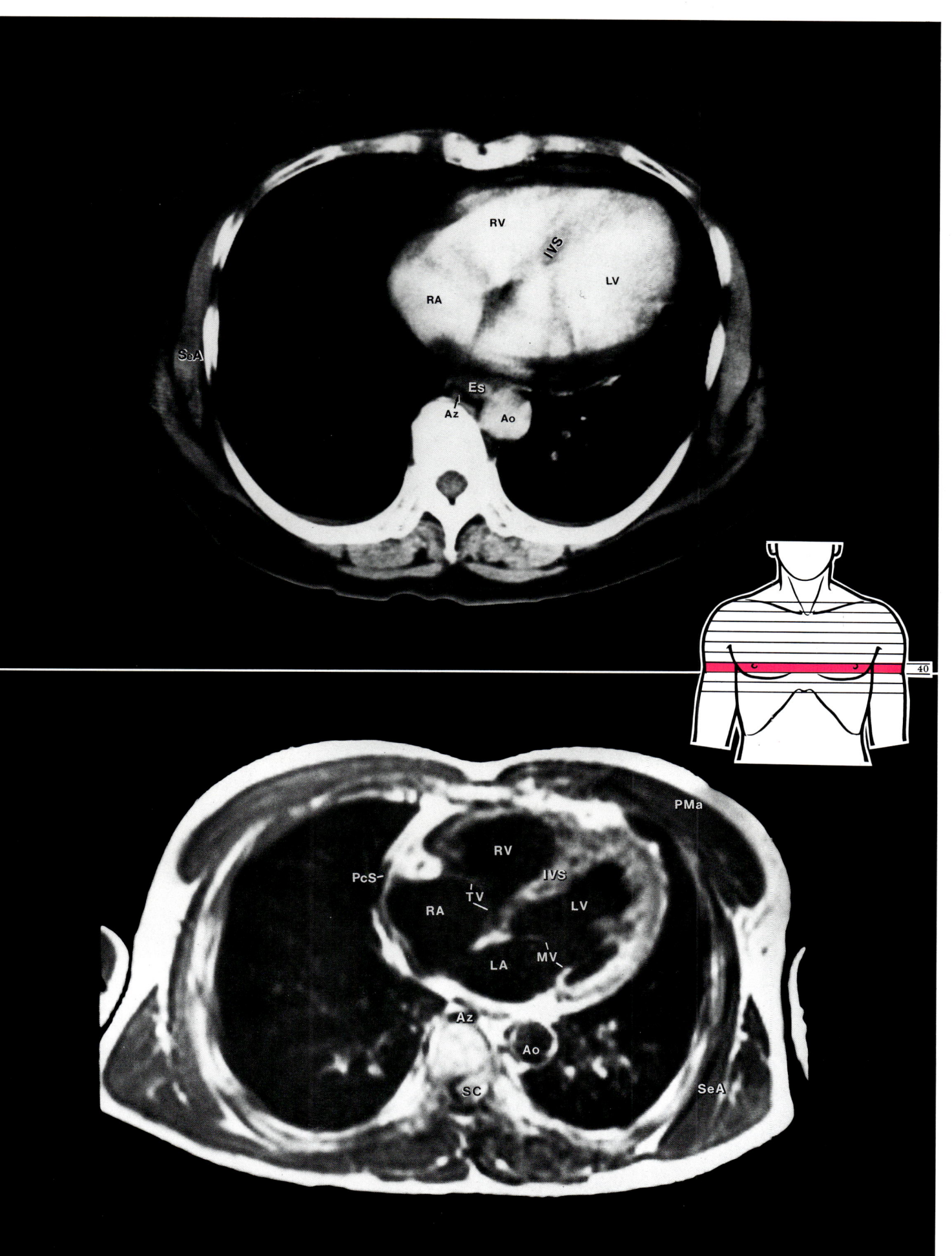

Plate 41. Transverse CHEST

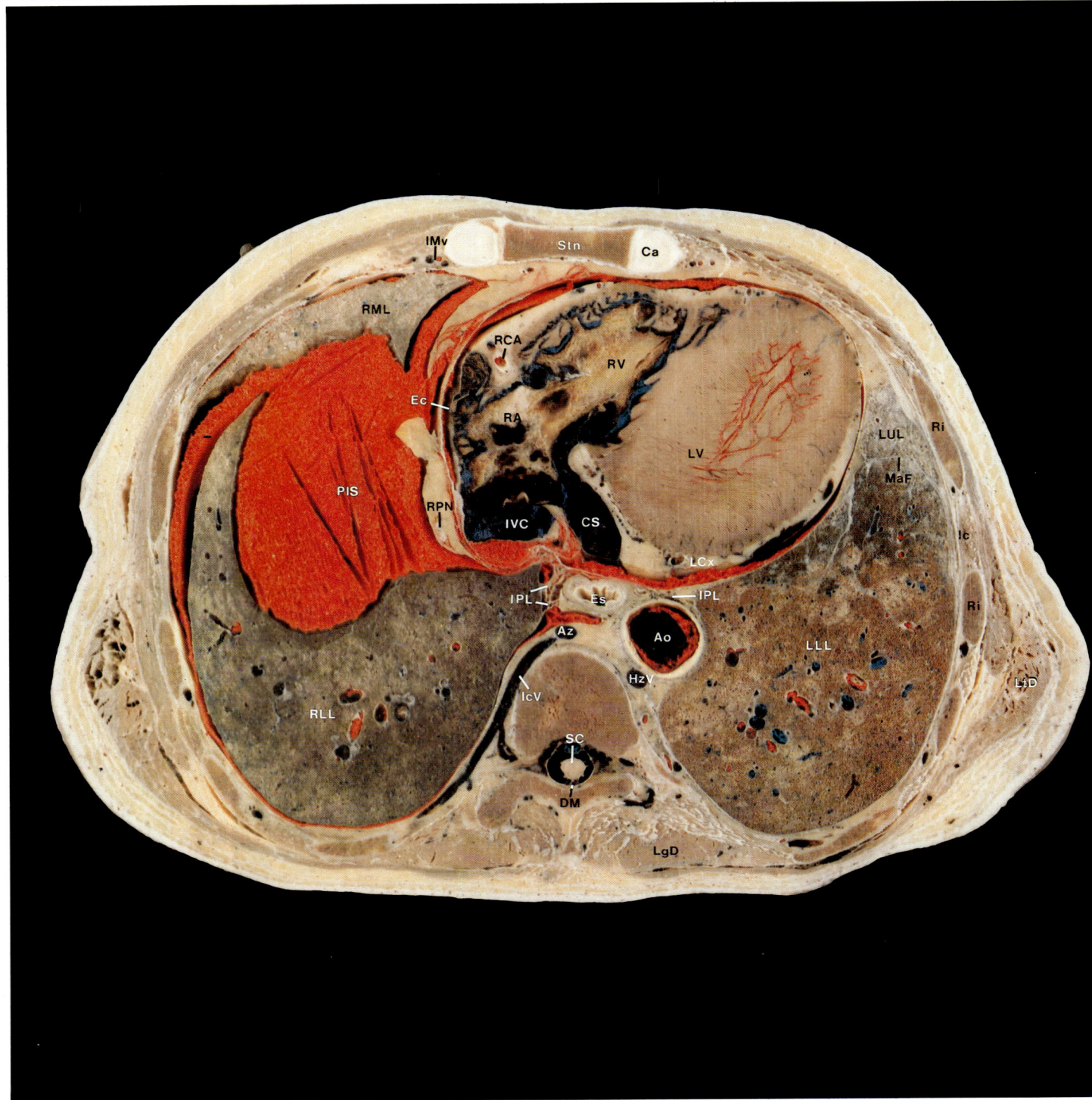

Ao	Aorta	LgD	Longissimus dorsi muscle
Az	Azygos vein	LtD	Latissimus dorsi muscle
CS	Coronary sinus	MaF	Major fissure
Ca	Cartilage	PlS	Pleural space
DM	Dura mater	RA	Right atrium of heart
Ec	Epicardium	RCA	Right coronary artery
Es	Esophagus	RLL	Right lower lobe of lung
HzV	Hemiazygos vein	RML	Right middle lobe of lung
IMv	Internal mammary vessel	RPN	Right phrenic nerve
IPL	Inferior pulmonary ligament	RV	Right ventricle of heart
IVC	Inferior vena cava	Ri	Rib
IVS	Interventricular septum	SC	Spinal cord
Ic	Intercostal muscle	SeA	Serratus anteior muscle
IcV	Intercostal vein	Stn	Sternum
LCx	Left circumflex artery		
LLL	Left lower lobe of lung		
LUL	Left upper lobe of lung		
LV	Left ventricle of heart		

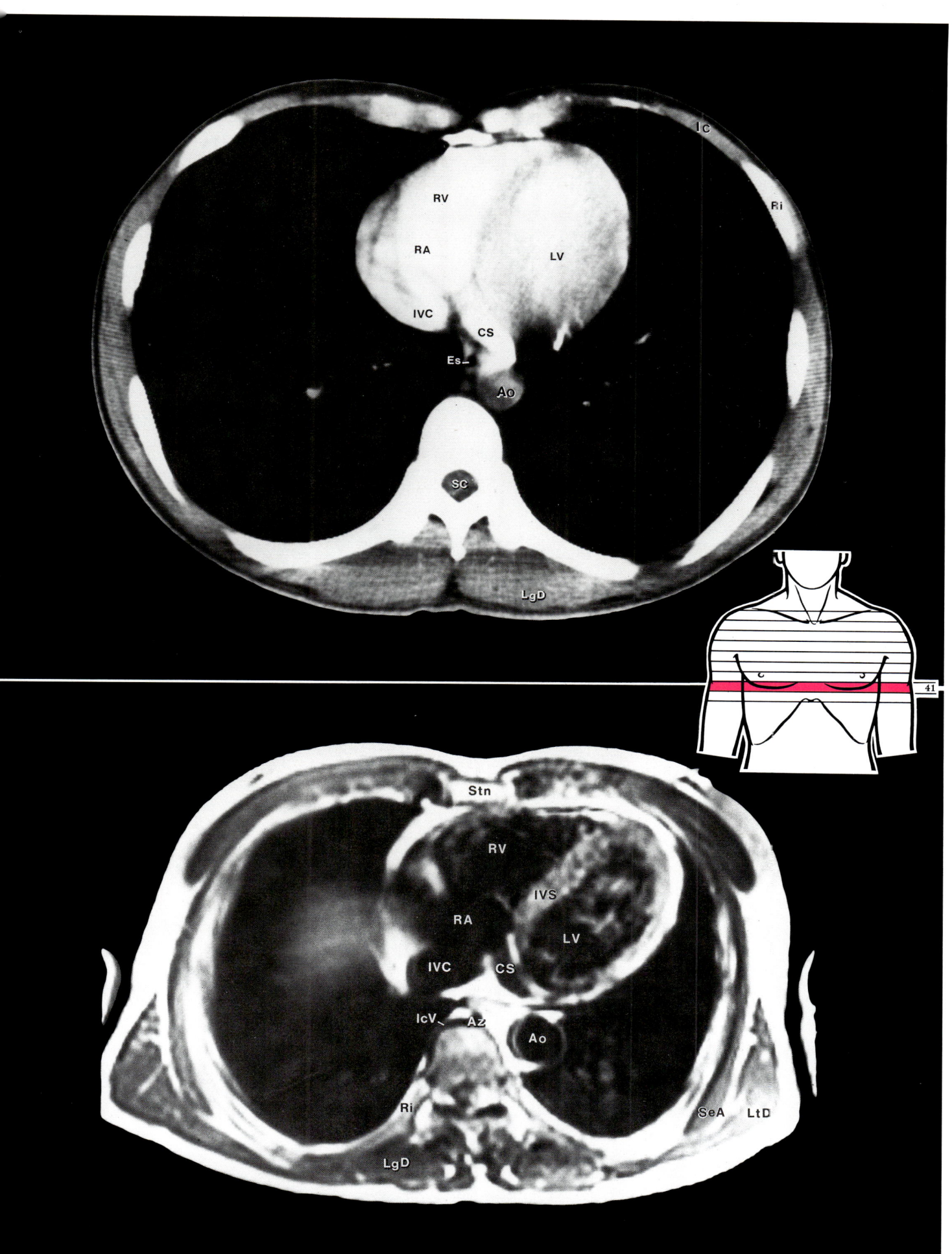

Plate 42. TRANSVERSE CHEST

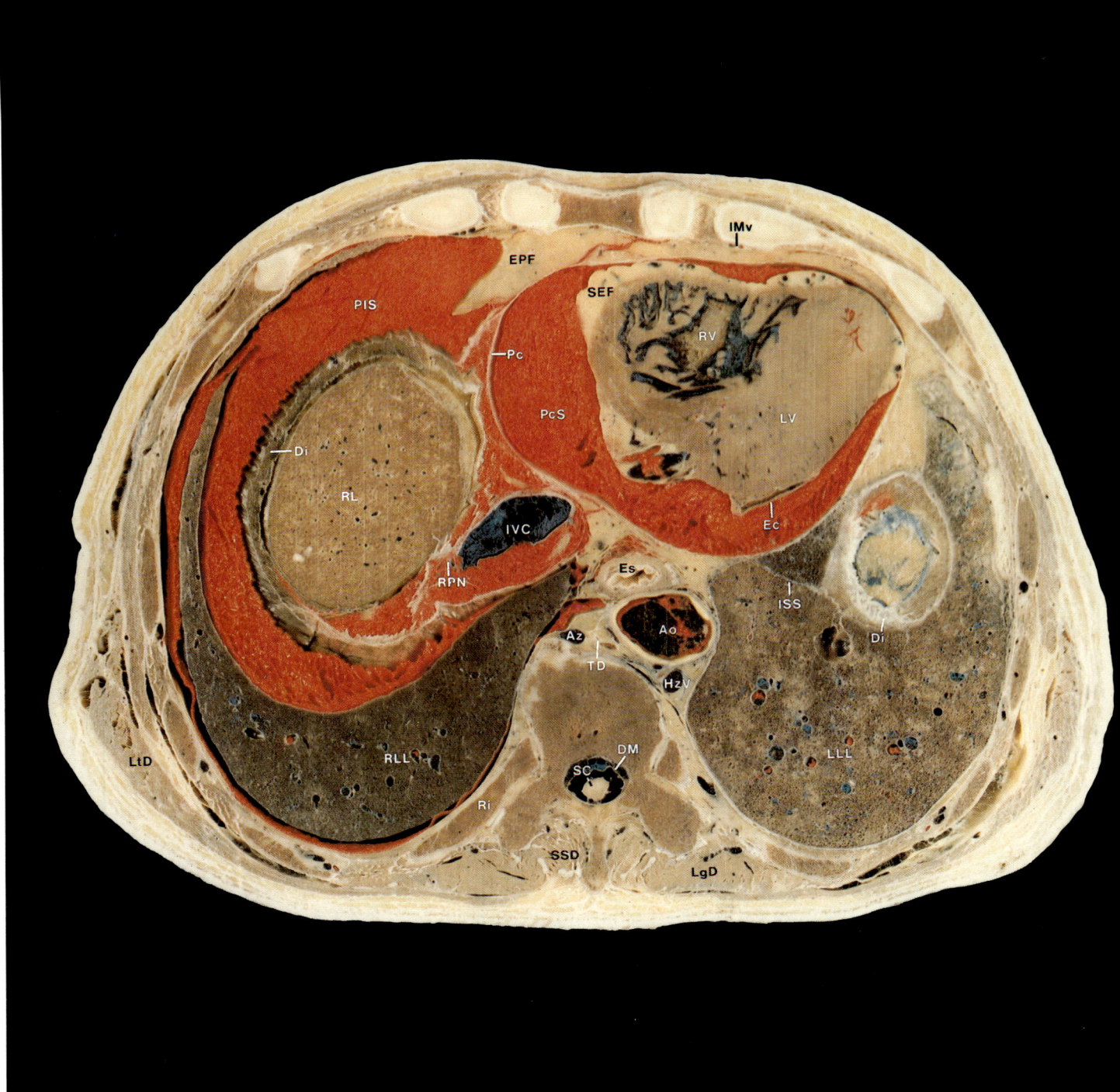

Ao	Aorta	MHV	Middle hepatic vein
Az	Azygos vein	Pc	Pericardium
CS	Coronary sinus	PcS	Pericardial space
Ca	Cartilage	PlS	Pleural space
DM	Dura mater	RHV	Right hepatic vein
Di	Diaphragm	RL	Right lobe of liver
EPF	Extrapericardial fat	RLL	Right lower lobe of lung
Ec	Epicardium	RPN	Right phrenic nerve
Es	Esophagus	RV	Right ventricle of heart
HzV	Hemiazygos vein	Ri	Rib
IMv	Internal mammary vessel	SC	Spinal cord
ISS	Intersublobar septum	SEF	Subepicardial fat
IVC	Inferior vena cava	SSD	Semispinalis dorsi muscle
IcV	Intercostal vein	TD	Thoracic duct
LLL	Left lower lobe of lung		
LV	Left ventricle of heart		
LgD	Longissimus dorsi muscle		
LtD	Latissimus dorsi muscle		

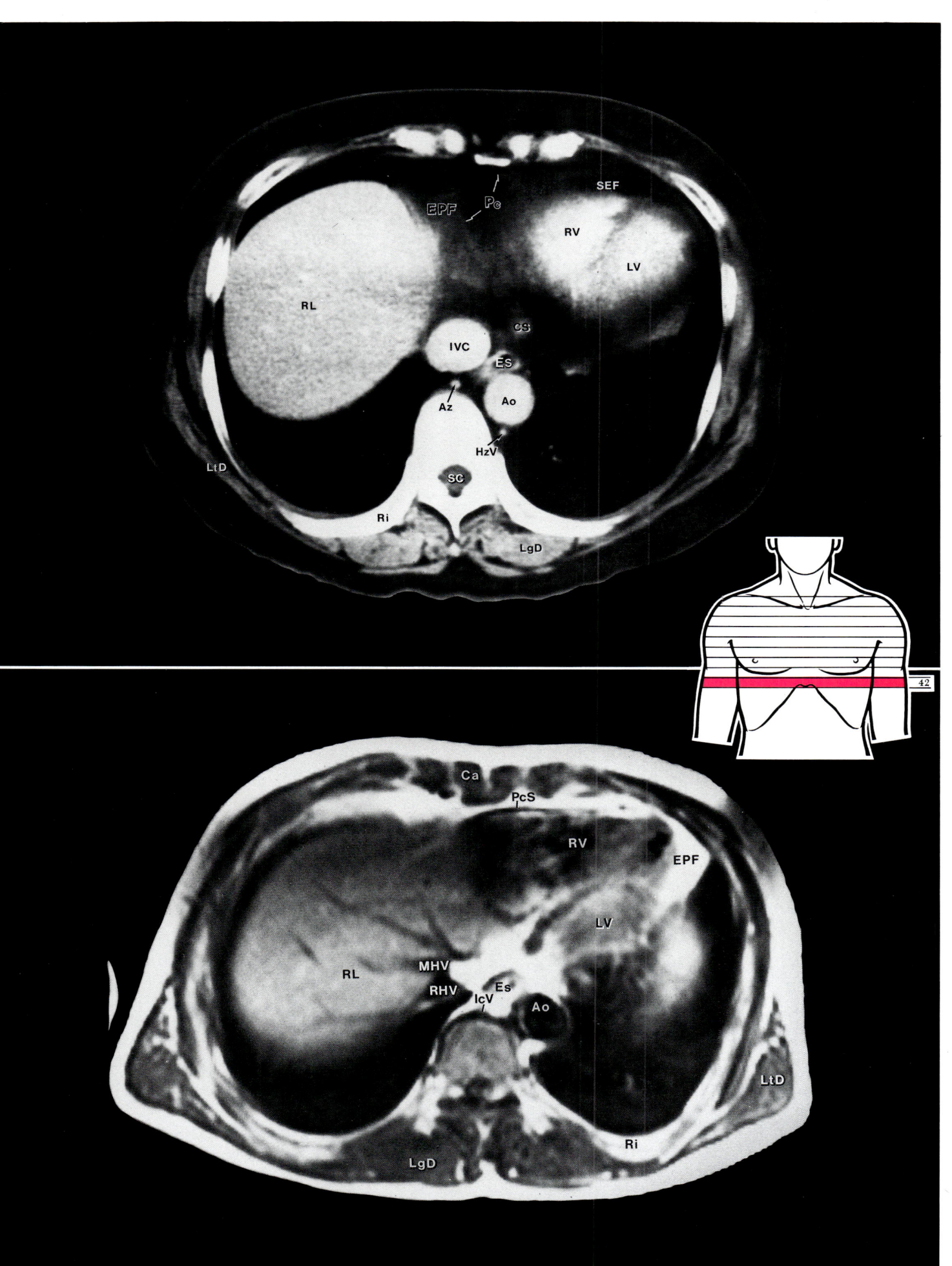

Sagittal Section-female (Cadaver & MRI) Plate 43-48

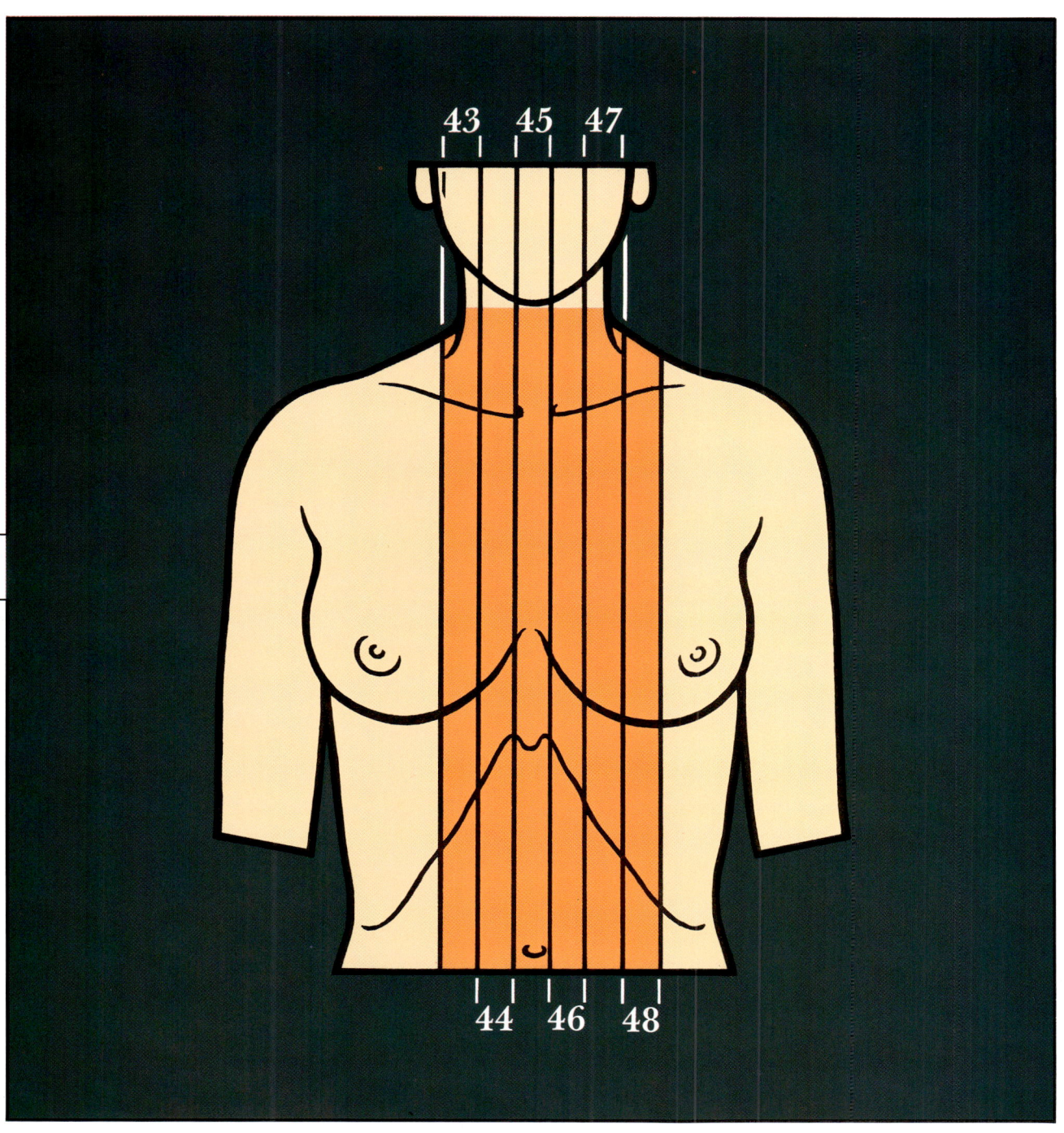

Plate 43. SAGITTAL CHEST

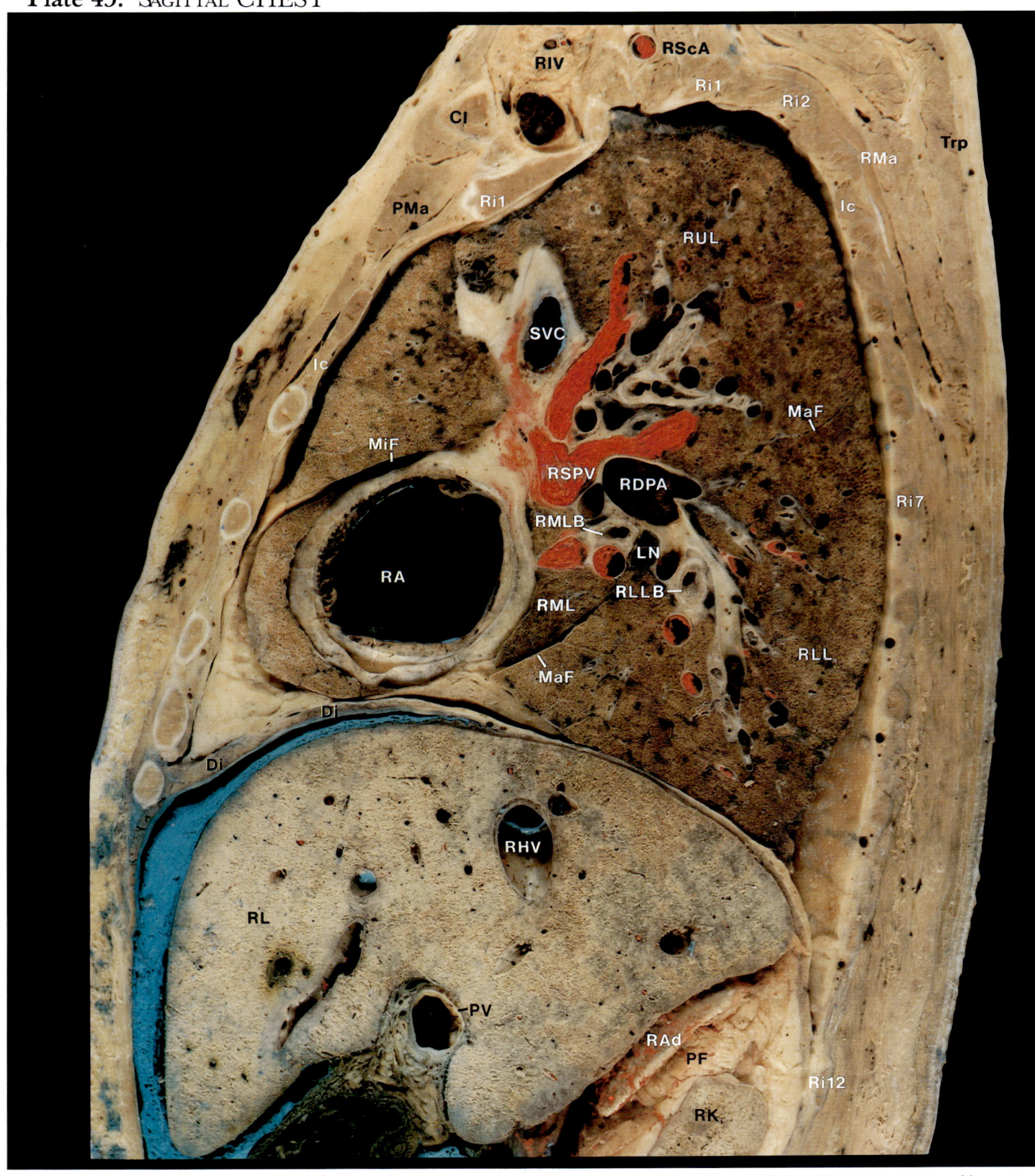

Cl	Clavicle	RDPA	Right descending pulmonary artery	RUL	Right upper lobe of lung
Di	Diaphragm	RHV	Right hepatic vein	Ri	Rib
HV	Hepatic vein	RIV	Right innominate vein	Ri1	1st rib
Ic	Intercostal muscle	RK	Right kidney	Ri2	2nd rib
LN	Lymph node	RL	Right lobe of liver	Ri7	7th rib
MaF	Major fissure	RLL	Right lower lobe of lung	Ri12	12th rib
MiF	Minor fissure	RLLB	Right lower lobe bronchus	SVC	Superior vena cava
PF	Perirenal fat	RML	Right middle lobe of lung	Trp	Trapezius muscle
PMa	Pectoralis major muscle	RMLB	Right middle lobe bronchus		
PV	Portal vein	RMa	Rhomboideus major muscle		
RA	Right atrium of heart	RSPV	Right superior pulmonary vein		
RAd	Right adrenal gland	RScA	Right subclavian artery		

— 98 —

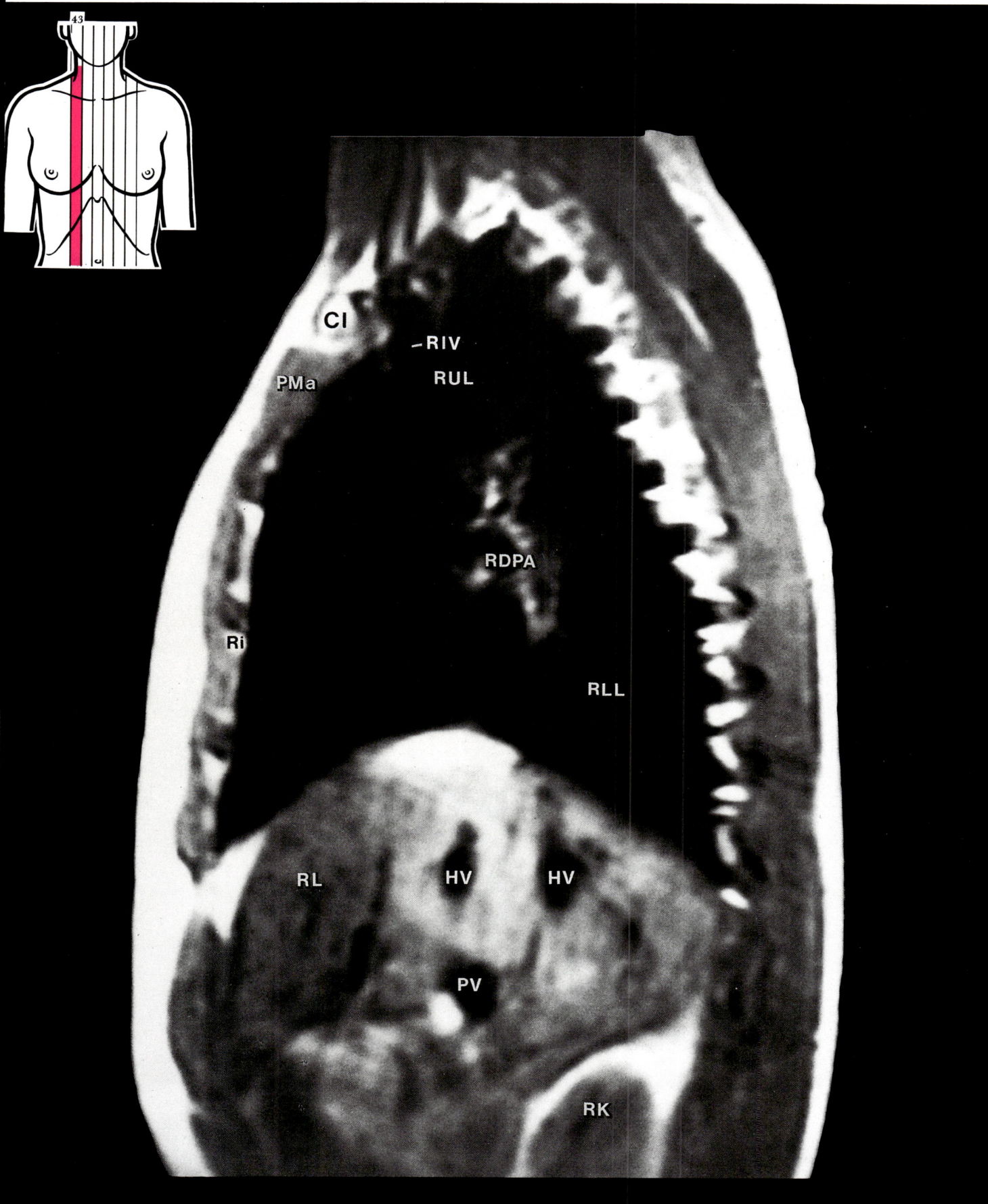

— 99 —

Plate 44. SAGITTAL CHEST

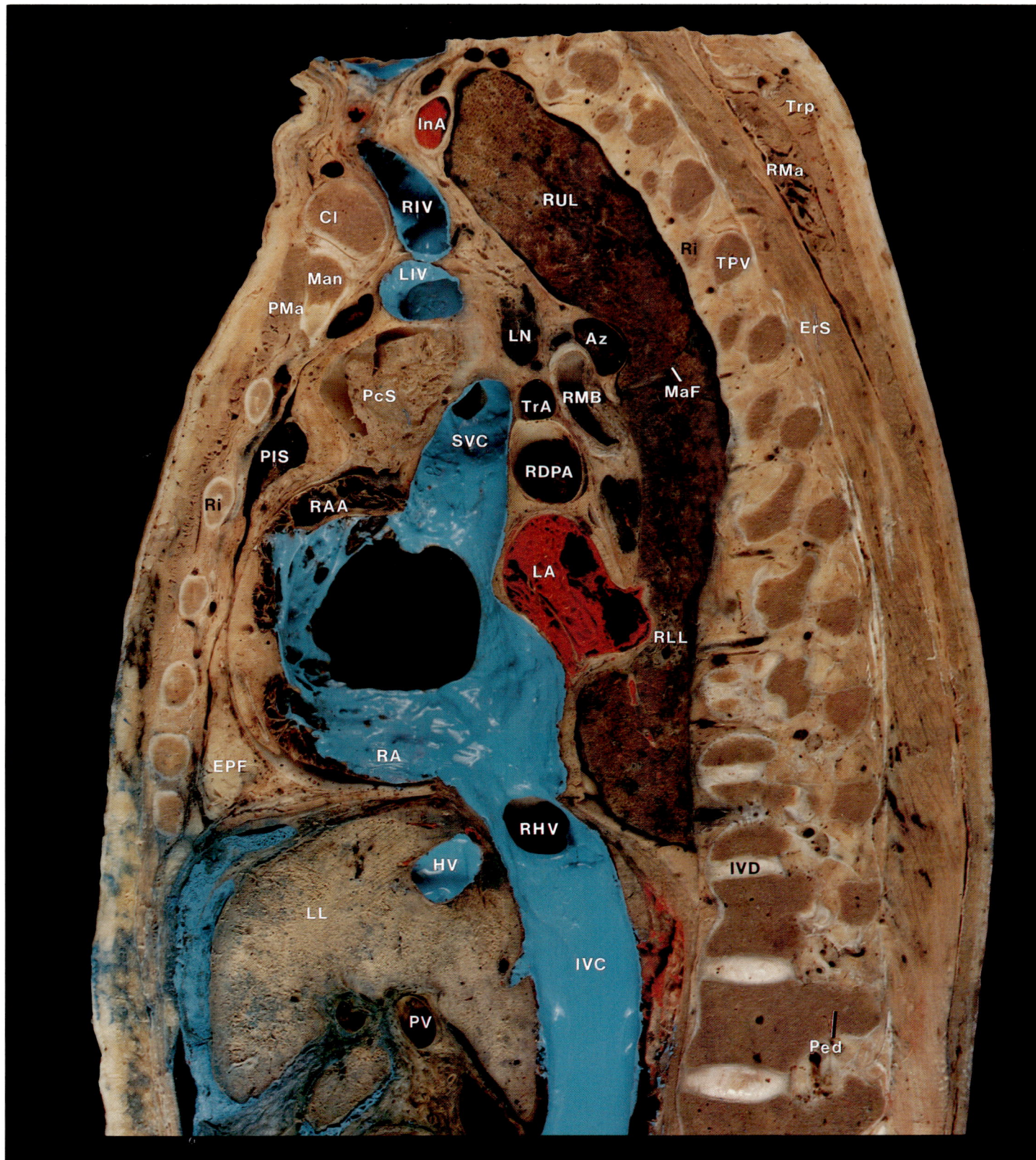

Az	Azygos vein	MaF	Major fissure	RLL	Right lower lobe of lung
Cl	Clavicle	Man	Manubrium	RMB	Right main bronchus
EPF	Extrapericardial fat	PMa	Pectoralis major muscle	RMa	Rhomboideus major muscle
ErS	Erector spinae muscle	PV	Portal vein	RPA	Right pulmonary artery
HV	Hepatic vein	PcS	Pericardial space	RUL	Right upper lobe of lung
IVC	Inferior vena cava	Ped	Pedicle	Ri	Rib
IVD	Intervertebral disc	PlS	Pleural space	SC	Spinal cord
InA	Innominate artery	RA	Right atrium of heart	SVC	Superior vena cava
LA	Left atrium of heart	RAA	Right atrial appendage of heart	TPV	Transverse process of vertebra
LIV	Left innominate vein	RDPA	Right descending pulmonary artery	Tr	Trachea
LL	Left lobe of liver	RHV	Right hepatic vein	TrA	Truncus anterior
LN	Lymph node	RIV	Right innominate vein	Trp	Trapezius muscle

— 100 —

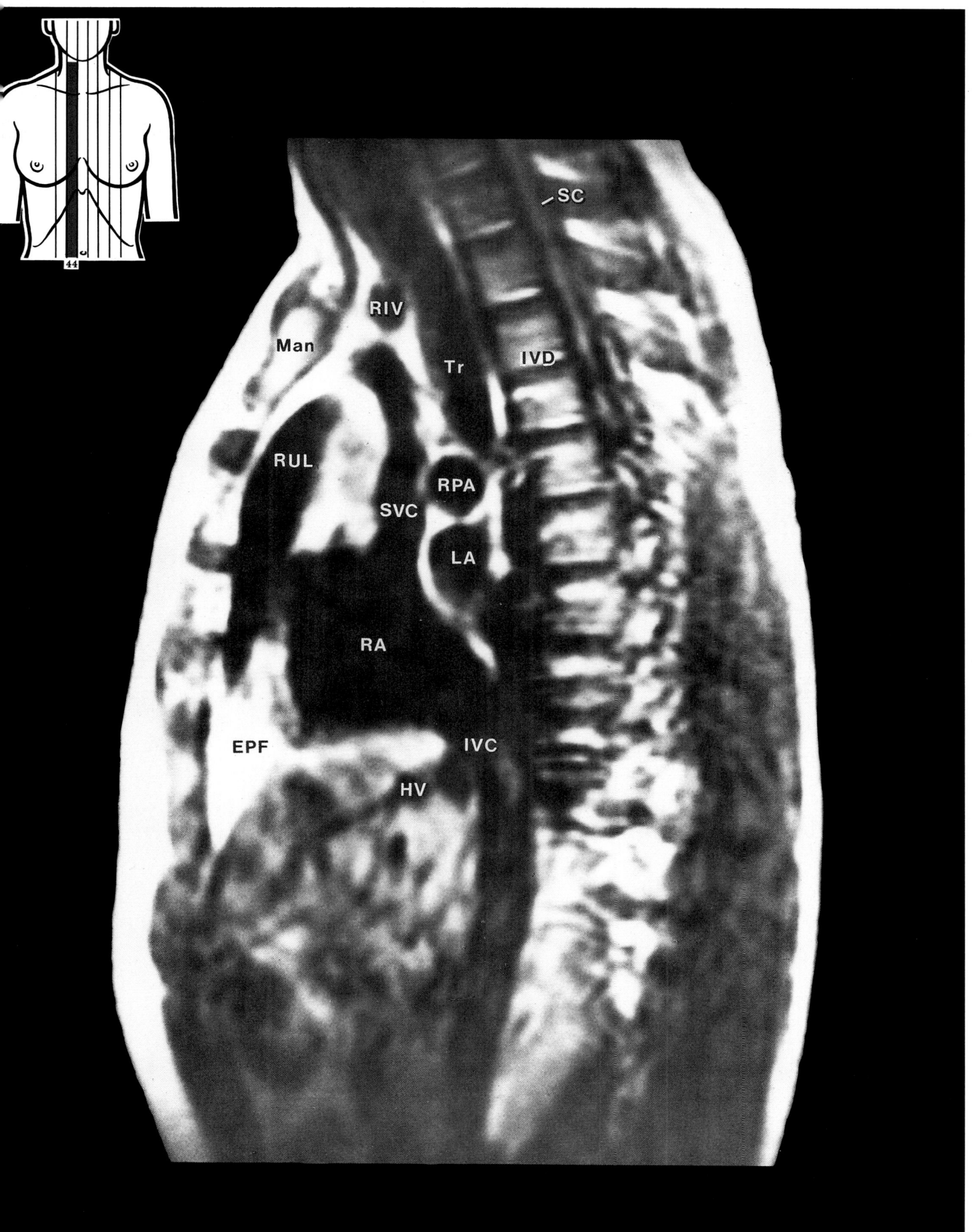

Plate 45. Sagittal CHEST

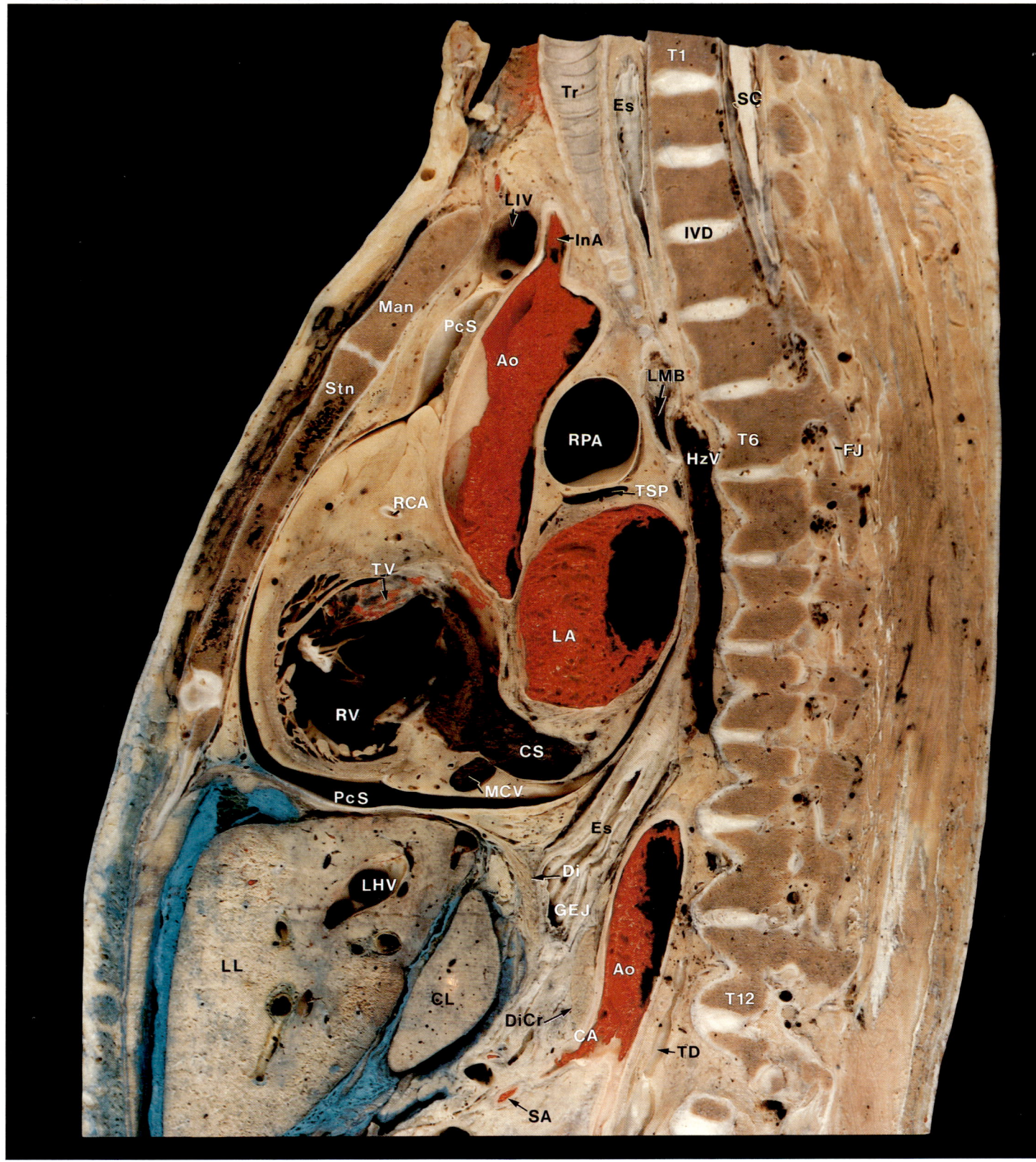

Ao	Aorta	InA	Innominate artery	SA	Splenic artery
CA	Celiac axis	LA	Left atrium of heart	SC	Spinal cord
CL	Caudate lobe of liver	LHV	Left hepatic vein	Stn	Sternum
CS	Coronary sinus	LIV	Left innominate vein	T1	T1 vertebral body
Di	Diaphragm	LL	Left lobe of liver	T6	T6 vertebral body
DiCr	Diaphragmatic crus	LMB	Left main bronchus	TD	Thoracic duct
EPF	Extrapericardial fat	MCV	Middle cardiac vein	TSP	Transverse sinus of pericardium
Es	Esophagus	Man	Manubrium	TV	Tricuspid valve
FJ	Facet joint of thoracic spine	PcS	Pericardial space	Tr	Trachea
GEJ	Gastroesophageal junction	RCA	Right coronary artery		
HzV	Hemiazygos vein	RPA	Right pulmonary artery		
IVD	Intervertebral disc	RV	Right ventricle of heart		

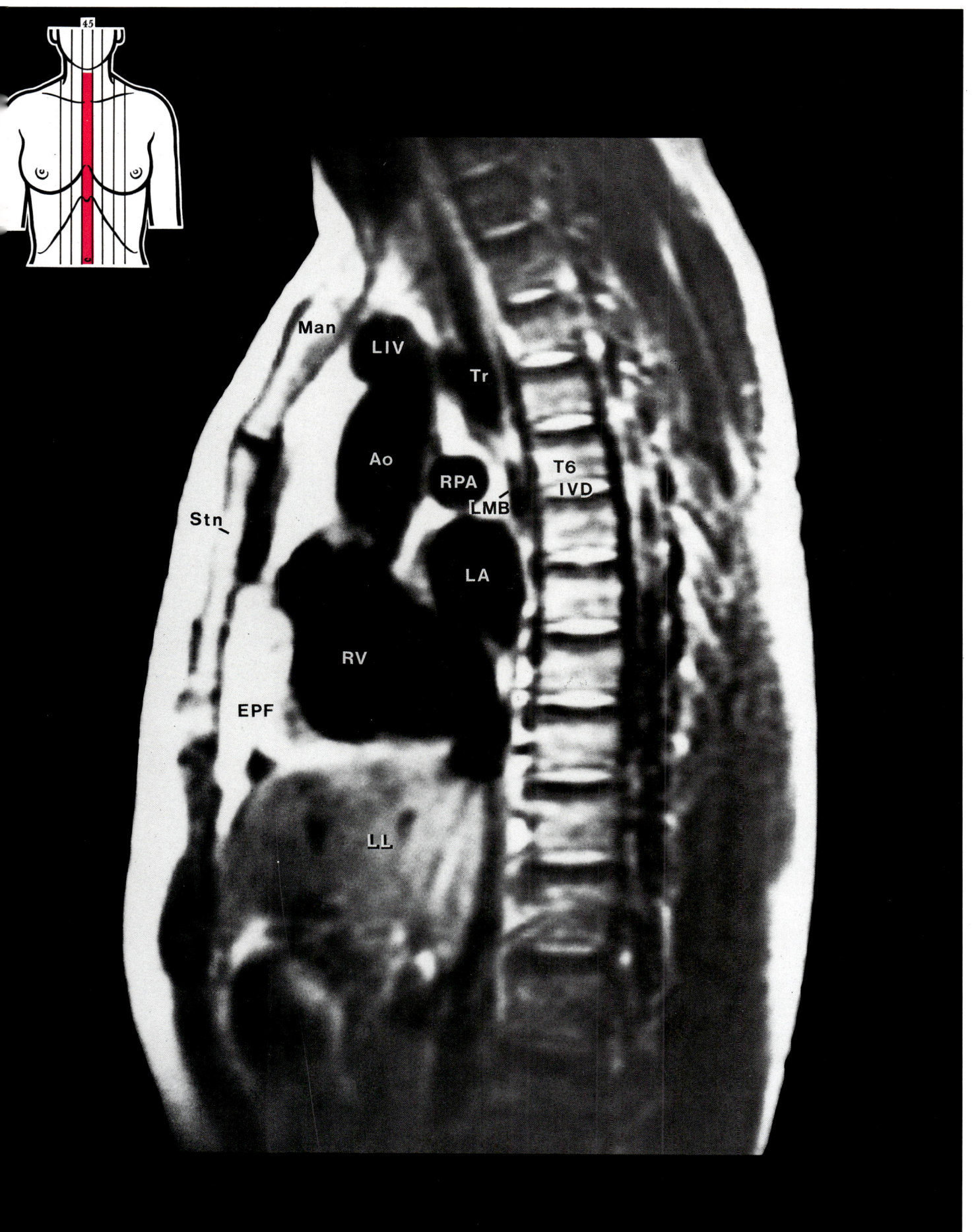

Plate 46. SAGITTAL CHEST

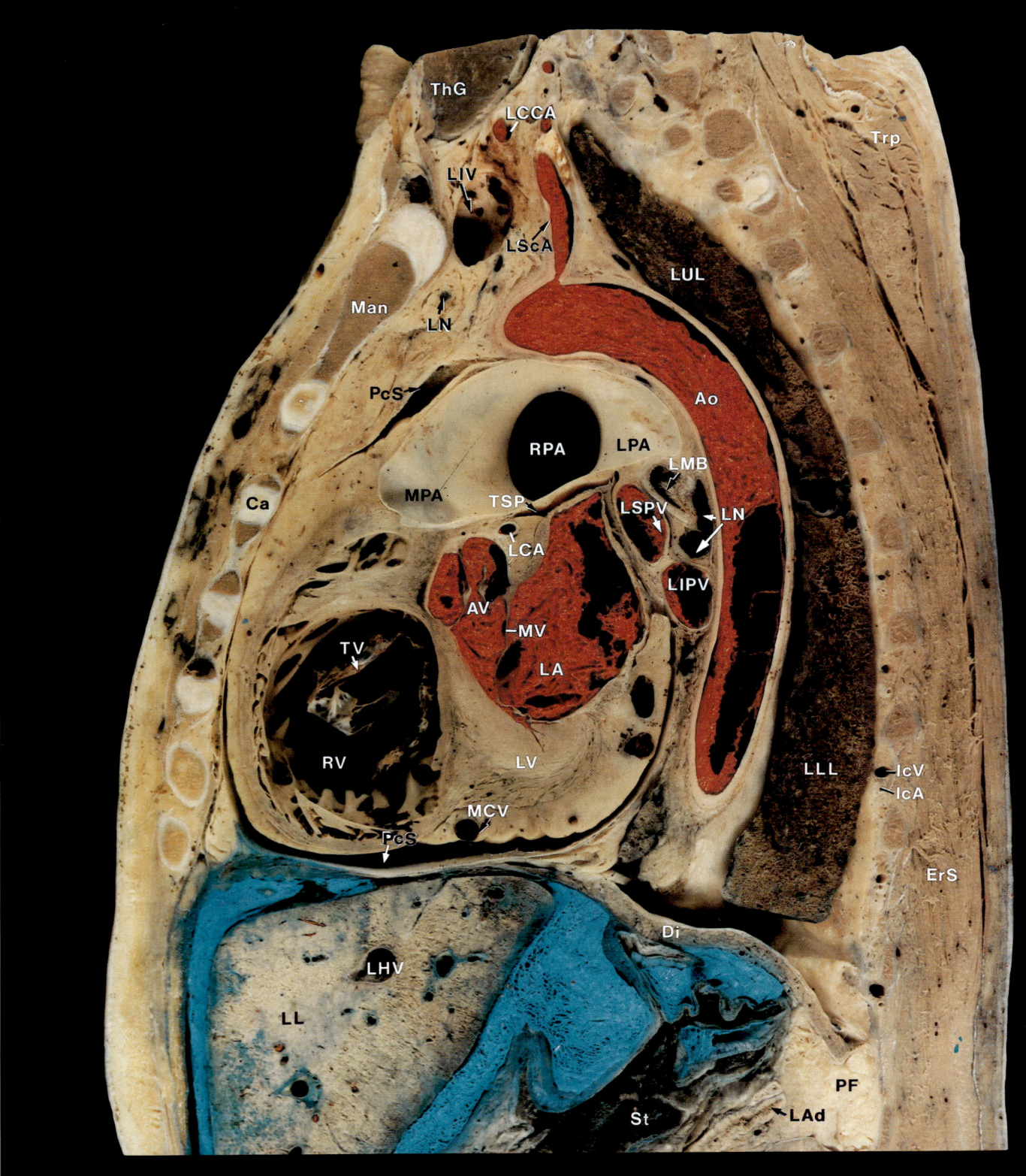

AV	Aortic valve	LIPV	Left inferior pulmonary vein	MPA	Main pulmonary artery
Ao	Aorta	LIV	Left innominate vein	MV	Mitral valve
Ca	Cartilage	LL	Left lobe of liver	Man	Manubrium
Di	Diaphragm	LLL	Left lower lobe of lung	PF	Perirenal fat
ErS	Erector spinae muscle	LMB	Left main bronchus	PcS	Pericardial space
IcA	Intercostal artery	LN	Lymph node	RPA	Right pulmonary artery
IcV	Intercostal vein	LPA	Left pulmonary artery	RV	Right ventricle of heart
LA	Left atrium of heart	LSPV	Left superior pulmonary vein	St	Stomach
LAd	Left adrenal gland	LScA	Left subclavian artery	TSP	Transverse sinus of pericardium
LCA	Left coronary artery	LUL	Left upper lobe of lung	TV	Tricuspid valve
LCCA	Left common carotid artery	LV	Left ventricle of heart	ThG	Thyroid gland
LHV	Left hepatic vein	MCV	Middle cardiac vein	Trp	Trapezius muscle

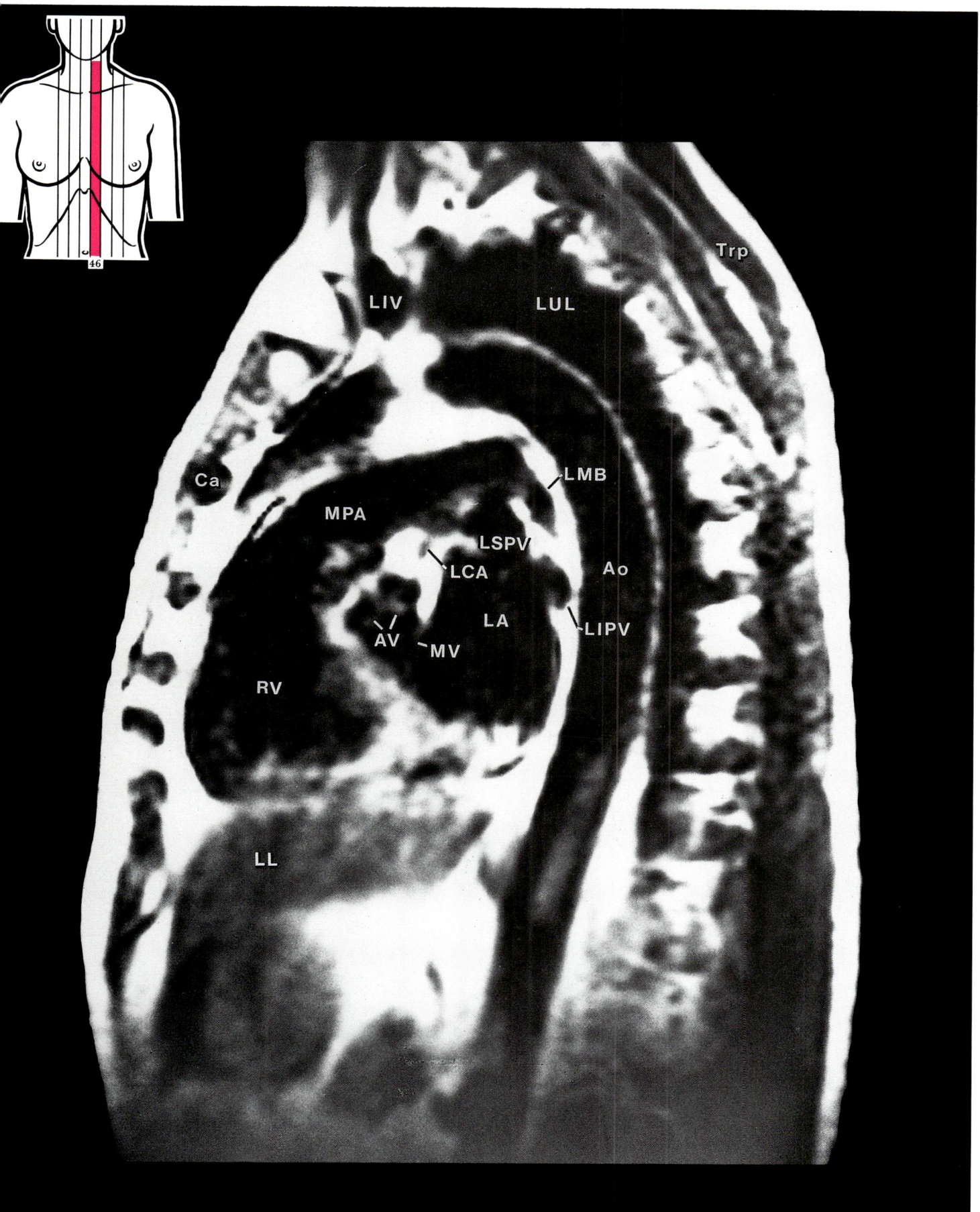

— 105 —

Plate 47. Sagittal CHEST

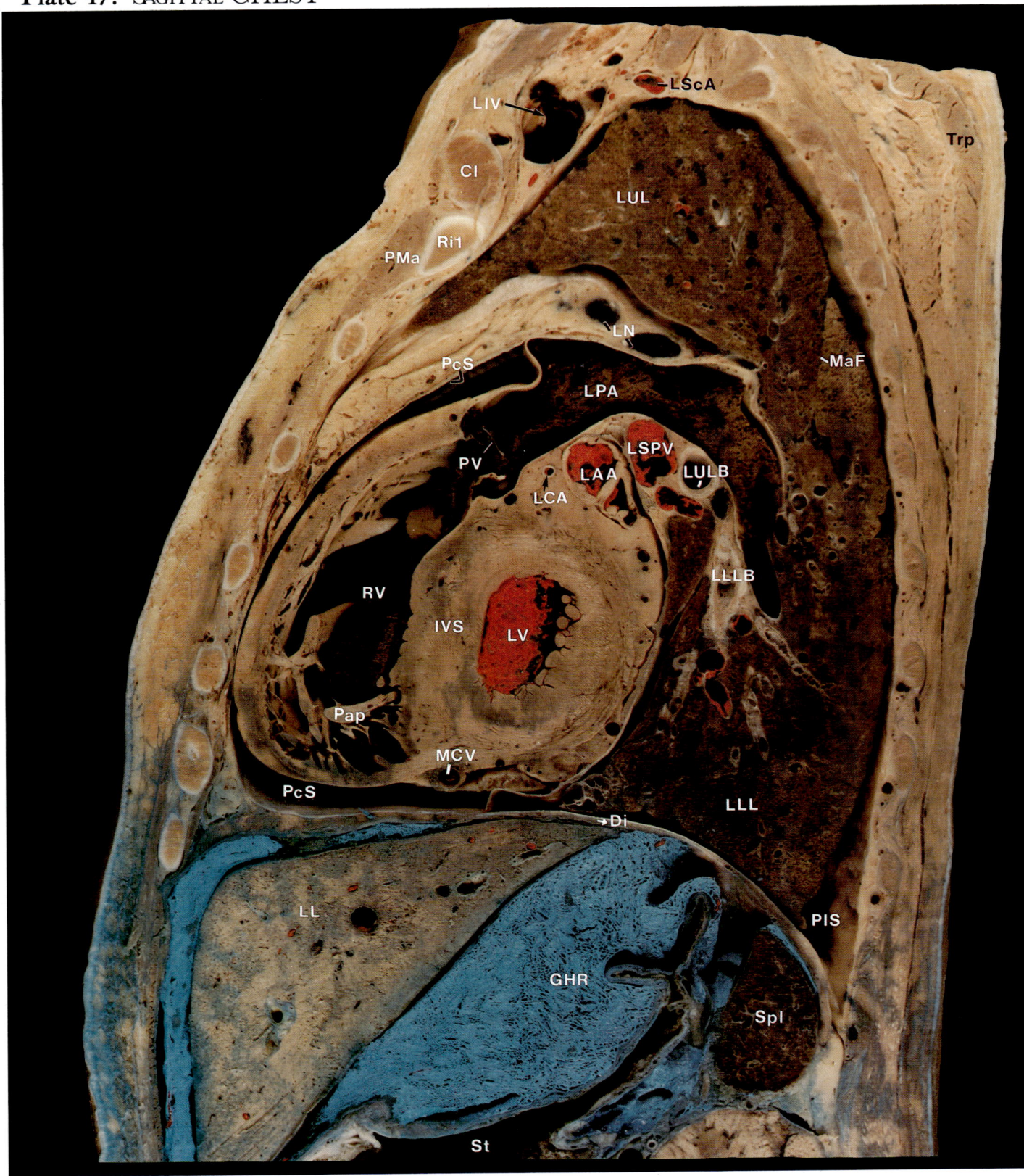

Ca	Cartilage	LN	Lymph node	PcS	Pericardial space
Cl	Clavicle	LPA	Left pulmonary artery	PlS	Pleural space
Di	Diaphragm	LSPV	Left superior pulmonary vein	RV	Right ventricle of heart
EPF	Extrapericardial fat	LScA	Left subclavian artery	Ri1	1st rib
GHR	Gastrohepatic recess	LUL	Left upper lobe of lung	Spl	Spleen
IVS	Interventricular septum	LULB	Left upper lobe bronchus	St	Stomach
LAA	Left atrial appendage of heart	LV	Left ventricle of heart	Trp	Trapezius muscle
LCA	Left coronary artery	MCV	Middle cardiac vein		
LIV	Left innominate vein	MaF	Major fissure		
LL	Left lobe of liver	PMa	Pectoralis major muscle		
LLL	Left lower lobe of lung	PV	Pulmonic valve		
LLLB	Left lower lobe bronchus	Pap	Papillary muscle		

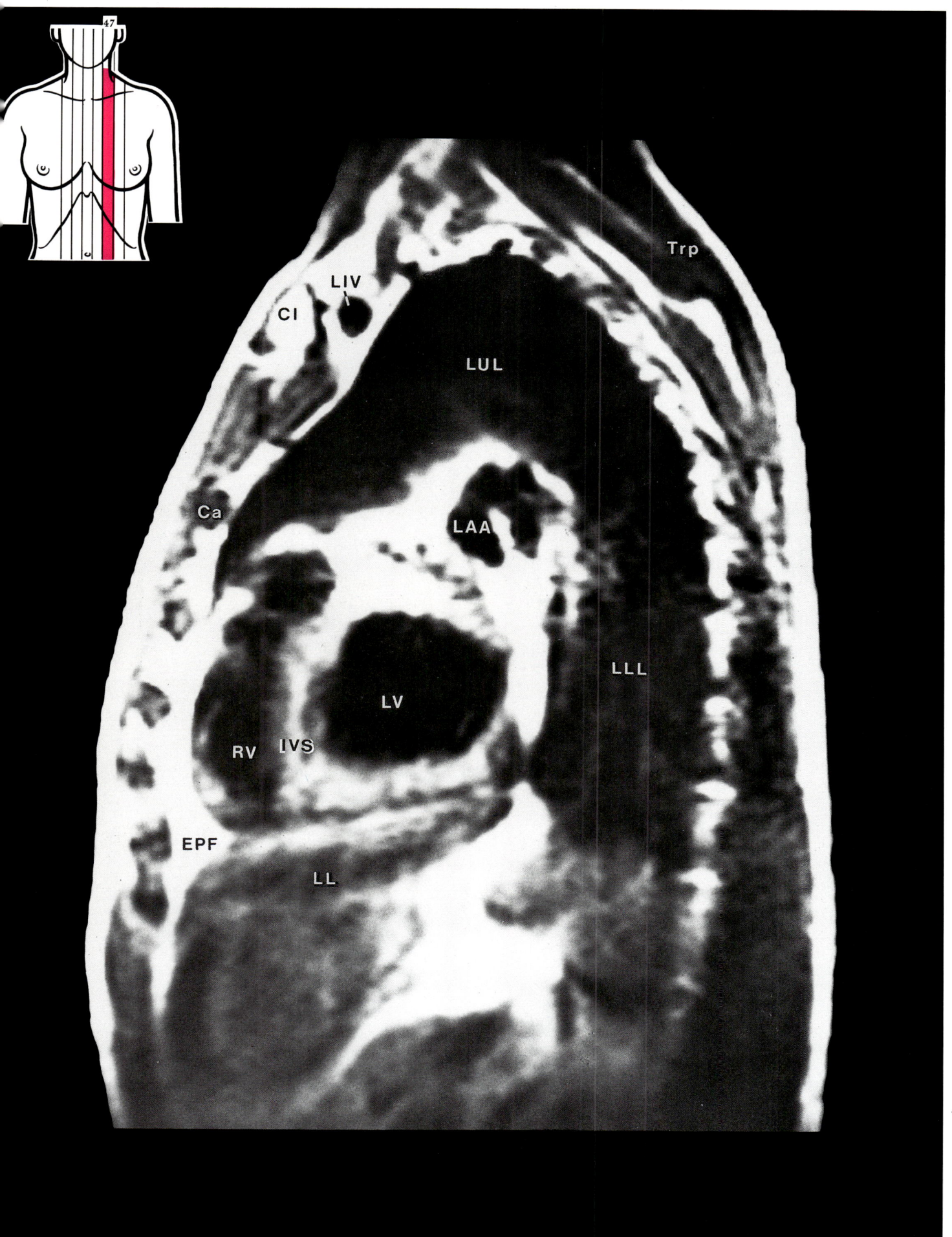

Plate 48. Sagittal CHEST

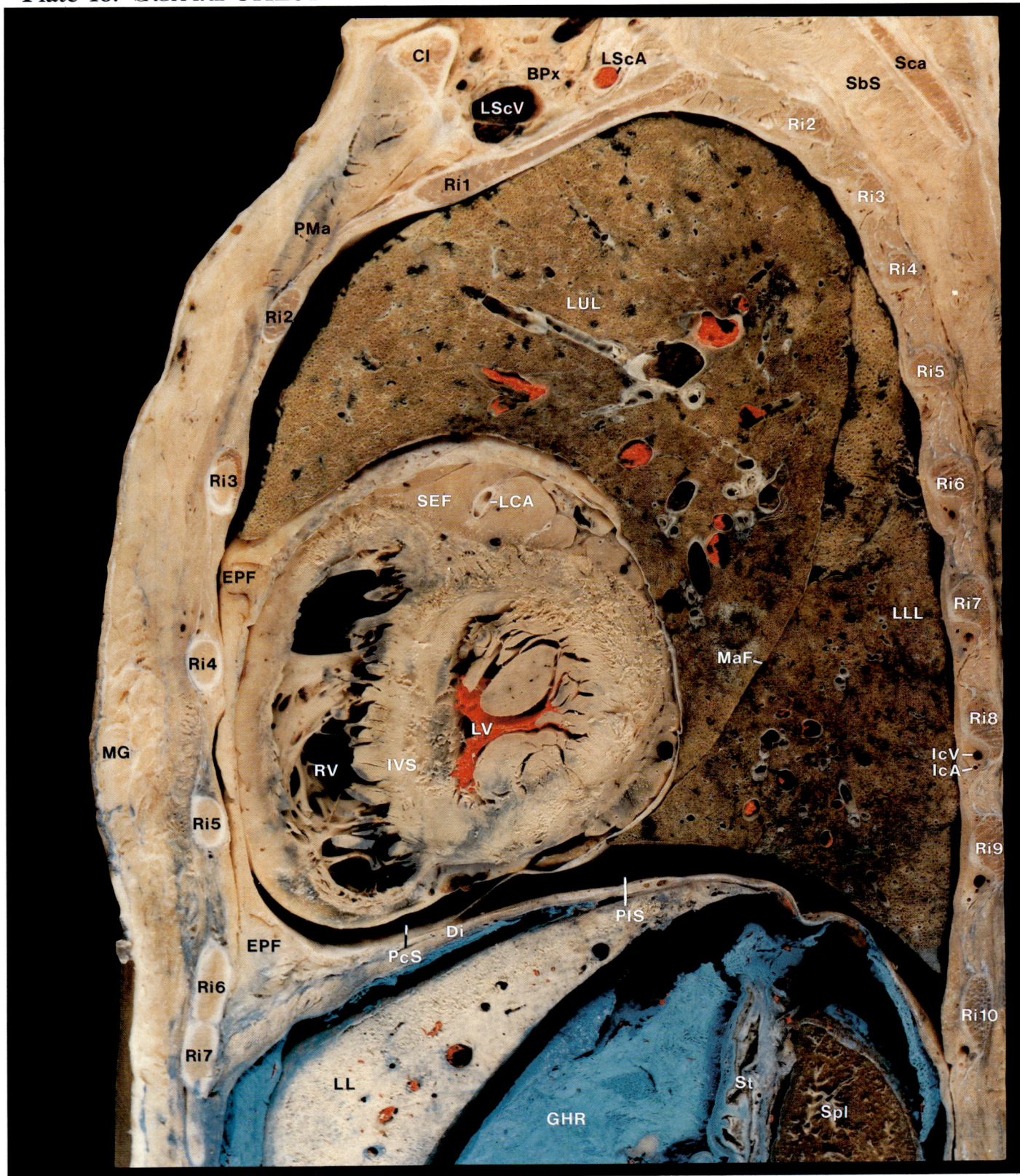

BPx	Brachial plexus	LScV	Left subclavian vein	SbS	Subscapularis muscle
Cl	Clavicle	LUL	Left upper lobe of lung	Sca	Scapula
Di	Diaphragm	LV	Left ventricle of heart	Spl	Spleen
EPF	Extrapericardial fat	MG	Mammary gland	St	Stomach
GHR	Gastrohepatic recess	MaF	Major fissure		
IVS	Interventricular septum	PMa	Pectoralis major muscle		
IcA	Intercostal artery	PcS	Pericardial space		
IcV	Intercostal vein	PlS	Pleural space		
LCA	Left coronary artery	RV	Right ventricle of heart		
LL	Left lobe of liver	Ri1	1st rib		
LLL	Left lower lobe of lung	Ri10	10th rib		
LScA	Left subclavian artery	SEF	Subepicardial fat		

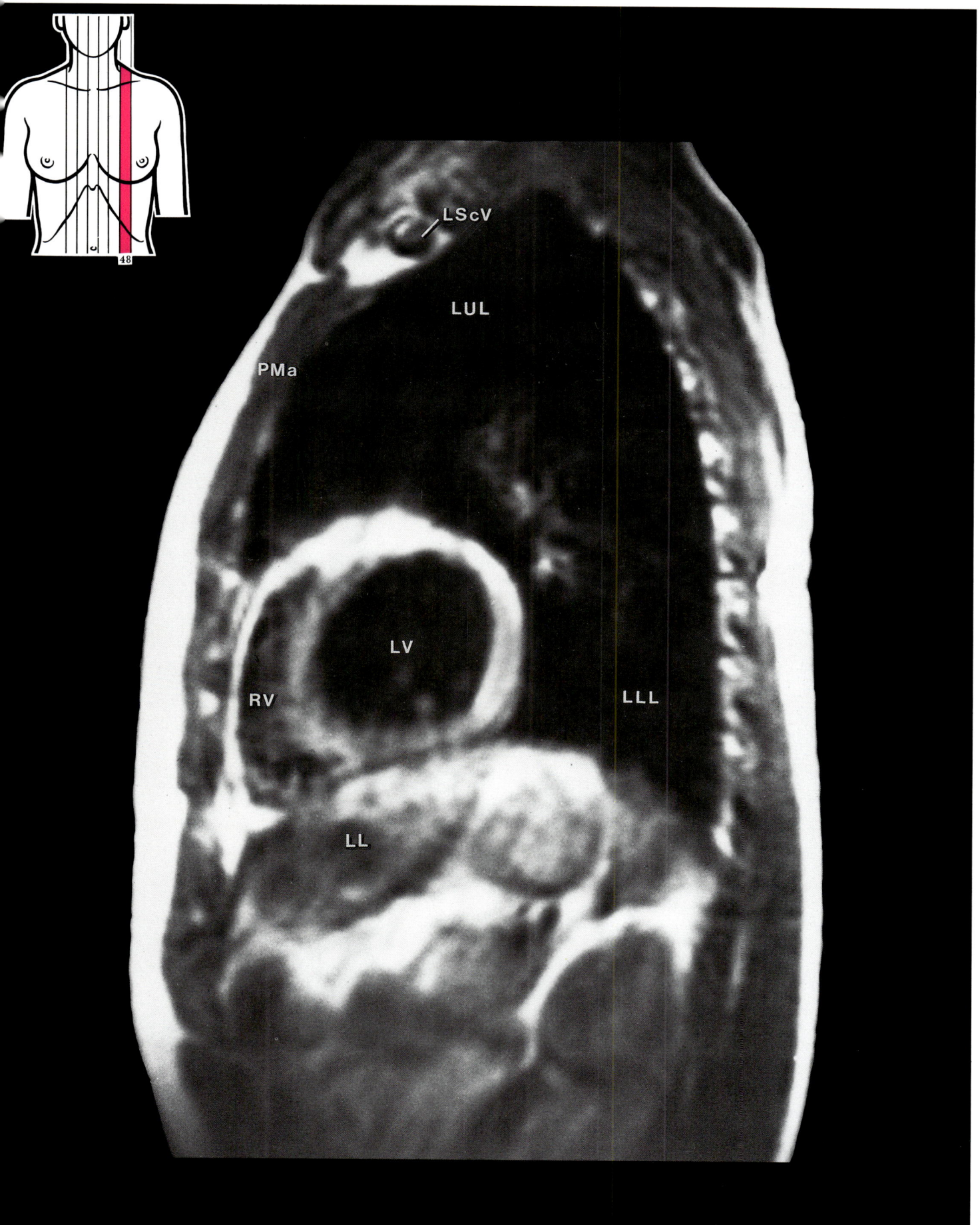

PART 3
ABDOMEN AND PELVIS

Transverse Section-male (Cadaver, CT & MRI) Plate 49-80

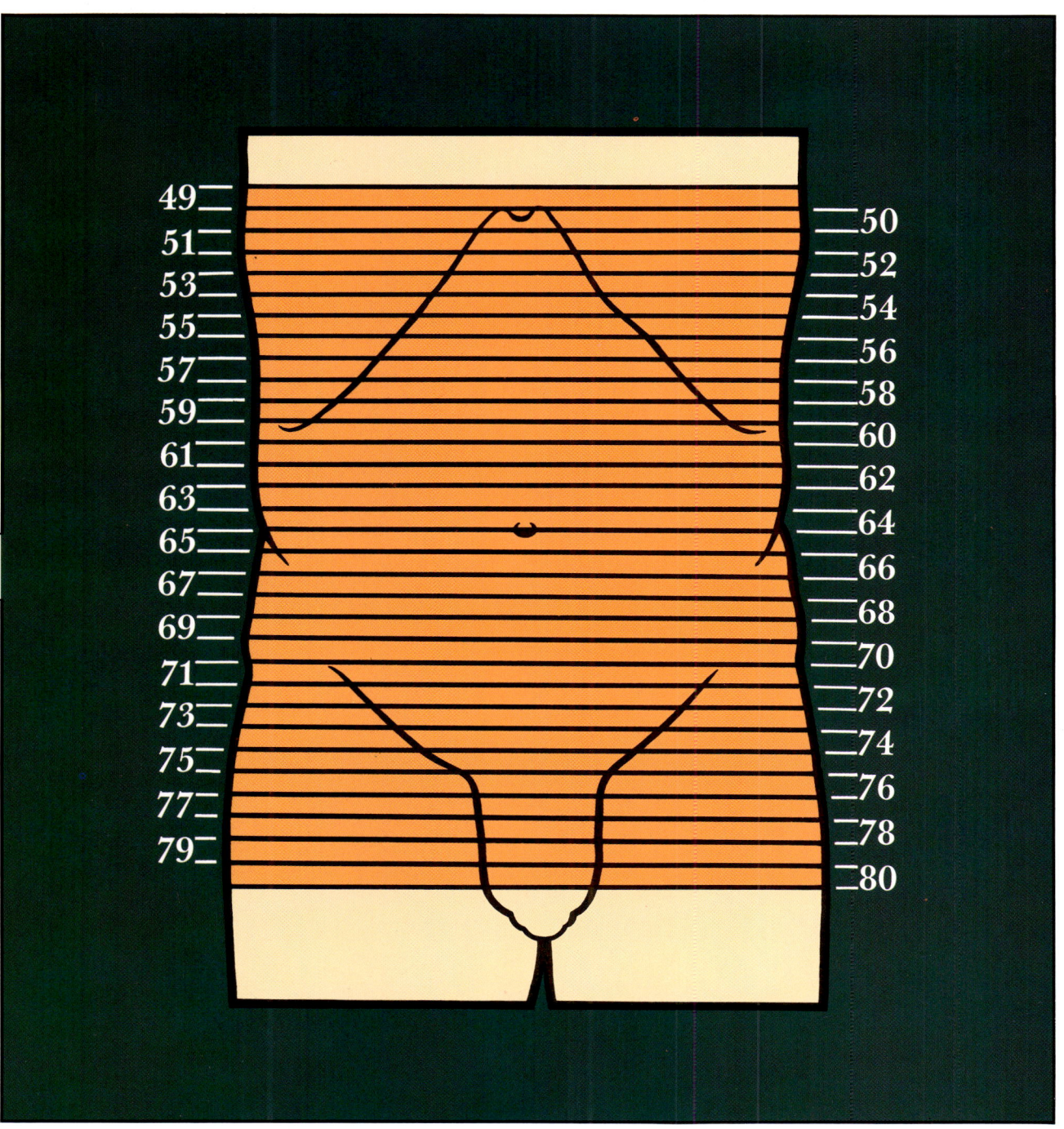

Plate 49. Transverse ABDOMEN

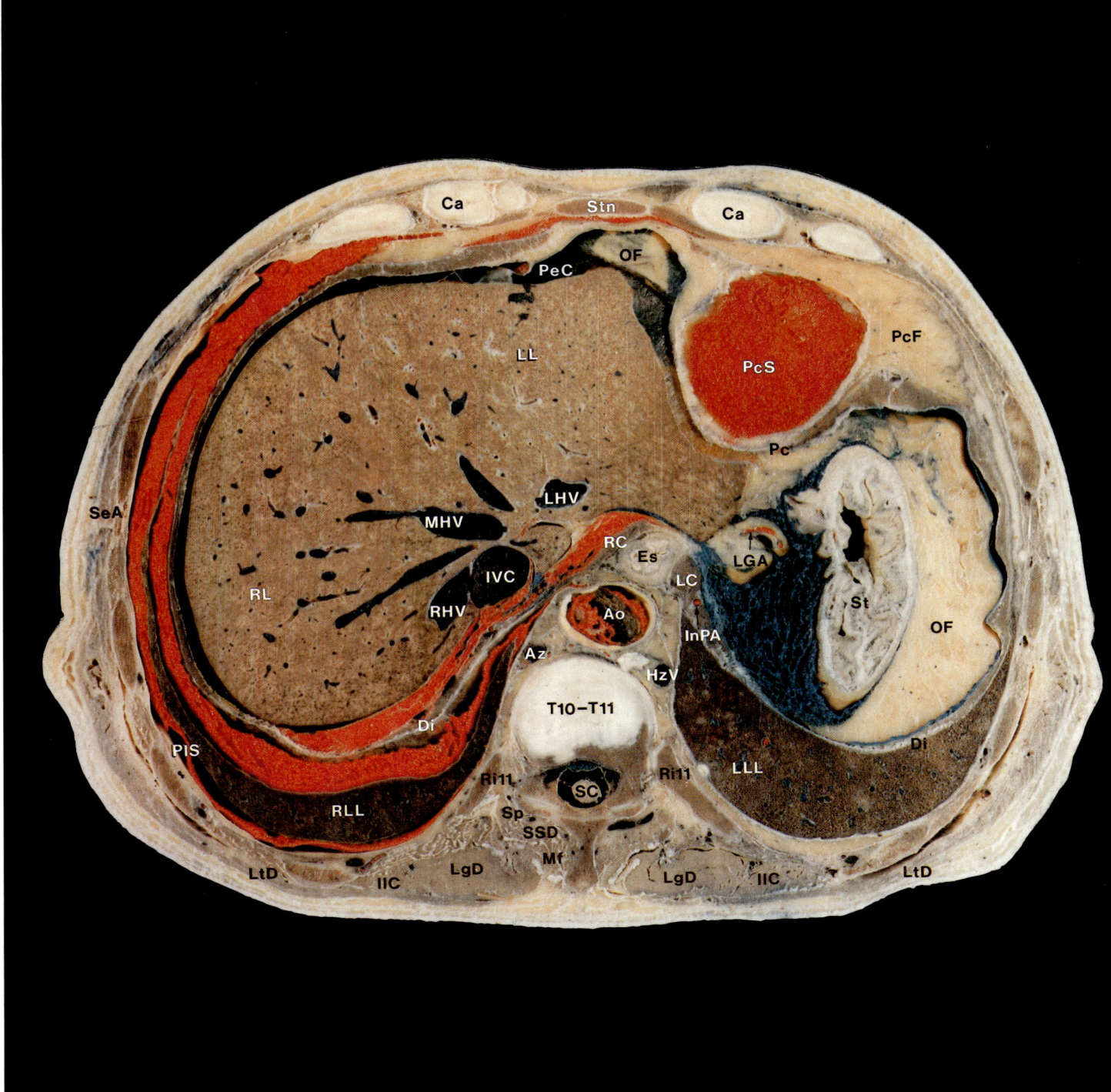

Ao	Aorta	OF	Omental fat	St	Stomach
Az	Azygos vein	Pc	Pericardium	Stn	Sternum
Ca	Cartilage	PcF	Pericardial fat	T10-11	T10-11 intervertebral disc
Di	Diaphragm	PcS	Pericardial space	T11	T11 vertebral body
Es	Esophagus	PeC	Peritoneal cavity	XP	Xiphoid process
HzV	Hemiazygos vein	PlS	Pleural space		
IVC	Inferior vena cava	RC	Right diaphragmatic crus		
IlC	Iliocostalis muscle	RHV	Right hepatic vein		
InPA	Inferior phrenic artery	RL	Right lobe of liver		
LC	Left diaphragmatic crus	RLL	Right lower lobe of lung		
LGA	Left gastric artery	RPV	Right portal vein		
LHV	Left hepatic vein	Ri	Rib		
LL	Left lobe of liver	Ri11	11th rib		
LLL	Left lower lobe of lung	SC	Spinal cord		
LgD	Longissimus dorsi muscle	SSD	Semispinalis dorsi muscle		
LtD	Latissimus dorsi muscle	SeA	Serratus anterior muscle		
MHV	Middle hepatic vein	Sp	Spinalis muscle		
Mf	Multifidus muscle	Spl	Spleen		

— 114 —

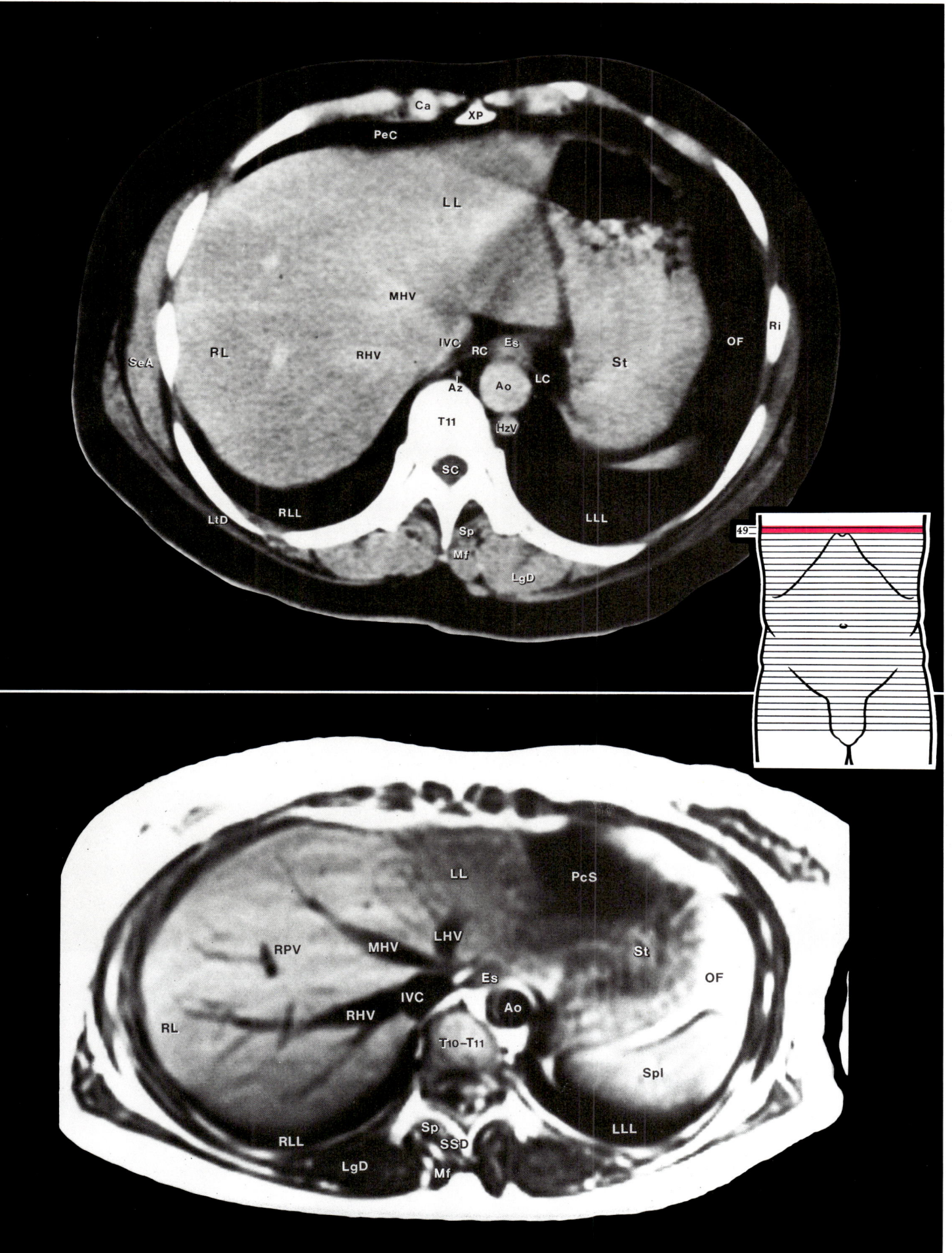

Plate 50. Transverse ABDOMEN

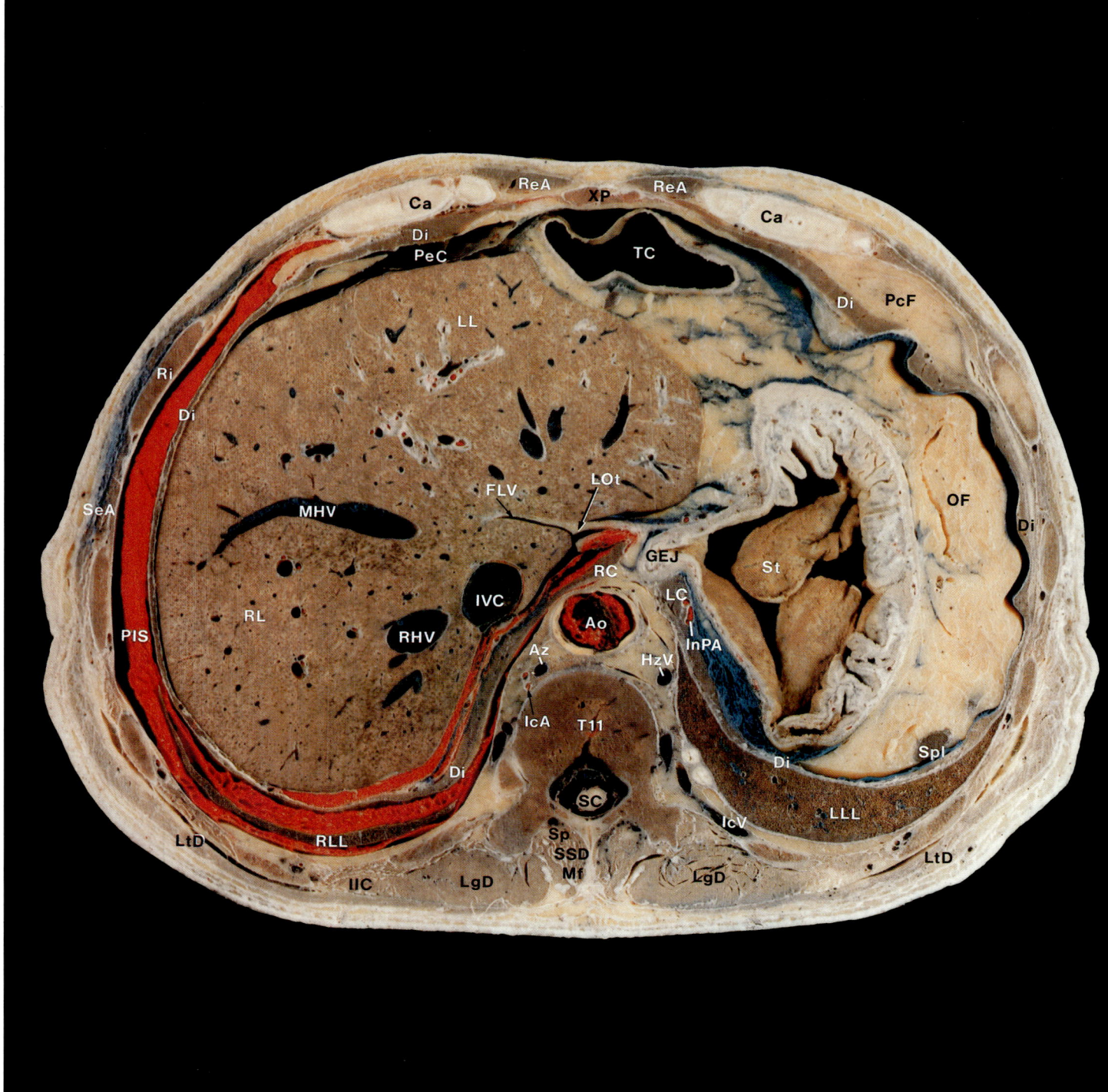

Ao	Aorta	LtD	Latissimus dorsi muscle	Spl	Spleen
Az	Azygos vein	MHV	Middle hepatic vein	St	Stomach
Ca	Cartilage	Mf	Multifidus muscle	T11	T11 vertebral body
Di	Diaphragm	OF	Omental fat	T11-12	T11-12 intervertebral disc
FLV	Fissure for ligamentum venosum	PcF	Pericardial fat	TC	Transverse colon
GEJ	Gastroesophageal junction	PeC	Peritoneal cavity	XP	Xiphoid process
HzV	Hemiazygos vein	PlS	Pleural space		
IVC	Inferior vena cava	RC	Right diaphragmatic crus		
IcA	Intercostal artery	RHV	Right hepatic vein		
IcV	Intercostal vein	RL	Right lobe of liver		
IlC	Iliocostalis muscle	RLL	Right lower lobe of lung		
InPA	Inferior phrenic artery	RPV	Right portal vein		
LC	Left diaphragmatic crus	ReA	Rectus abdominis muscle		
LHV	Left hepatic vein	Ri	Rib		
LL	Left lobe of liver	SC	Spinal cord		
LLL	Left lower lobe of lung	SSD	Semispinalis dorsi muscle		
LOt	Lesser omentum	SeA	Serratus anterior muscle		
LgD	Longissimus dorsi muscle	Sp	Spinalis muscle		

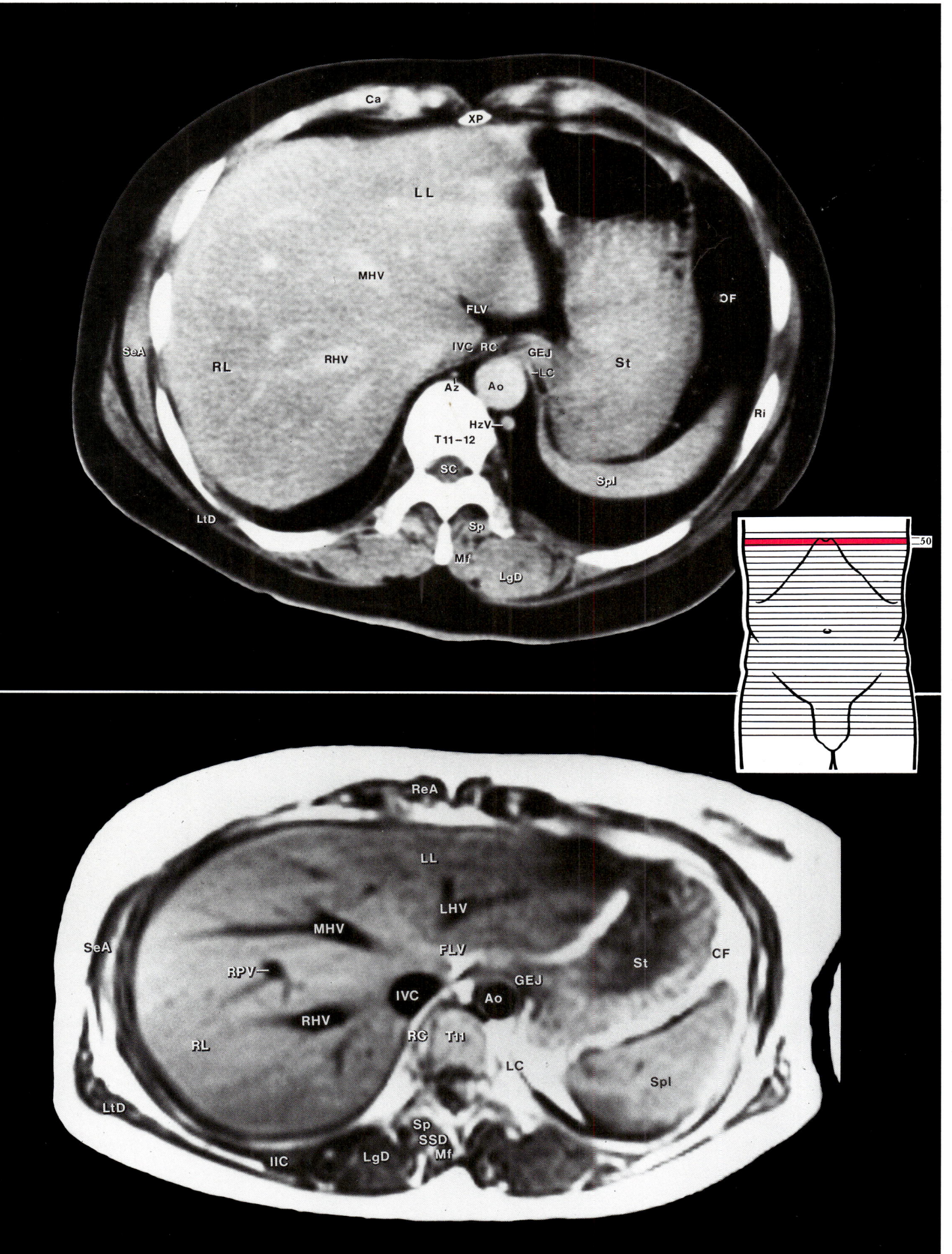

Plate 51. Transverse ABDOMEN

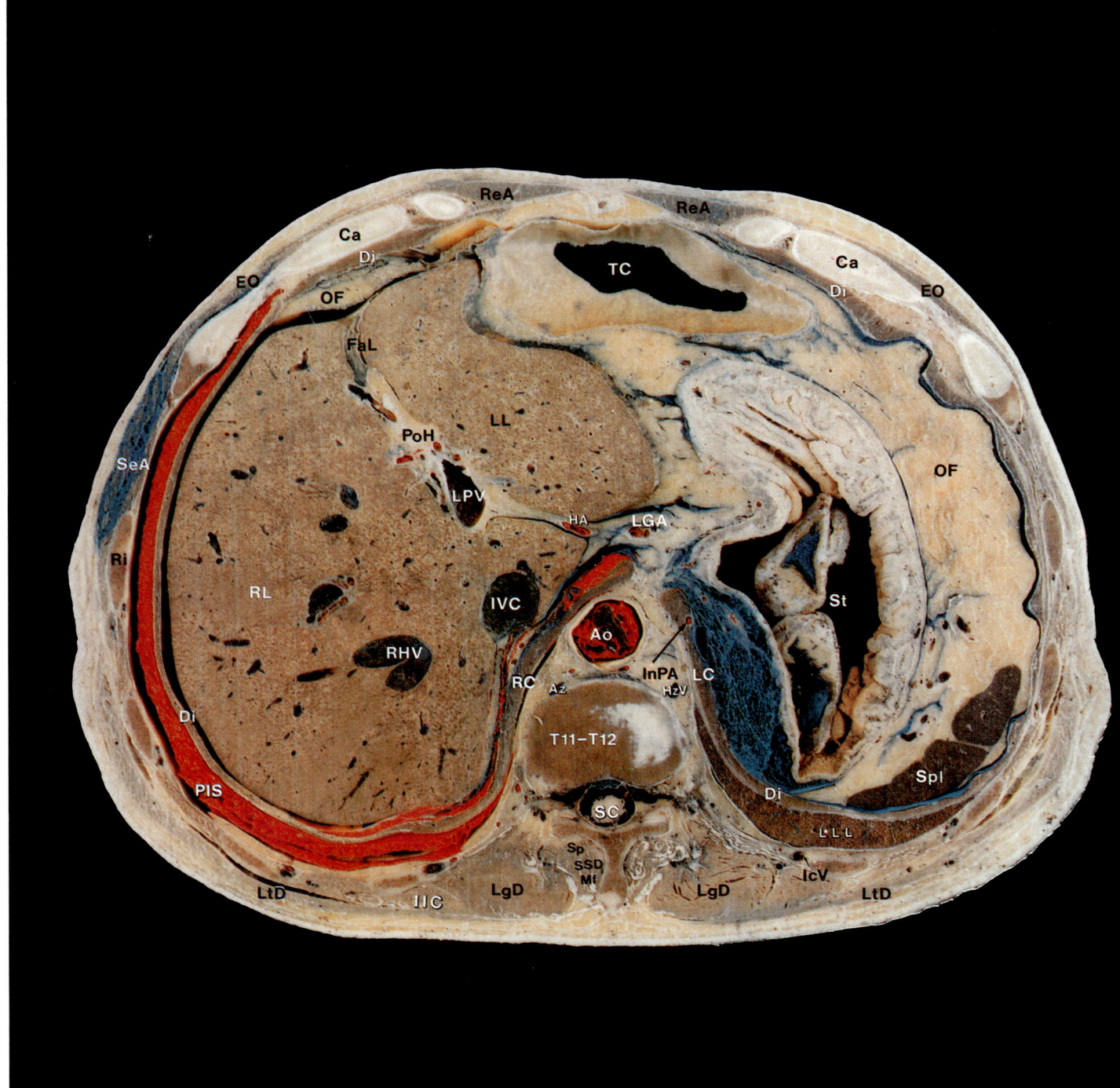

Ao	Aorta	LLL	Left lower lobe of lung	Sp	Spinalis muscle
Az	Azygos vein	LPV	Left portal vein	Spl	Spleen
CL	Caudate lobe of liver	LgD	Longissimus dorsi muscle	St	Stomach
Ca	Cartilage	LtD	Latissimus dorsi muscle	T11-12	T11-12 intervertebral disc
Di	Diaphragm	MHV	Middle hepatic vein	TC	Transverse colon
EO	External oblique muscle	Mf	Multifidus muscle	XP	Xiphoid process
FLV	Fissure for ligamentum venosum	OF	Omental fat		
FaL	Falciform ligament	PlS	Pleural space		
HA	Hepatic artery	PoH	Porta hepatis		
HzV	Hemiazygos vein	RC	Right diaphragmatic crus		
IVC	Inferior vena cava	RHV	Right hepatic vein		
IcV	Intercostal vein	RL	Right lobe of liver		
IlC	Iliocostalis muscle	RPV	Right portal vein		
InPA	Inferior phrenic artery	ReA	Rectus abdominis muscle		
LC	Left diaphragmatic crus	Ri	Rib		
LGA	Left gastric artery	SC	Spinal cord		
LHV	Left hepatic vein	SSD	Semispinalis dorsi muscle		
LL	Left lobe of liver	SeA	Serratus anterior muscle		

— 118 —

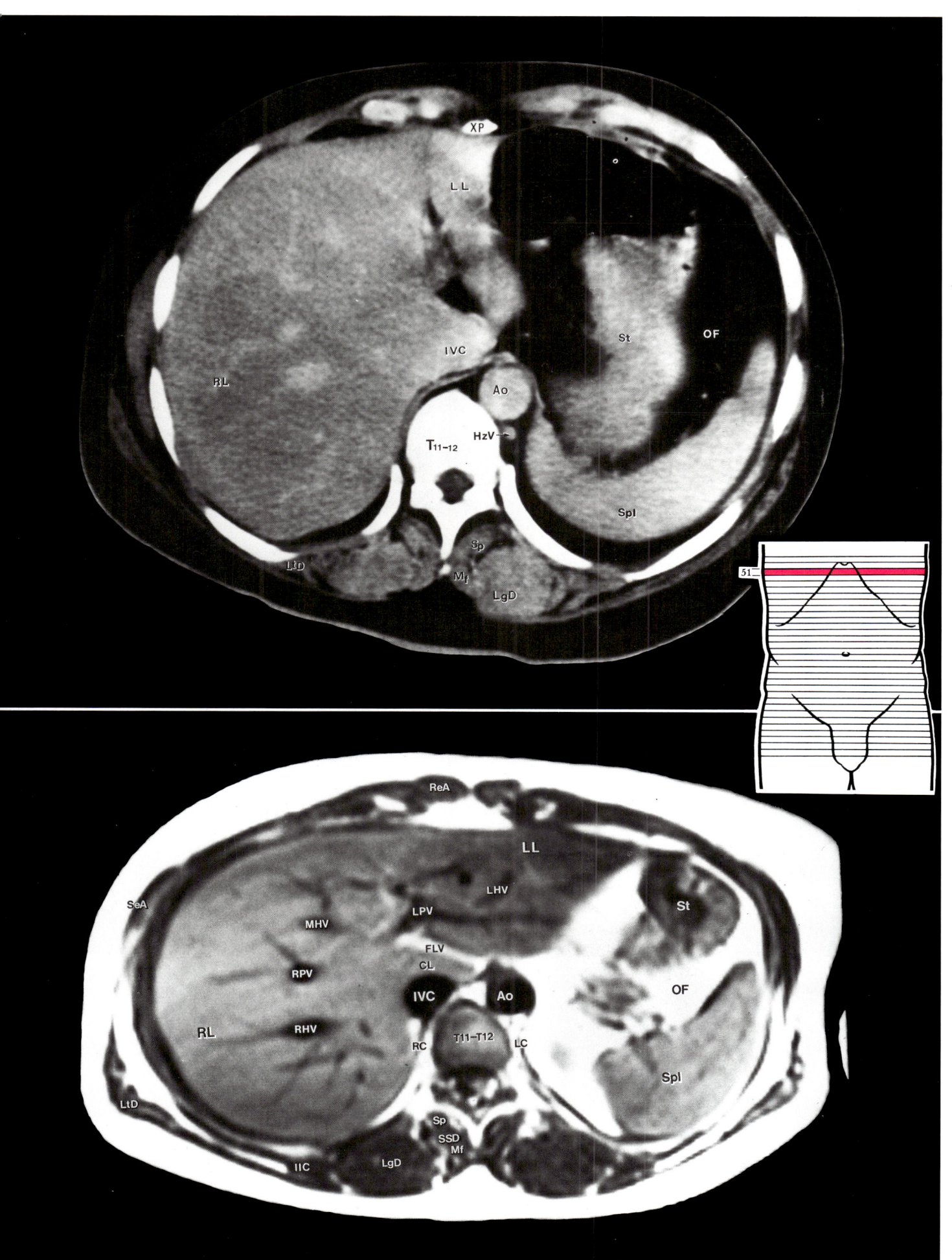

Plate 52. Transverse ABDOMEN

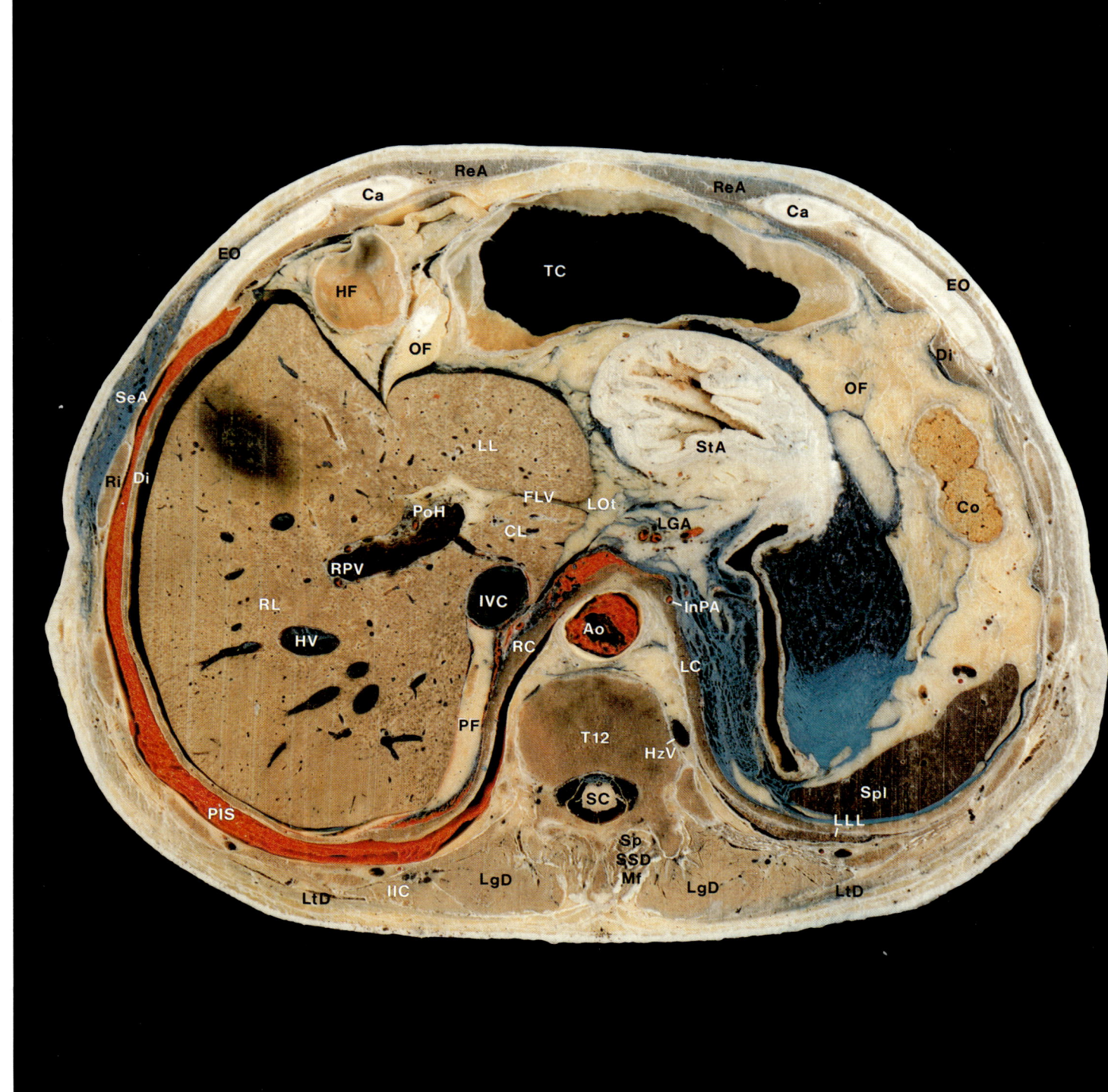

Ao	Aorta	LOt	Lesser omentum	SSD	Semispinalis dorsi muscle
CL	Caudate lobe of liver	LgD	Longissimus dorsi muscle	SV	Splenic vein
Ca	Cartilage	LtD	Latissimus dorsi muscle	SeA	Serratus anterior muscle
Co	Colon	Mf	Multifidus muscle	Sp	Spinalis muscle
Di	Diaphragm	OF	Omental fat	Spl	Spleen
EO	External oblique muscle	PB	Pancreas, body	St	Stomach
FLV	Fissure for ligamentum venosum	PF	Perirenal fat	StA	Stomach, antrum
HF	Hepatic flexure of colon	PT	Pancreas, tail	T12	T12 vertebral body
HV	Hepatic vein	PV	Portal vein	TC	Transverse colon
HzV	Hemiazygos vein	PlS	Pleural space		
IVC	Inferior vena cava	PoH	Porta hepatis		
IlC	Iliocostalis muscle	RC	Right diaphragmatic crus		
InPA	Inferior phrenic artery	RHV	Right hepatic vein		
LC	Left diaphragmatic crus	RL	Right lobe of liver		
LGA	Left gastric artery	RPV	Right portal vein		
LK	Left kidney	ReA	Rectus abdominis muscle		
LL	Left lobe of liver	Ri	Rib		
LLL	Left lower lobe of lung	SC	Spinal cord		

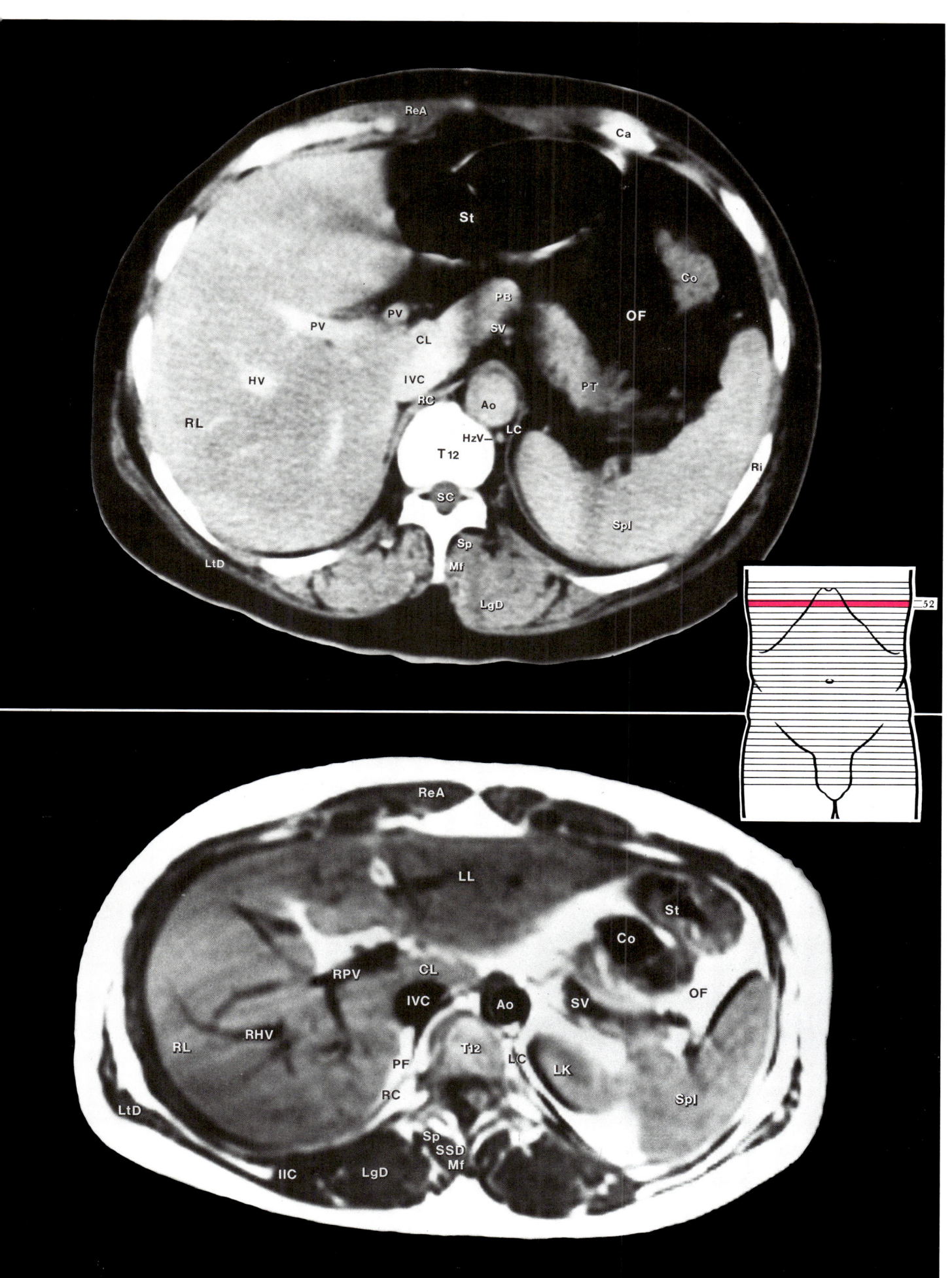

Plate 53. Transverse ABDOMEN

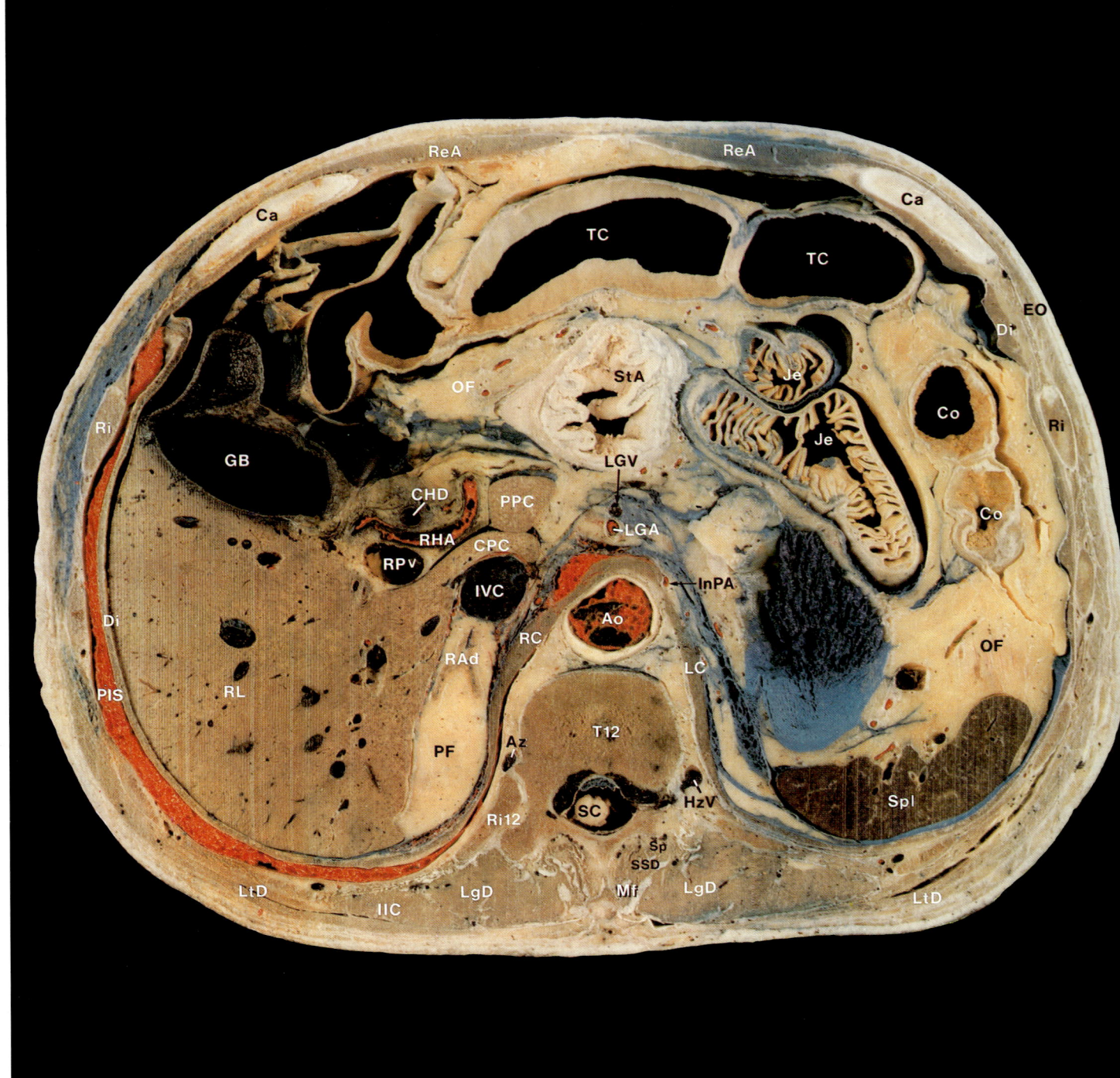

Ao	Aorta	LGV	Left gastric vein	ReA	Rectus abdominis muscle
Az	Azygos vein	LL	Left lobe of liver	Ri	Rib
CHD	Common hepatic duct	LgD	Longissimus dorsi muscle	SC	Spinal cord
CL	Caudate lobe of liver	LtD	Latissimus dorsi muscle	SSD	Semispinalis dorsi muscle
CPC	Caudate process of caudate lobe	MeF	Mesenteric fat	SV	Splenic vein
Ca	Cartilage	Mf	Multifidus muscle	Sp	Spinalis muscle
Co	Colon	OF	Omental fat	Spl	Spleen
DB	Duodenal bulb	PB	Pancreas, body	St	Stomach
Di	Diaphragm	PF	Perirenal fat	StA	Stomach, antrum
EO	External oblique muscle	PPC	Papillary process of caudate lobe	T12	T12 vertebral body
GB	Gall bladder	PT	Pancreas, tail	TC	Transverse colon
HzV	Hemiazygos vein	PV	Portal vein		
IVC	Inferior vena cava	PlS	Pleural space		
IlC	Iliocostalis muscle	RAd	Right adrenal gland		
InPA	Inferior phrenic artery	RC	Right diaphragmatic crus		
Je	Jejunum	RHA	Right hepatic artery		
LC	Left diaphragmatic crus	RL	Right lobe of liver		
LGA	Left gastric artery	RPV	Right portal vein		

— 122 —

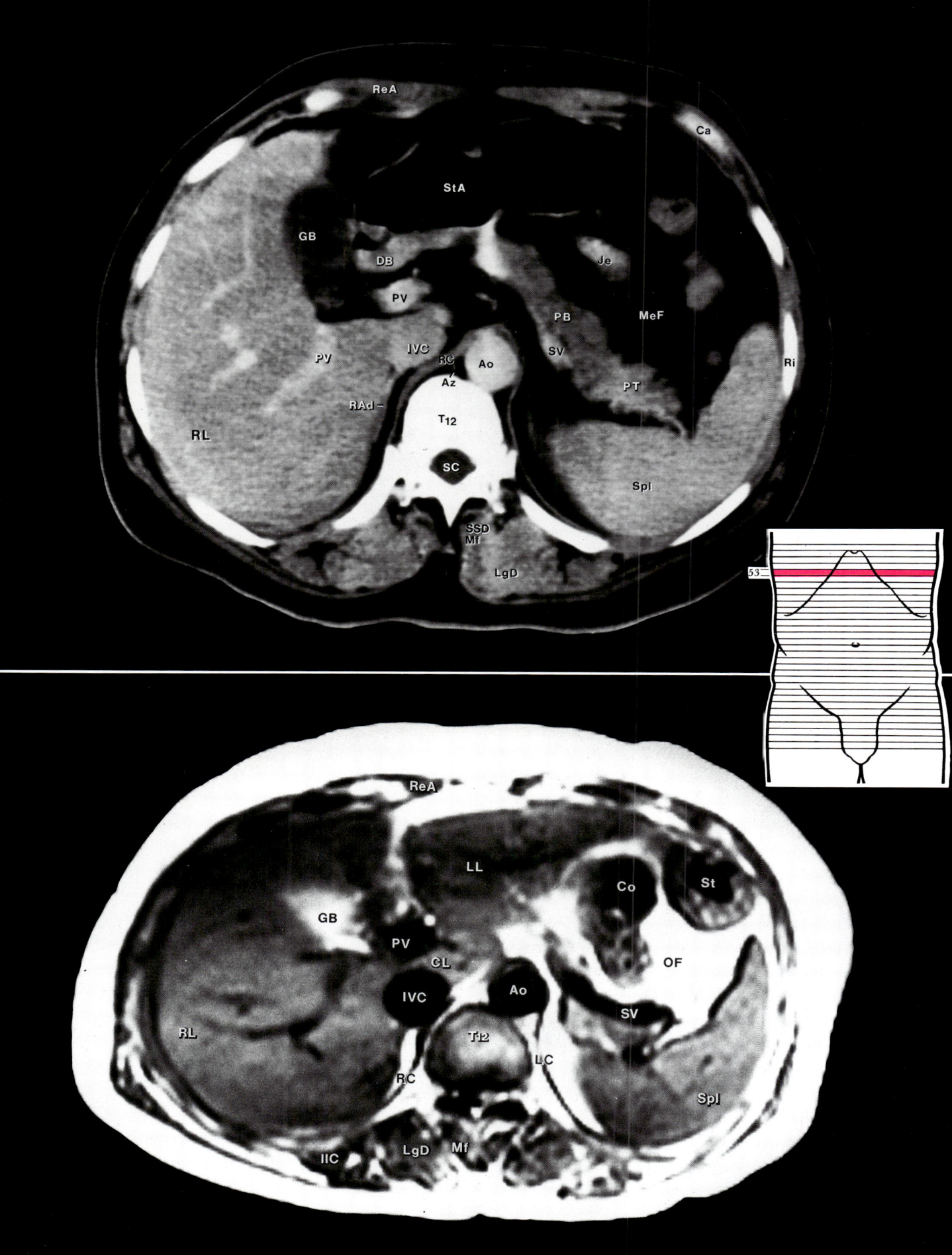

Plate 54. Transverse ABDOMEN

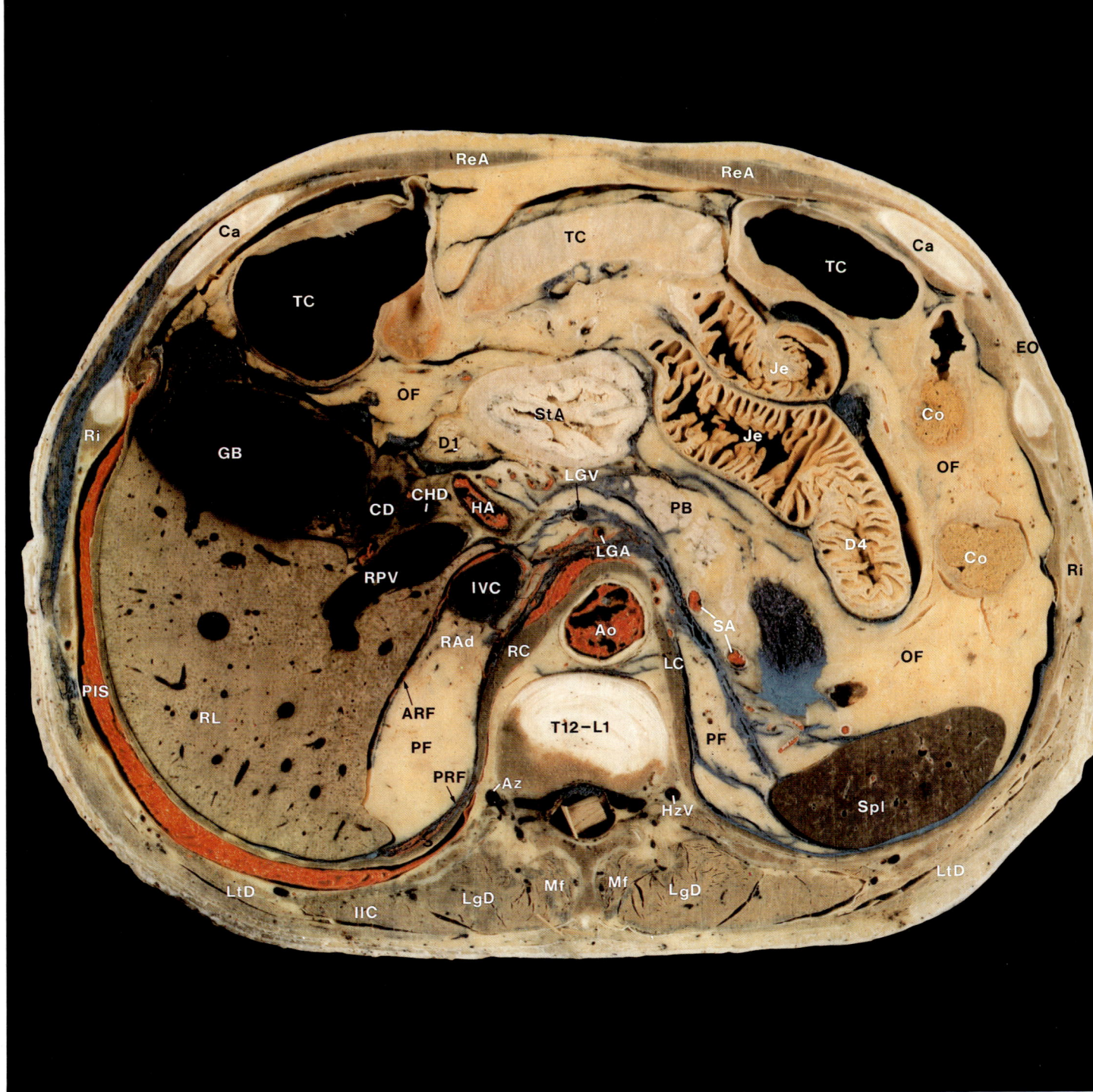

ARF	Anterior renal fascia	LAd	Left adrenal gland	RPV	Right portal vein
Ao	Aorta	LC	Left diaphragmatic crus	ReA	Rectus abdominis muscle
Az	Azygos vein	LGA	Left gastric artery	Ri	Rib
CD	Cystic duct	LGV	Left gastric vein	SA	Splenic artery
CHD	Common hepatic duct	LK	Keft kidney	SC	Spinal cord
Ca	Cartilage	LL	Left lobe of liver	SV	Splenic vein
Co	Colon	LgD	Longissimus dorsi muscle	Spl	Spleen
Dl	First portion of duodenum	LtD	Latissimus dorsi muscle	St	Stomach
D4	Fourth protion of duodenum	Mf	Multifidus muscle	StA	Stomach, antrum
DB	Duodenal bulb	OF	Omental fat	T12-L1	T12-L1 intervertebral disc
EO	External oblique muscle	PB	Pancreas, body	TC	Transverse colon
GB	Gall bladder	PF	Perirenal fat		
HA	Hepatic artery	PRF	Posterior renal fascia		
HzV	Hemiazygos vein	PV	Portal vein		
IVC	Inferior vena cava	PlS	Pleural space		
IlC	Iliocostalis muscle	RAd	Right adrenal gland		
Je	Jejunum	RC	Right diaphragmatic crus		
Ll	Ll vertebral body	RL	Right lobe of liver		

— 124 —

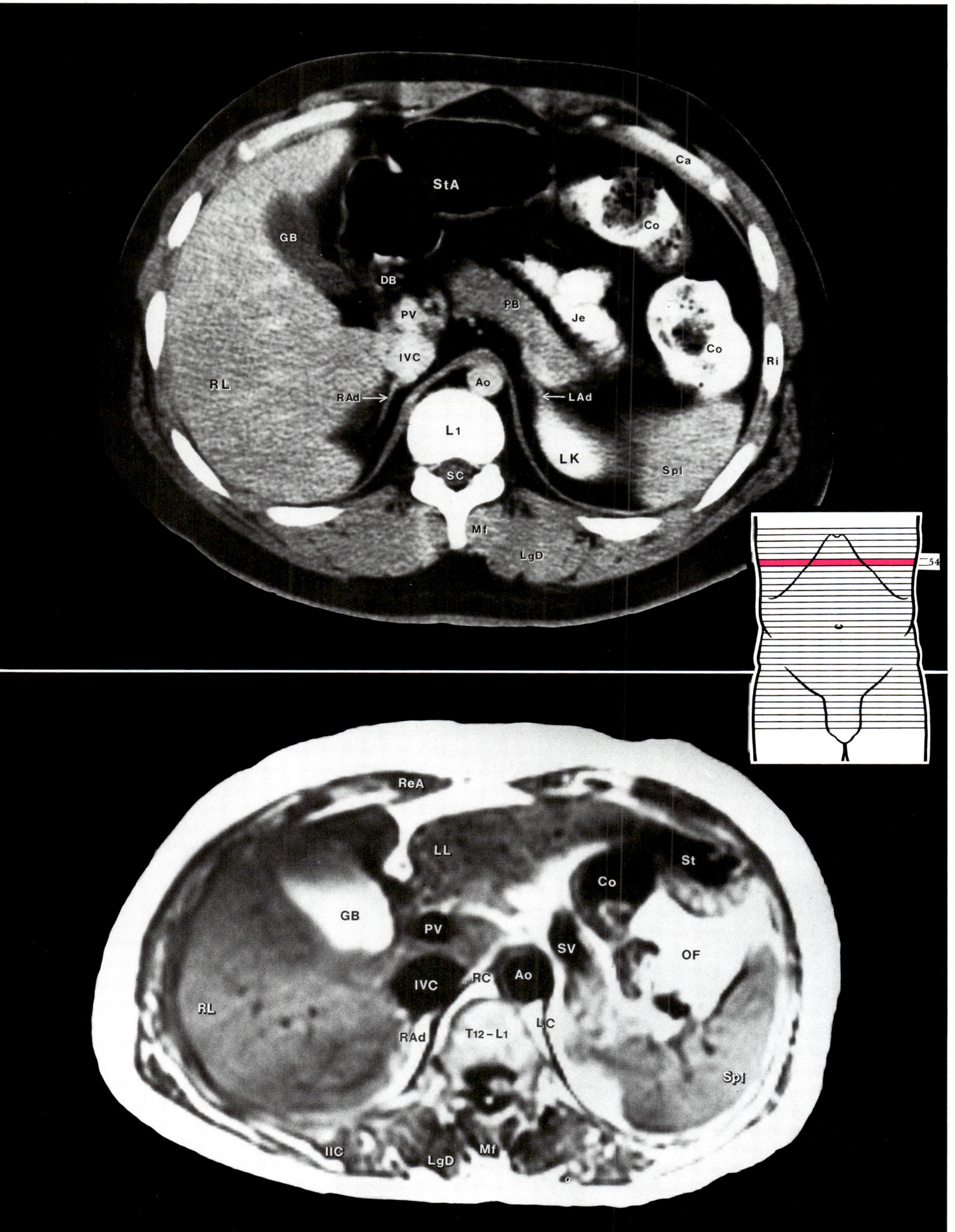

Plate 55. Transverse ABDOMEN

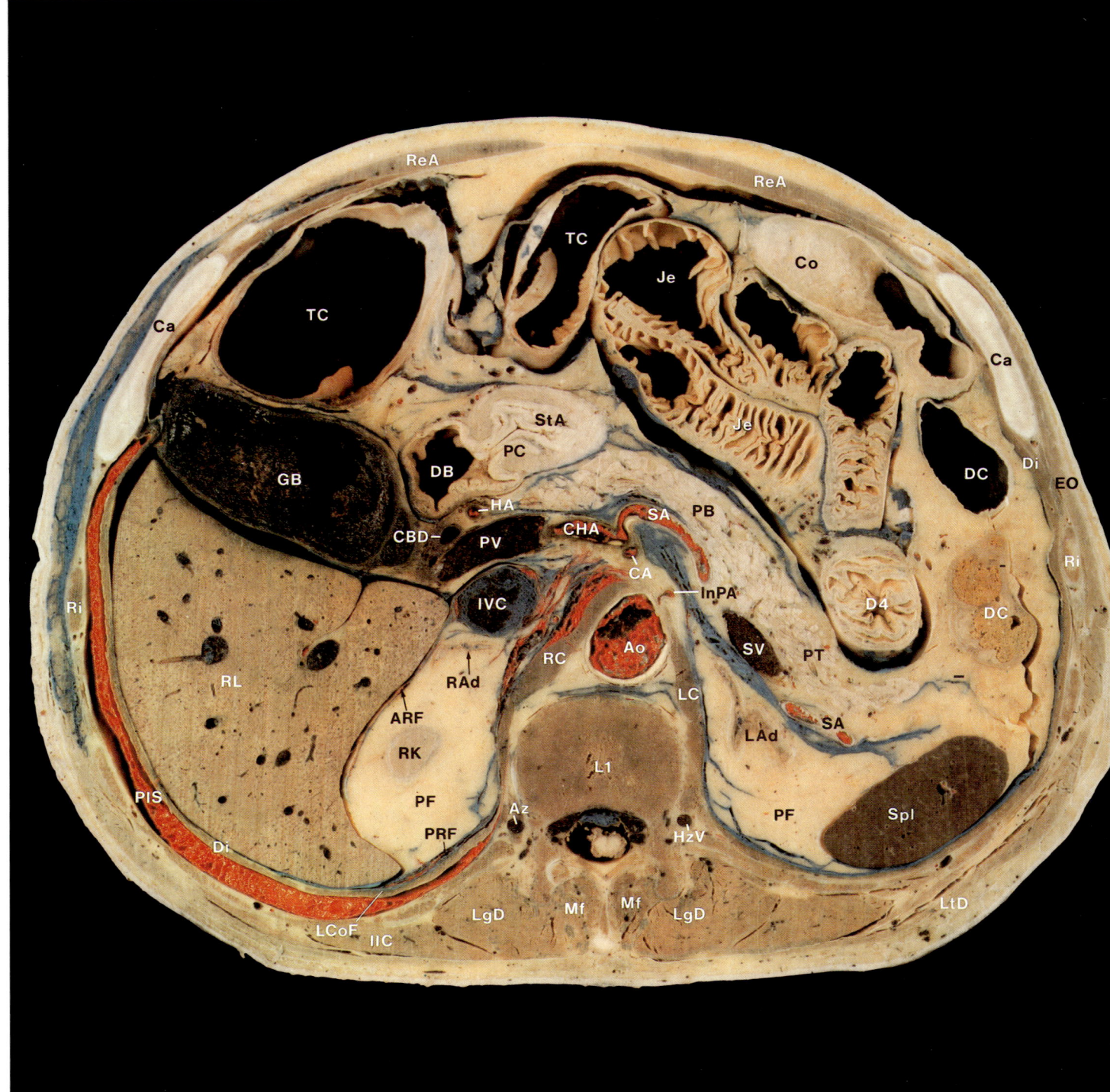

ARF	Anterior renal fascia	InPA	Inferior phrenic artery	RAd	Right adrenal gland
Ao	Aorta	Je	Jejunum	RC	Right diaphragmatic crus
Az	Azygos vein	Ll	Ll vertebral body	RK	Right kidney
CA	Celiac axis	LAd	Left adrenal gland	RL	Right lobe of liver
CBD	Common bile duct	LC	Left diaphragmatic crus	ReA	Rectus abdominis muscle
CHA	Common hepatic artery	LCoF	Lateroconal fascia	Ri	Rib
Ca	Cartilage	LK	Left kidney	SA	Splenic artery
Co	Colon	LL	Left lobe of liver	SC	Spinal cord
D4	Fourth portion of duodenum	LgD	Longissimus dorsi muscle	SV	Splenic vein
DB	Duodenal bulb	LtD	Latissimus dorsi muscle	Spl	Spleen
DC	Descending colon	Mf	Multifidus muscle	St	Stomach
Di	Diaphragm	PB	Pancreas, body	StA	Stomach, antrum
EO	External oblique muscle	PC	Pyloric canal of stomach	TC	Transverse colon
GB	Gall bladder	PF	Perirenal fat		
HA	Hepatic artery	PRF	Posterior renal fascia		
HzV	Hemiazygos vein	PT	Pancreas, tail		
IVC	Inferior vena cava	PV	Portal vein		
IlC	Iliocostalis muscle	PlS	Pleural space		

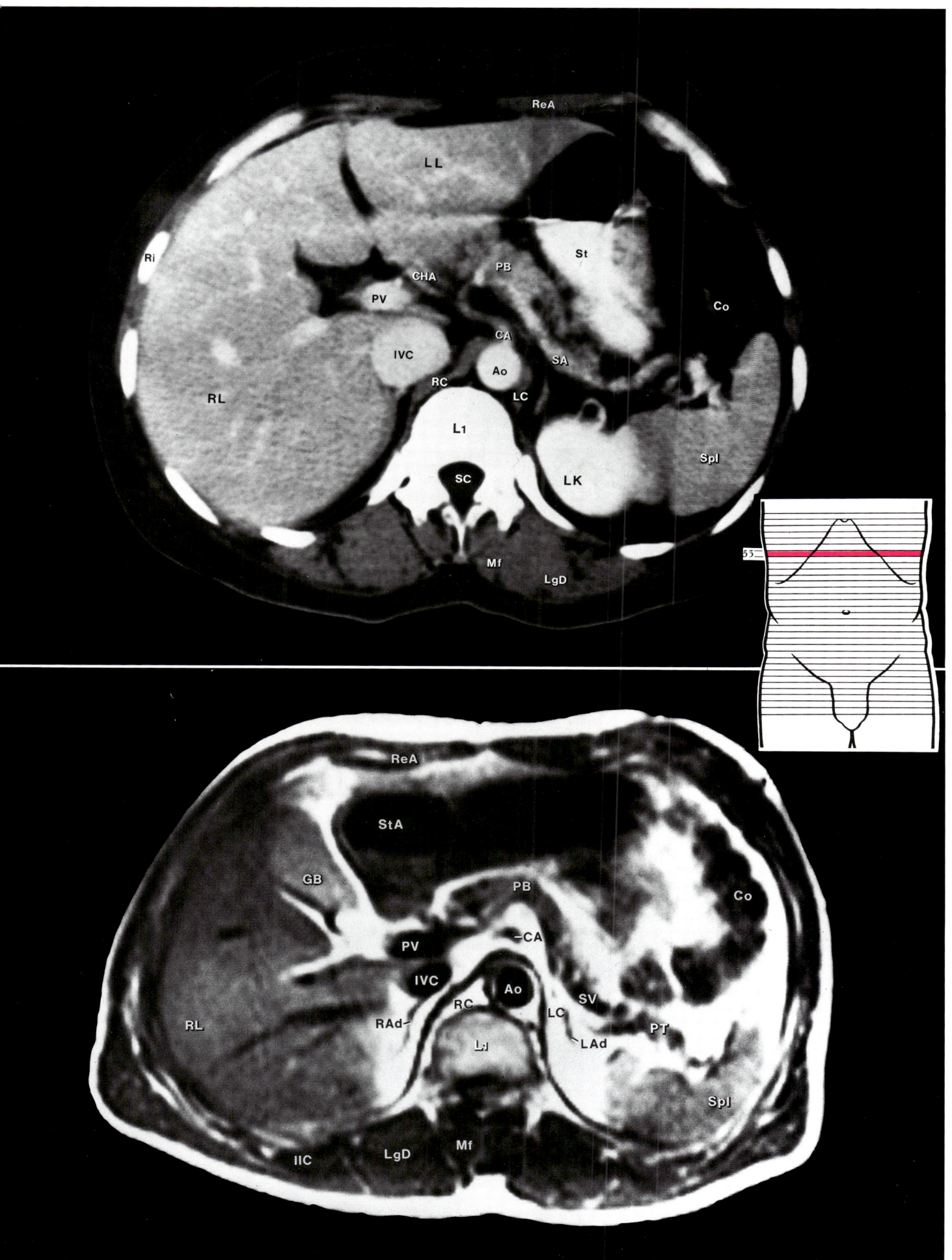

Plate 56. Transverse ABDOMEN

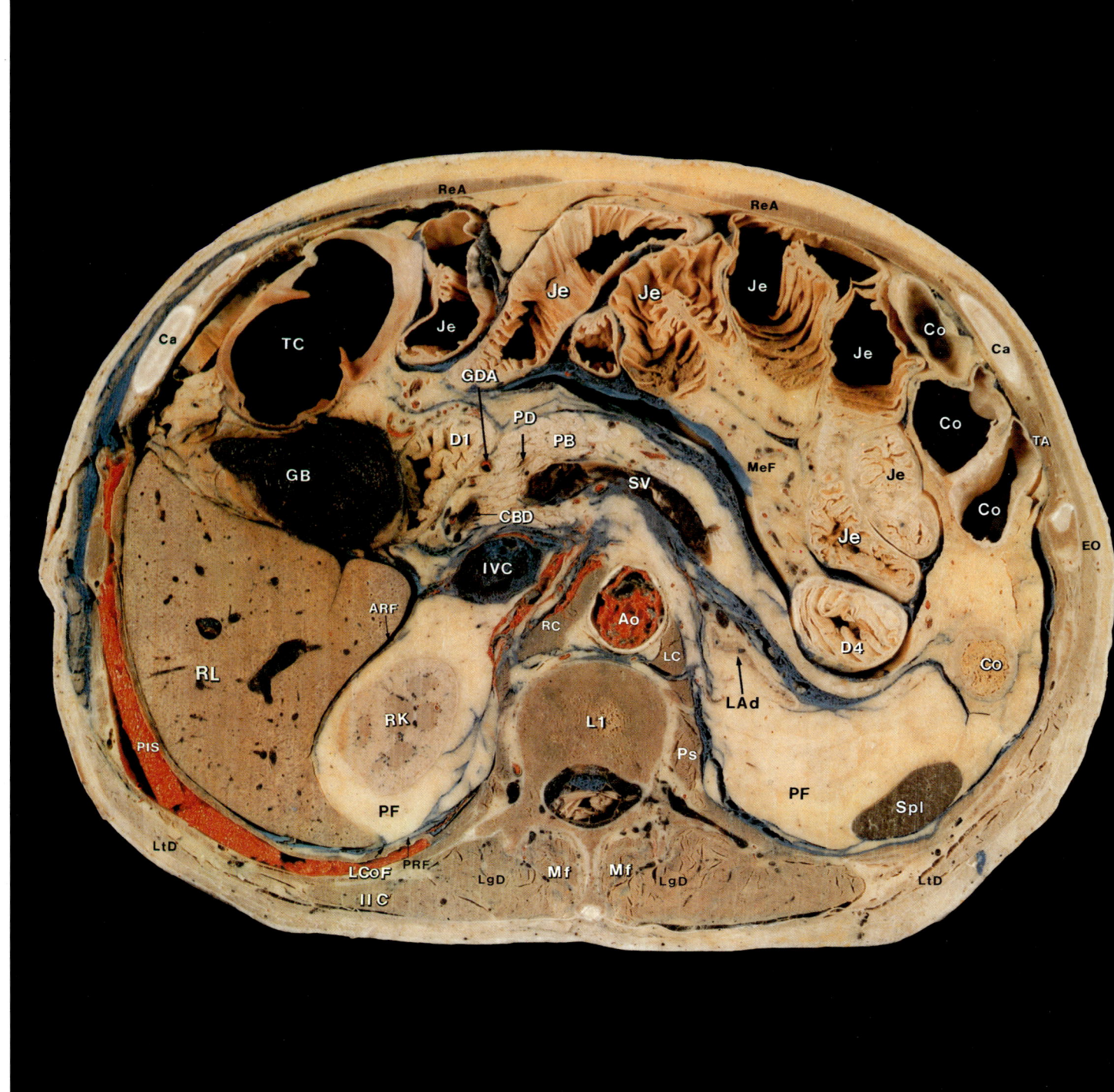

ARF	Anterior renal fascia	LAd	Left adrenal gland	RC	Right diaphragmatic crus
Ao	Aorta	LC	Left diaphragmatic crus	RK	Right kidney
Az	Azygos vein	LCoF	Lateroconal fascia	RL	Right lobe of liver
CA	Celiac axis	LK	Left kidney	RPV	Right portal vein
CBD	Common bile duct	LL	Left lobe of liver	ReA	Rectus abdominis muscle
Ca	Cartilage	LgD	Longissimus dorsi muscle	Ri	Rib
Co	Colon	LtD	Latissimus dorsi muscle	SC	Spinal cord
Dl	First portion of duodenum	MeF	Mesenteric fat	SV	Splenic vein
D4	Fourth portion of duodenum	Mf	Multifidus muscle	Spl	Spleen
DB	Duodenal bulb	PB	Pancreas, body	St	Stomach
DC	Descending colon	PD	Pancreatic duct	StA	Stomach, antrum
EO	External oblique muscle	PF	Perirenal fat	T12	T12 vertebral body
GB	Gall bladder	PRF	Posterior renal fascia	TA	Transversus abdominis muscle
GDA	Gastroduocenal artery	PT	Pancreas, tail	TC	Transverse colon
IVC	Inferior vena cava	PV	Portal vein		
IlC	Iliocostalis muscle	PlS	Pleural space		
Je	Jejunum	Ps	Psoas muscle		
Ll	Ll vertebral body	RAd	Right adrenal gland		

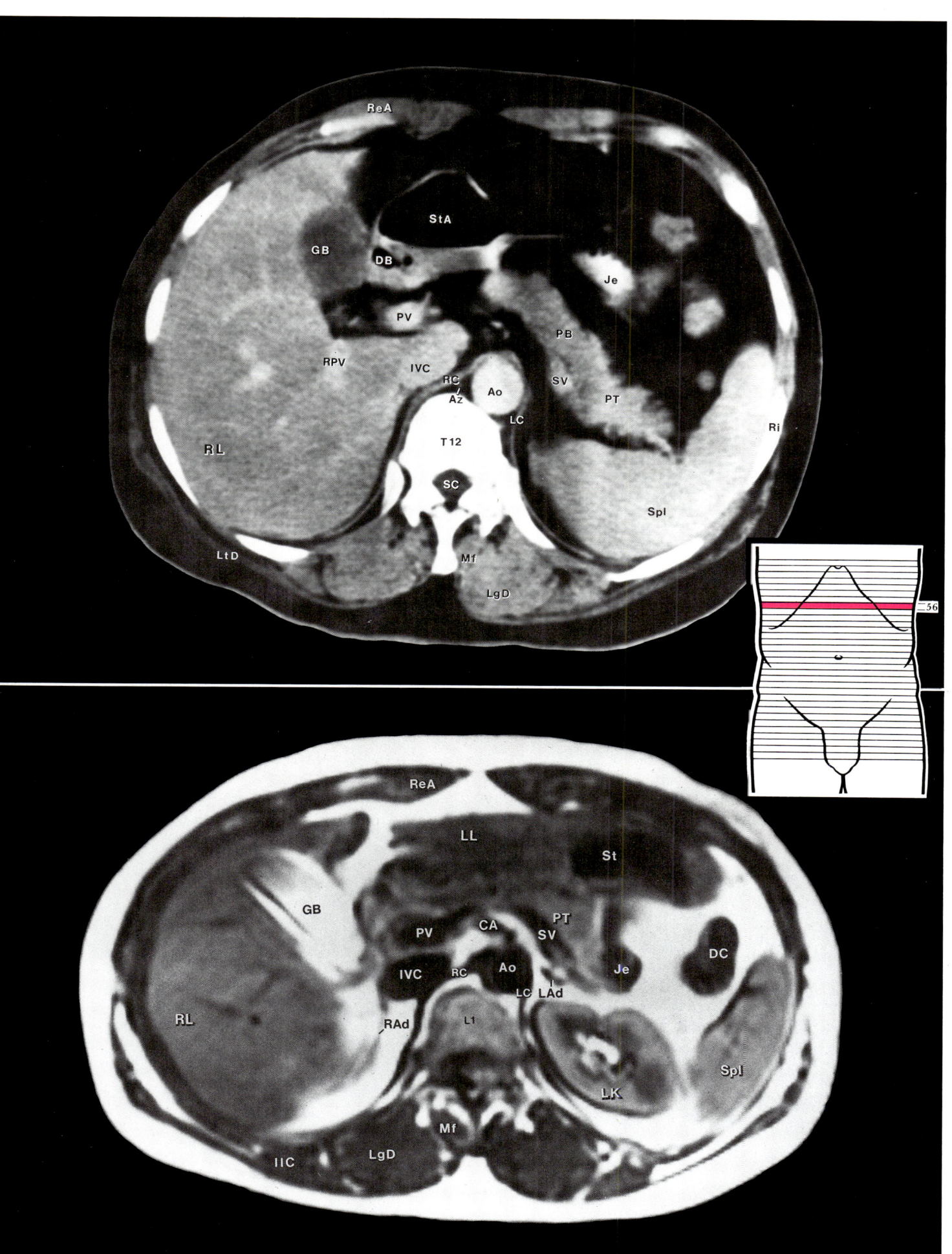

Plate 57. Transverse ABDOMEN

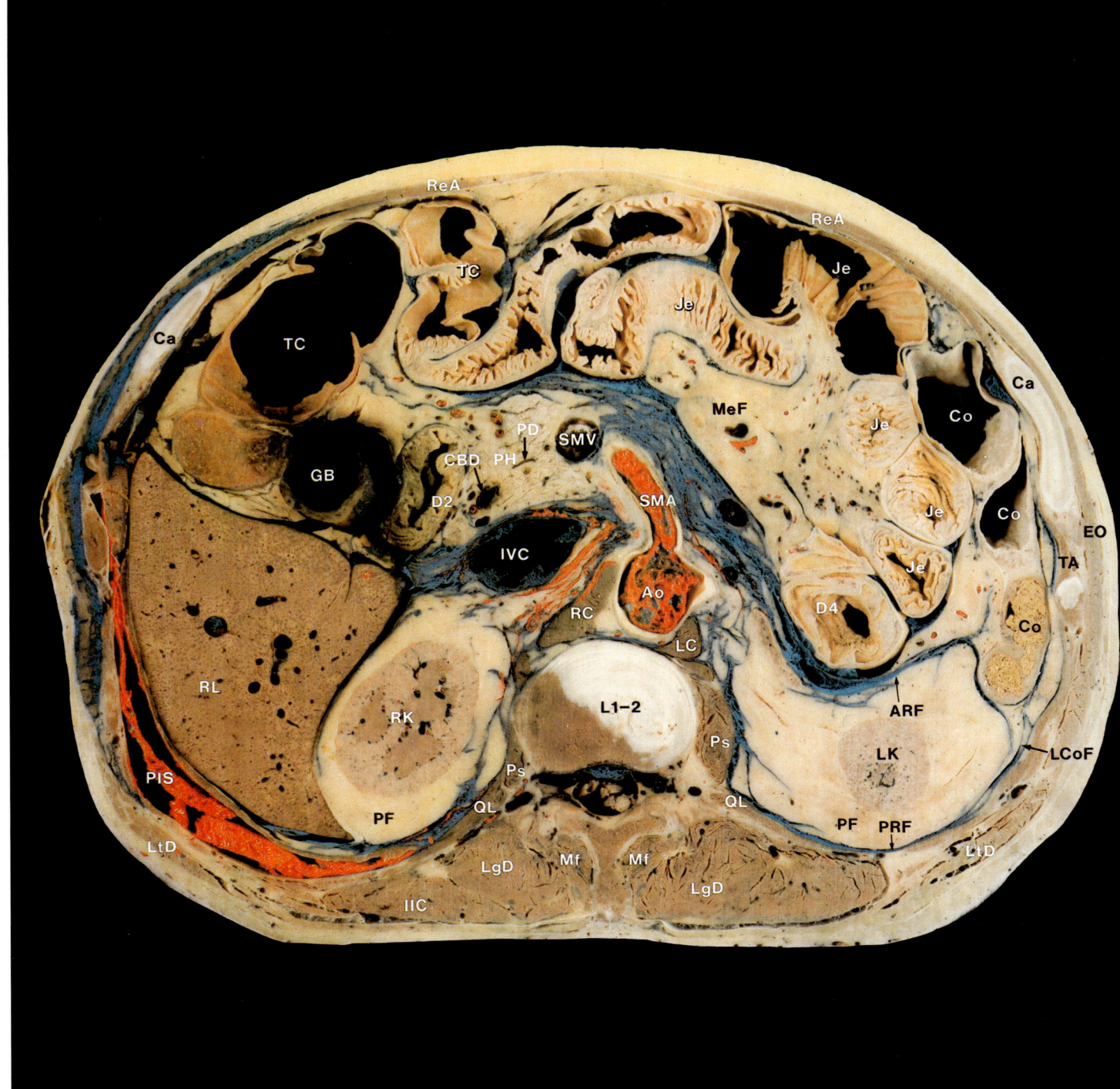

AC	Ascending colon	LC	Left diaphragmatic crus
ARF	Anterior renal fascia	LCoF	Lateroconal fascia
Ao	Aorta	LK	Left kidney
Az	Azygos vein	LgD	Longissimus dorsi muscle
CBD	Common bile duct	LtD	Latissimus dorsi muscle
Ca	Cartilage	MeF	Mesenteric fat
Co	Colon	Mf	Multifidus muscle
D2	Second portion of duodenum	PD	Pancreatic duct
D4	Fourth portion of duodenum	PF	Perirenal fat
DC	Descending colon	PH	Pancreas, head
EO	External oblique muscle	PRF	Posterior renal fascia
GB	Gall bladder	PlS	Pleural space
HzV	Hemiazygos vein	Ps	Psoas muscle
IVC	Inferior vena cava	QL	Quadratus lumborum muscle
IlC	Iliocostalis muscle	RC	Right diaphragmatic crus
Je	Jejunum	RCx	Renal cortex
L1	L1 vertebral body	RK	Right kidney
L1-2	L1-2 intervertebral disc	RL	Right lobe of liver
RM	Renal medulla		
ReA	Rectus abdominis muscle		
SC	Spinal cord		
SMA	Superior mesenteric artery		
SMV	Superior mesenteric vein		
Spl	Spleen		
St	Stomach		
TA	Transversus abdominis muscle		
TC	Transverse colon		

— 130 —

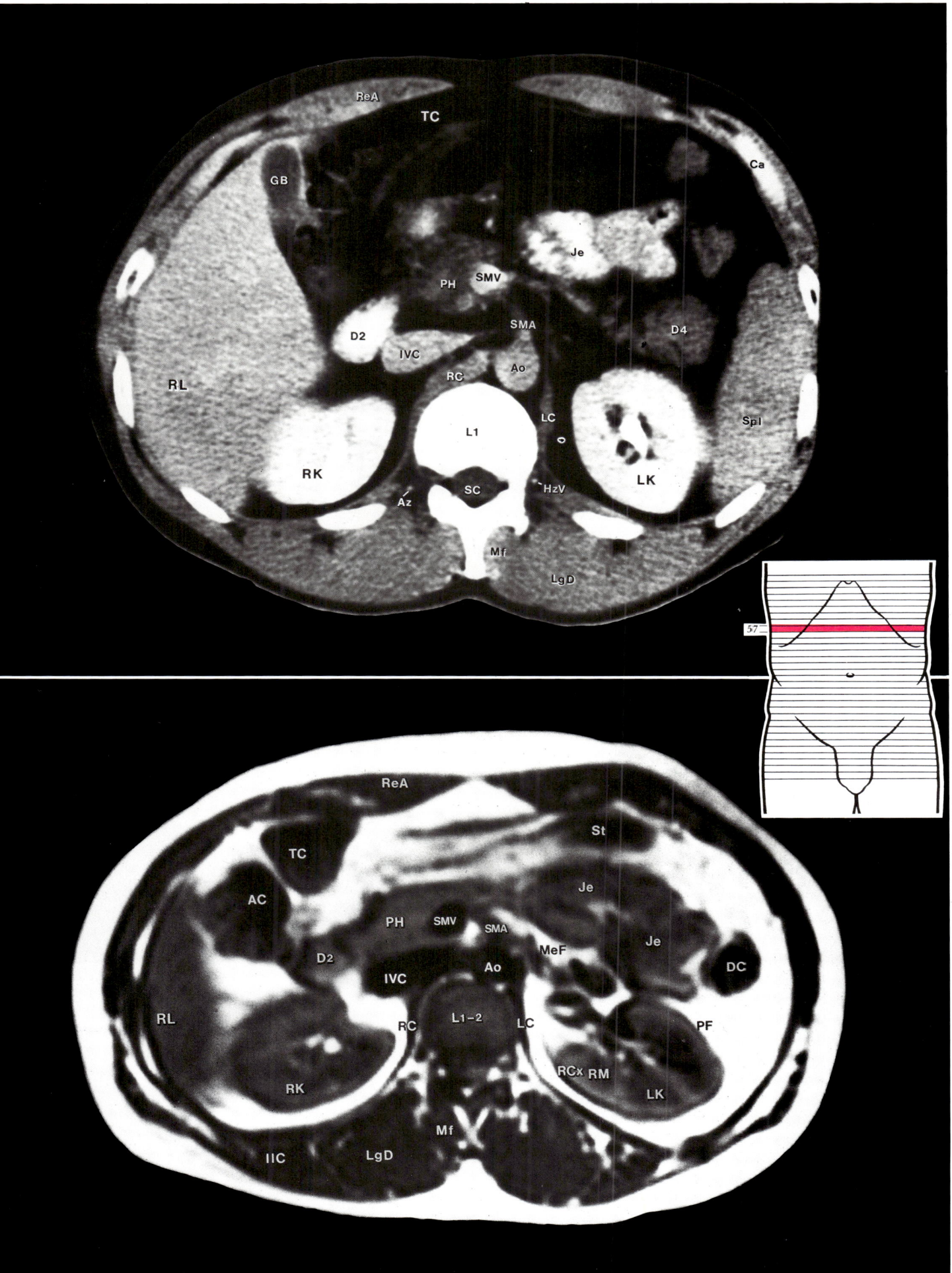

Plate 58. Transverse ABDOMEN

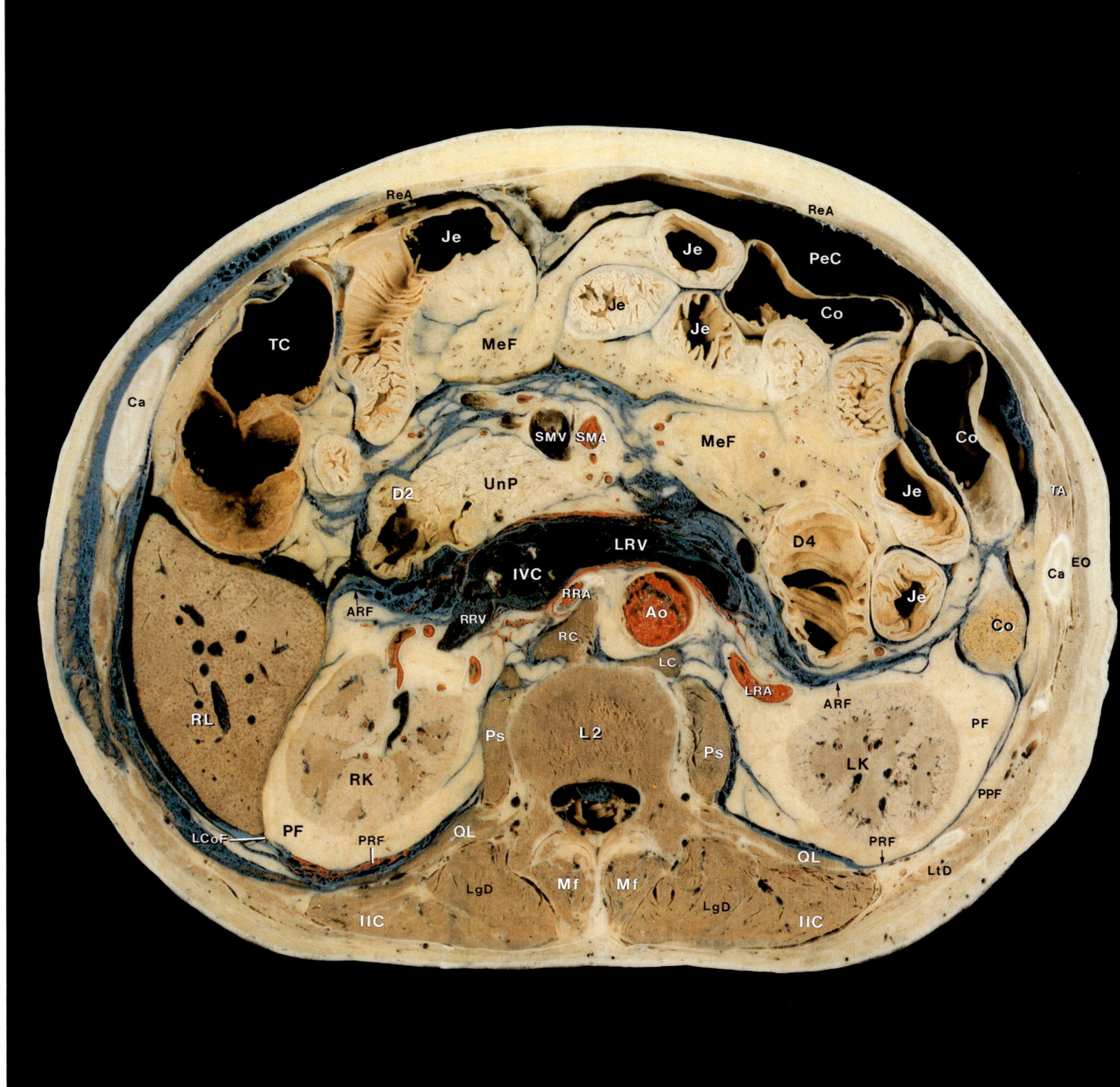

AC	Ascending colon	LRV	Left renal vein	SMV	Superior mesenteric vein
ARF	Anterior renal fascia	LgD	Longissimus dorsi muscle	TA	Transversus abdominis muscle
Ao	Aorta	LtD	Latissimus dorsi muscle	TC	Transverse colon
Ca	Cartilage	MeF	Mesenteric fat	UnP	Uncinate process of pancreas, hea
Co	Colon	Mf	Multifidus muscle	Ur	Ureter
D2	Second portion of duodenum	PF	Perirenal fat		
D4	Fourth portion of duodenum	PPF	Posterior pararenal fat		
DC	Descending colon	PRF	Posterior renal fascia		
EO	External oblique muscle	PeC	Peritoneal cavity		
IVC	Inferior vena cava	Ps	Psoas muscle		
IlC	Iliocostalis muscle	QL	Quadratus lumborum muscle		
Je	Jejunum	RC	Right diaphragmatic crus		
L1-2	L1-2 intervertebral disc	RK	Right kidney		
L2	L2 vertebral body	RL	Right lobe of liver		
LC	Left diaphragmatic crus	RRA	Right renal artery		
LCoF	Lateroconal fascia	RRV	Right renal vein		
LK	Left kidney	ReA	Rectus abdominis muscle		
LRA	Left renal artery	SMA	Superior mesenteric artery		

— 132 —

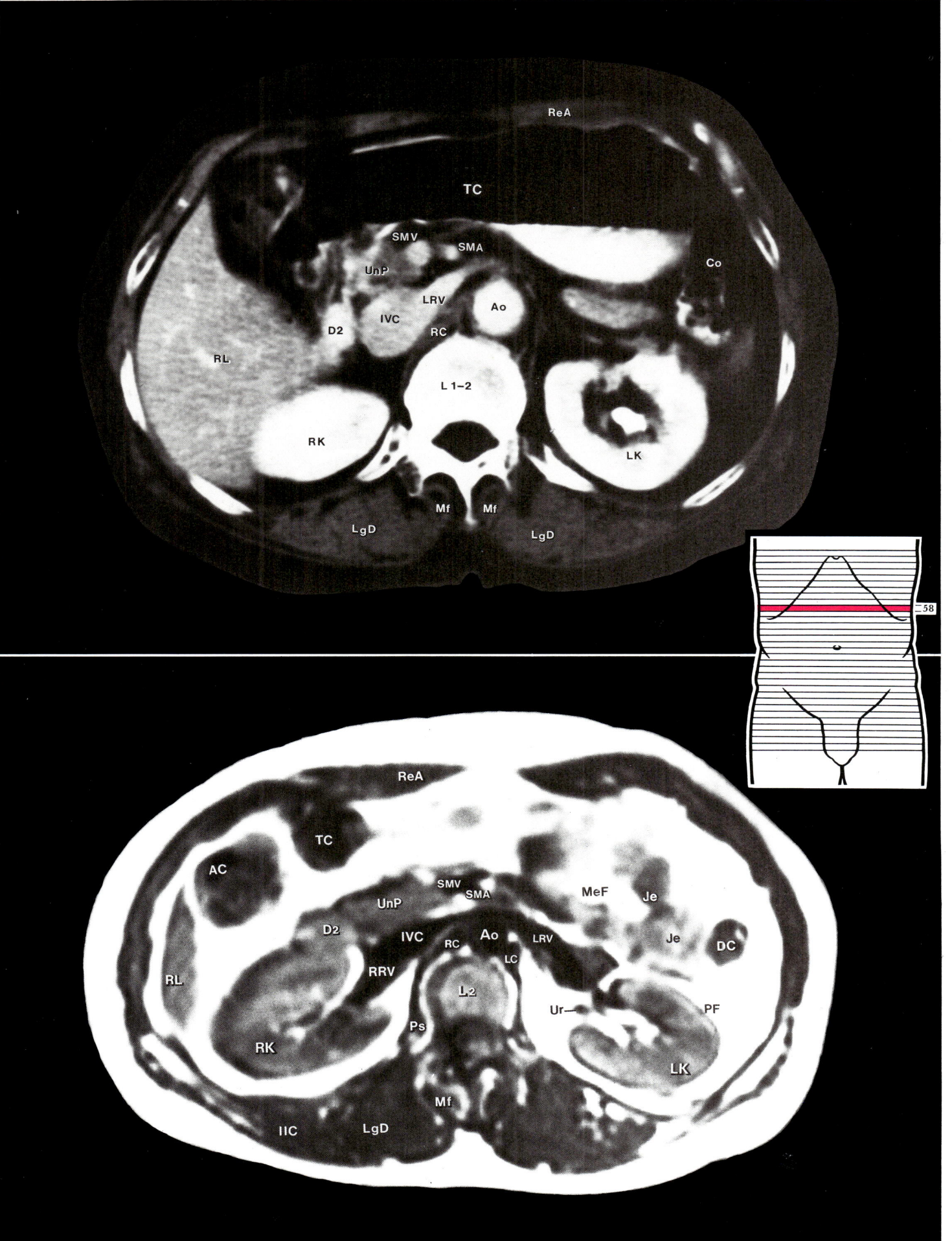

Plate 59. Transverse ABDOMEN

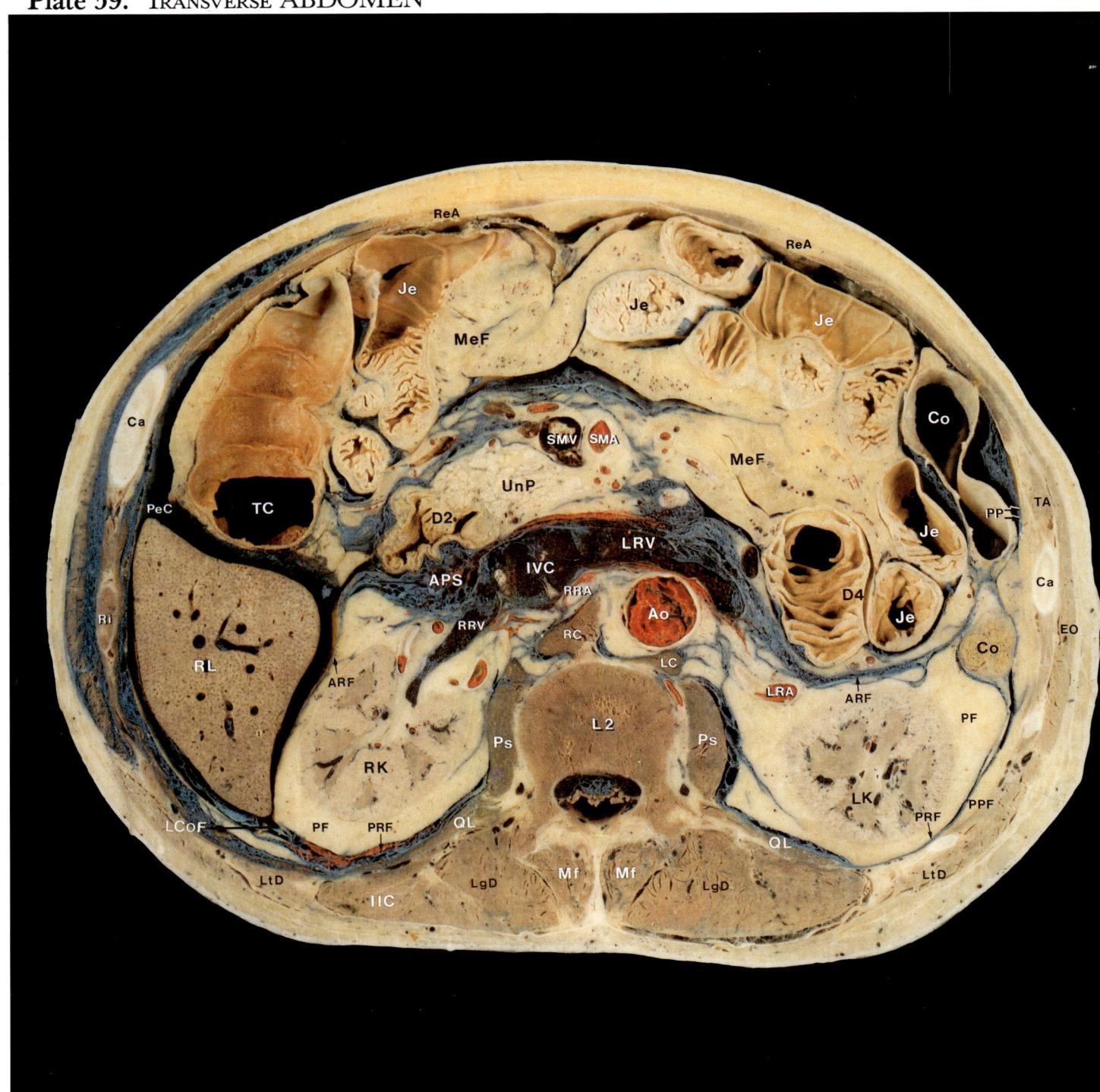

AC	Ascending colon	LRV	Left renal vein	RRA	Right renal artery
APS	Anterior pararenal space	LgD	Longissimus dorsi muscle	RRV	Right renal vein
ARF	Anterior renal fascia	LtD	Latissimus dorsi muscle	ReA	Rectus abdominis muscle
Ao	Aorta	MeF	Mesenteric fat	Ri	Rib
Ca	Cartilage	Mf	Multifidus muscle	SMA	Superior mesenteric artery
Co	Colon	PF	Perirenal fat	SMV	Superior mesenteric vein
D2	Second portion of duodenum	PP	Parietal peritoneum	Spl	Spleen
D4	Fourth portion of duodenum	PPF	Posterior paraenal fat	TA	Transversus abdominis muscle
DC	Descending colon	PRF	Posterior renal fascia	TC	Transverse colon
EO	External oblique muscle	PeC	Peritoneal cavity	UnP	Uncinate process of pancreas, he
IVC	Inferior vena cava	Ps	Psoas muscle	Ur	Ureter
IlC	Iliocostalis muscle	QL	Quadratus lumborum muscle		
Je	Jejunum	RC	Right diaphragmatic crus		
L2	L2 vertebral body	RCx	Renal cortex		
LC	Left diaphragmatic crus	RK	Right kidney		
LCoF	Lateroconal fascia	RL	Right lobe of liver		
LK	Left kidney	RM	Renal medulla		
LRA	Left renal artery	RP	Renal pelvis		

— 134 —

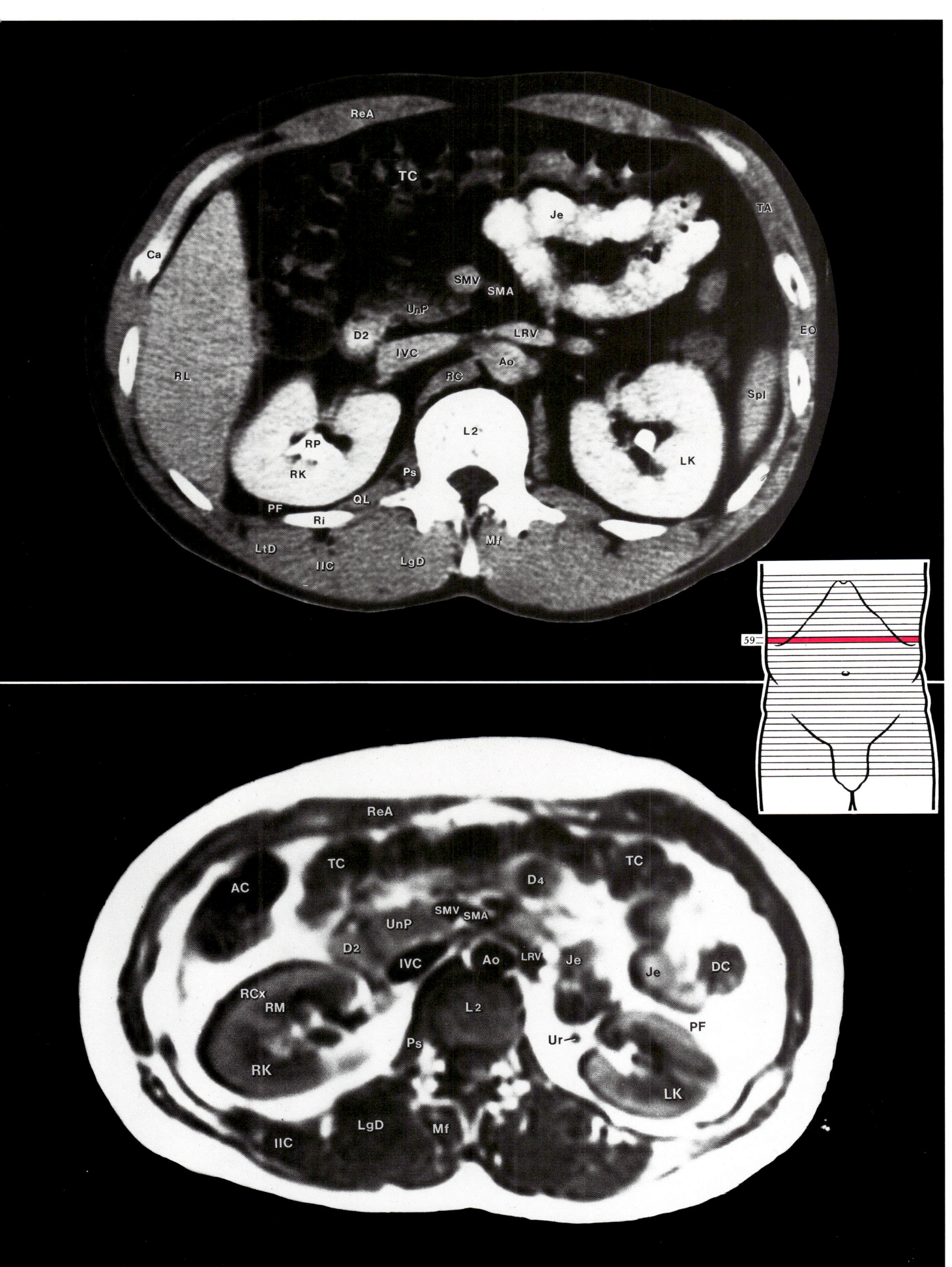

Plate 60. TRANSVERSE ABDOMEN

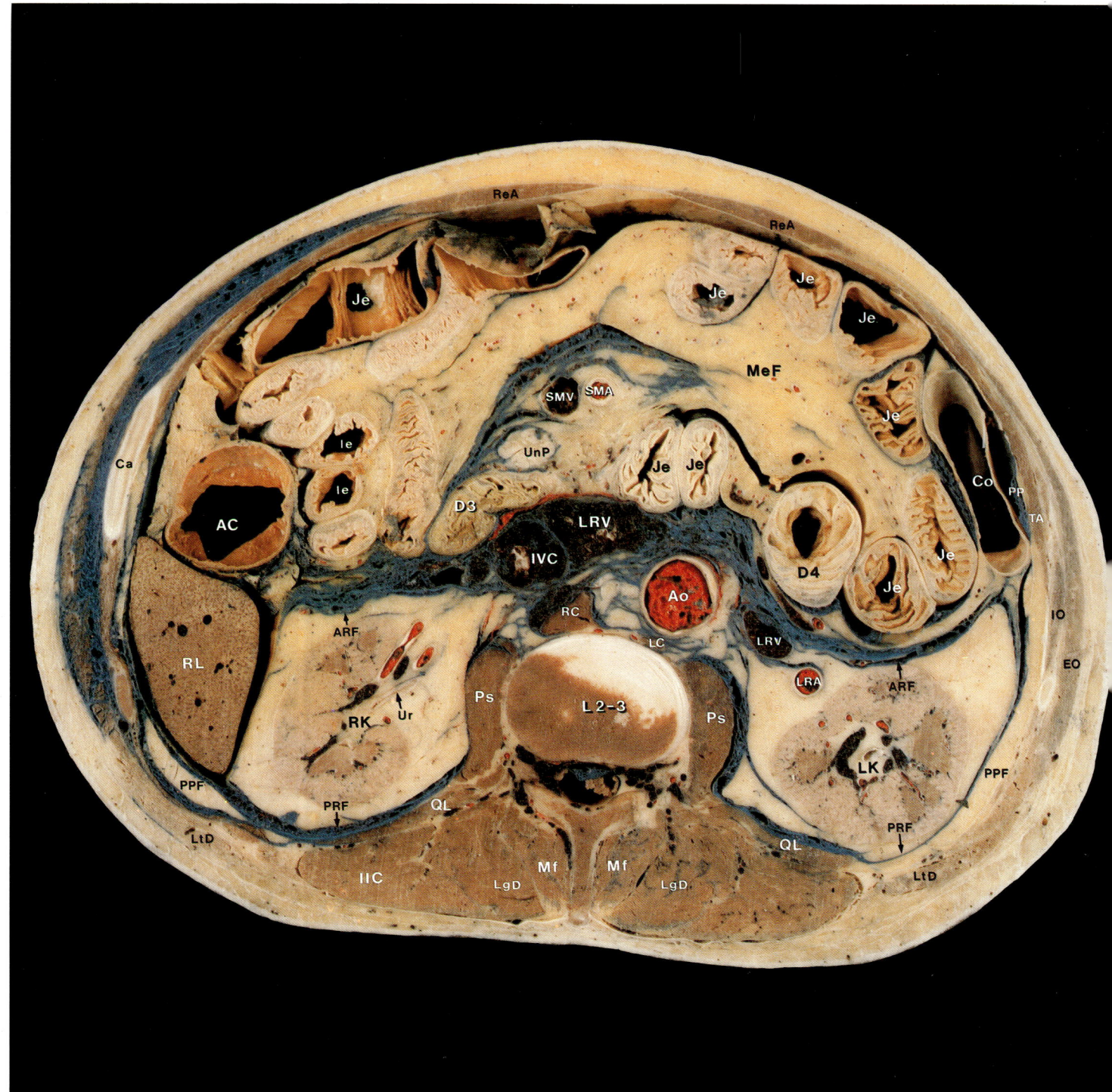

AC	Ascending colon	LRV	Left renal vein	SMA	Superior mesenteric artery
ARF	Anterior renal fascia	LgD	Longissimus dorsi muscle	SMV	Superior mesenteric vein
Ao	Aorta	LtD	Latissimus dorsi muscle	TA	Transversus abdominis muscle
Ca	Cartilage	MeF	Mesenteric fat	TC	Transverse colon
Co	Colon	Mf	Multifidus muscle	UnP	Uncinate process of pancreas, hea
D3	Third portion of duodenum	PF	Perirenal fat	Ur	Ureter
D4	Fourth portion of duodenum	PP	Parietal peritoneum		
DC	Descending colon	PPF	Posterior paraenal fat		
EO	External oblique muscle	PRF	Posterior renal fascia		
IO	Internal oblique muscle	Ps	Psoas muscle		
IVC	Inferior vena cava	QL	Quadratus lumborum muscle		
Ie	Ileum	RC	Right diaphragmatic crus		
IlC	Iliocostalis muscle	RK	Right kidney		
Je	Jejunum	RL	Right lobe of liver		
L2-3	L2-3 intervertebral disc	RP	Renal pelvis		
LC	Left diaphragmatic crus	RRA	Right renal artery		
LK	Left kidney	ReA	Rectus abdominis muscle		
LRA	Left renal artery	Ri	Rib		

— 136 —

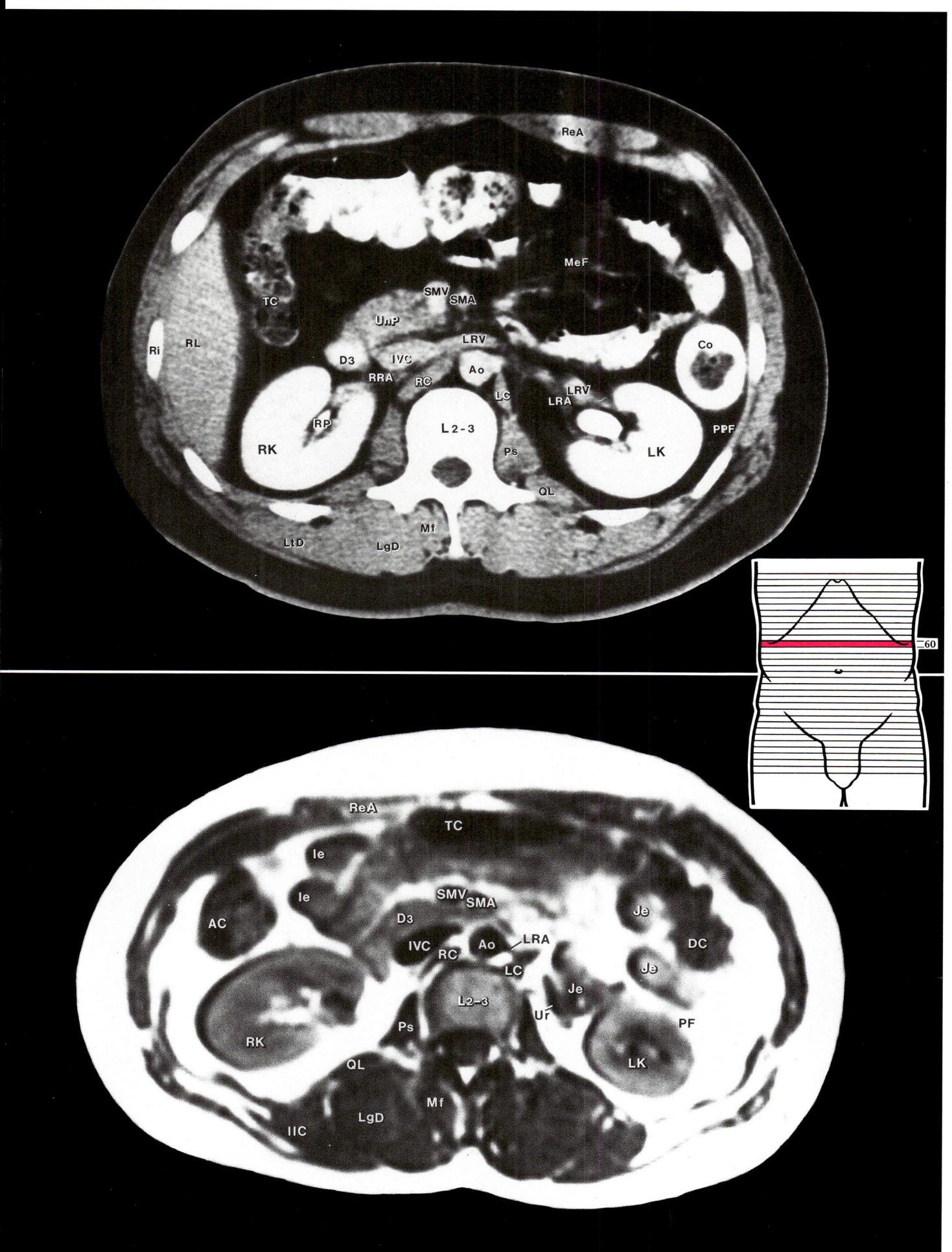

Plate 61. Transverse ABDOMEN

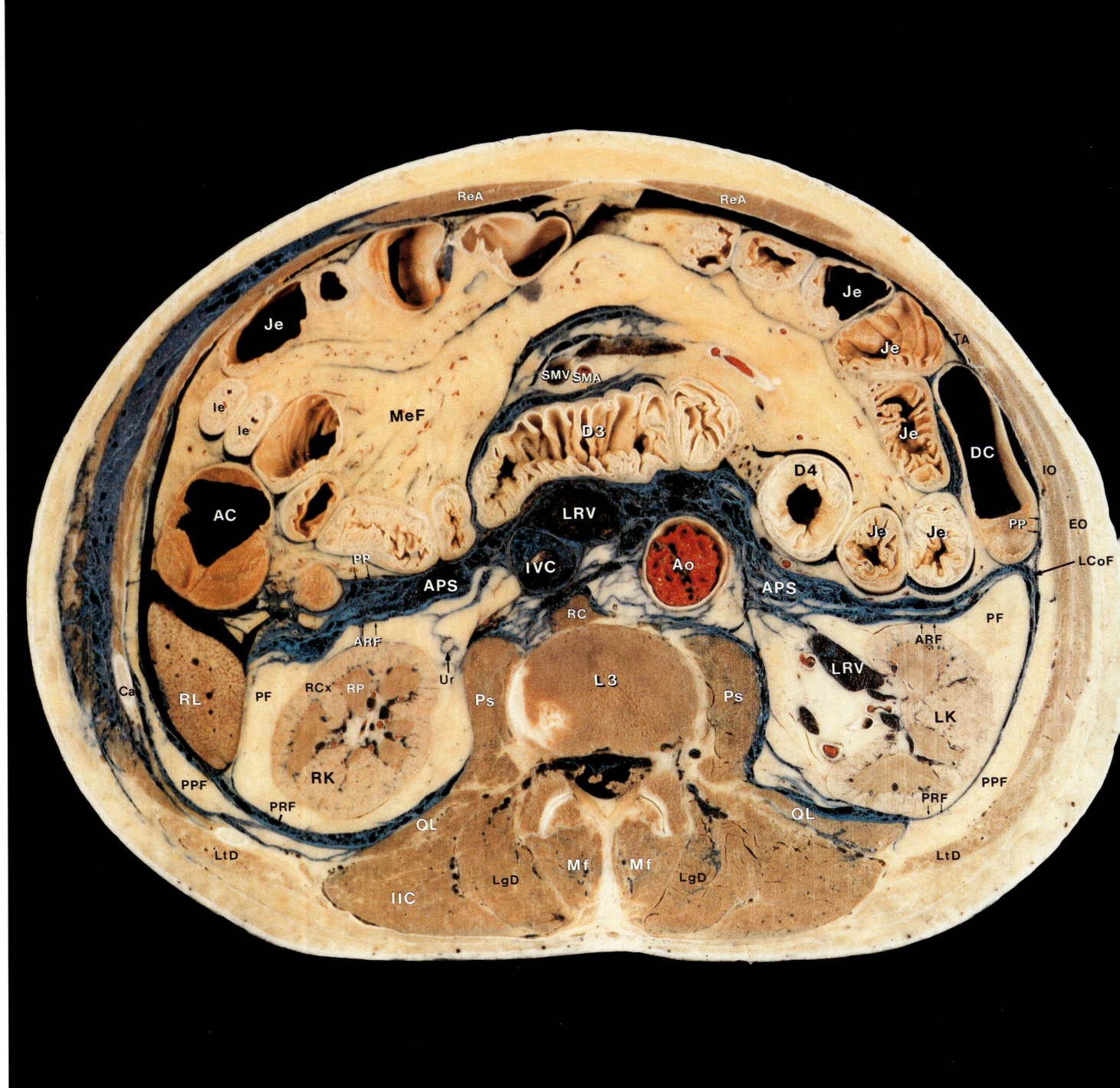

AC	Ascending colon	LRA	Left renal artery	Ri	Rib
APS	Anterior pararenal space	LRV	Left renal vein	SMA	Superior mesenteric artery
ARF	Anterior renal fascia	LgD	Longissimus dorsi muscle	SMV	Superior mesenteric vein
Ao	Aorta	LtD	Latissimus dorsi muscle	TA	Transversus abdominis muscle
Ca	Cartilage	MeF	Mesenteric fat	Ur	Ureter
D3	Third portion of duodenum	Mf	Multifidus muscle		
D4	Fourth portion of duodenum	PF	Perirenal fat		
DC	Descending colon	PP	Parietal peritoneum		
EO	External oblique muscle	PPF	Posterior pararenal fat		
IO	Internal oblique muscle	PRF	Posterior renal fascia		
IVC	Inferior vena cava	Ps	Psoas muscle		
Ie	Ileum	QL	Quadratus lumborum muscle		
IlC	Iliocostalis muscle	RC	Right diaphragmatic crus		
Je	Jejunum	RCx	Renal cortex		
L3	L3 vertebral body	RK	Right kidney		
LC	Left diaphragmatic crus	RL	Right lobe of liver		
LCoF	Lateroconal fascia	RP	Renal pelvis		
LK	Left kidney	ReA	Rectus abdominis muscle		

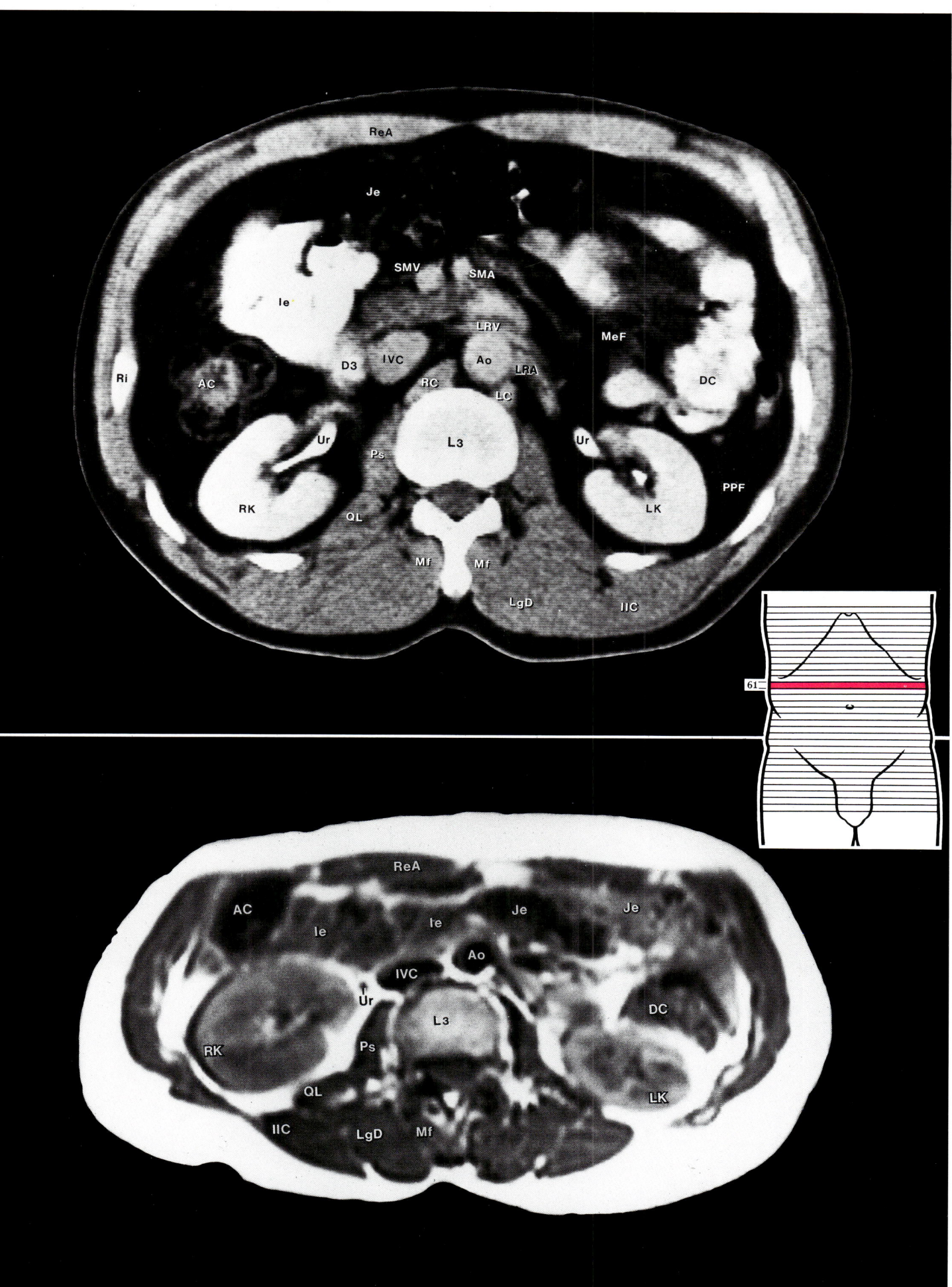

Plate 62. Transverse ABDOMEN

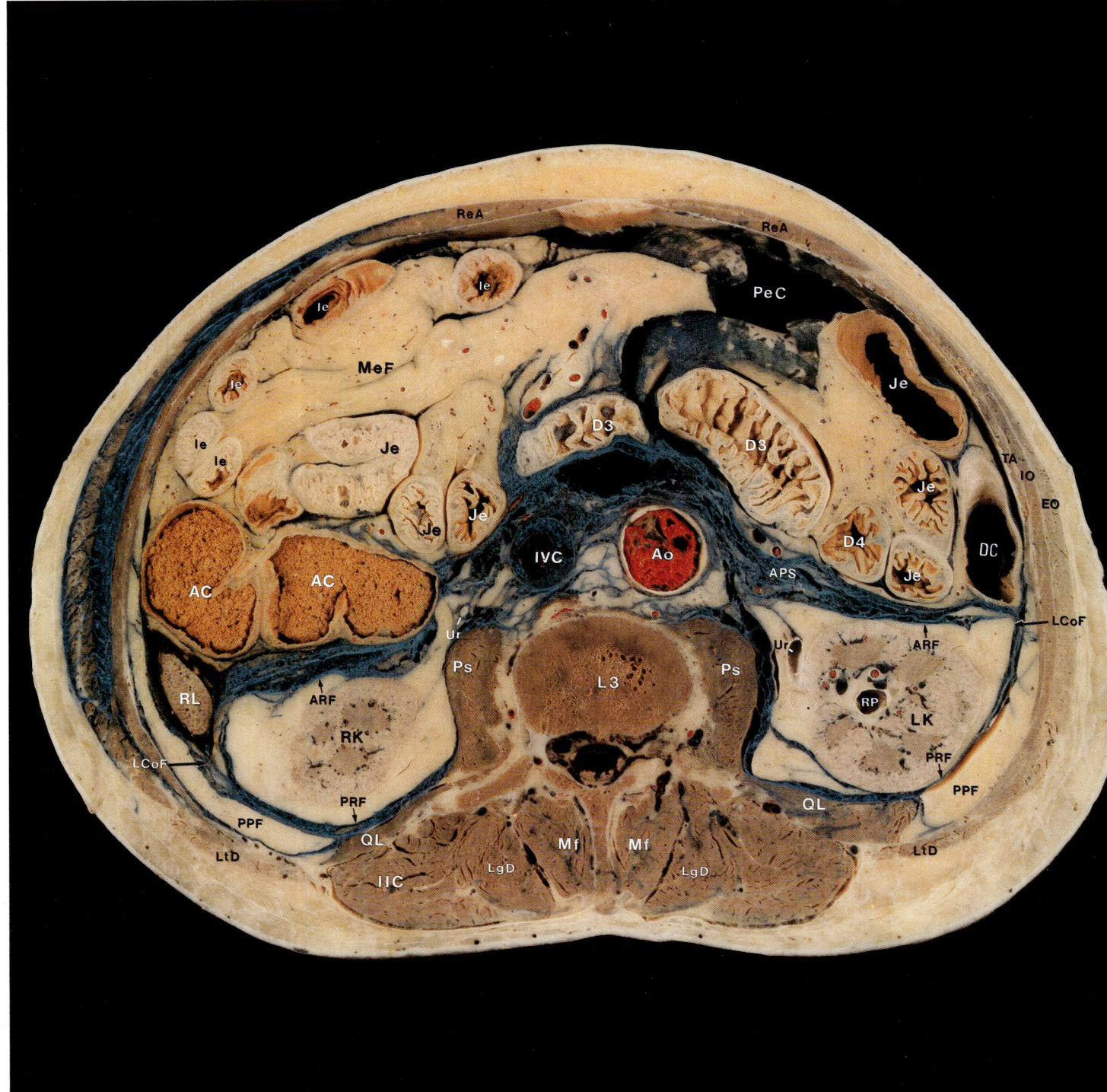

AC	Ascending colon	LtD	Latissimus dorsi muscle
APS	Anterior pararenal space	MeF	Mesenteric fat
ARF	Anterior renal fascia	Mf	Multifidus muscle
Ao	Aorta	PPF	Posterior pararenal fat
Ca	Cartilage	PRF	Posterior renal fascia
D3	Third portion of duodenum	PeC	Peritoneal cavity
D4	Fourth portion of duodenum	Ps	Psoas muscle
DC	Descending colon	QL	Quadratus lumborum muscle
EO	External oblique muscle	RK	Right kidney
IO	Internal oblique muscle	RL	Right lobe of liver
IVC	Inferior vena cava	RP	Renal pelvis
Ie	Ileum	ReA	Rectus abdominis muscle
IlC	Iliocostalis muscle	Ri	Rib
Je	Jejunum	SMA	Superior mesenteric artery
L3	L3 vertebral body	SMV	Superior mesenteric vein
LCoF	Lateroconal fascia	SiC	Sigmoid colon
LK	Left kidney	TA	Transversus abdominis muscle
LgD	Longissimus dorsi muscle	Ur	Ureter

— 140 —

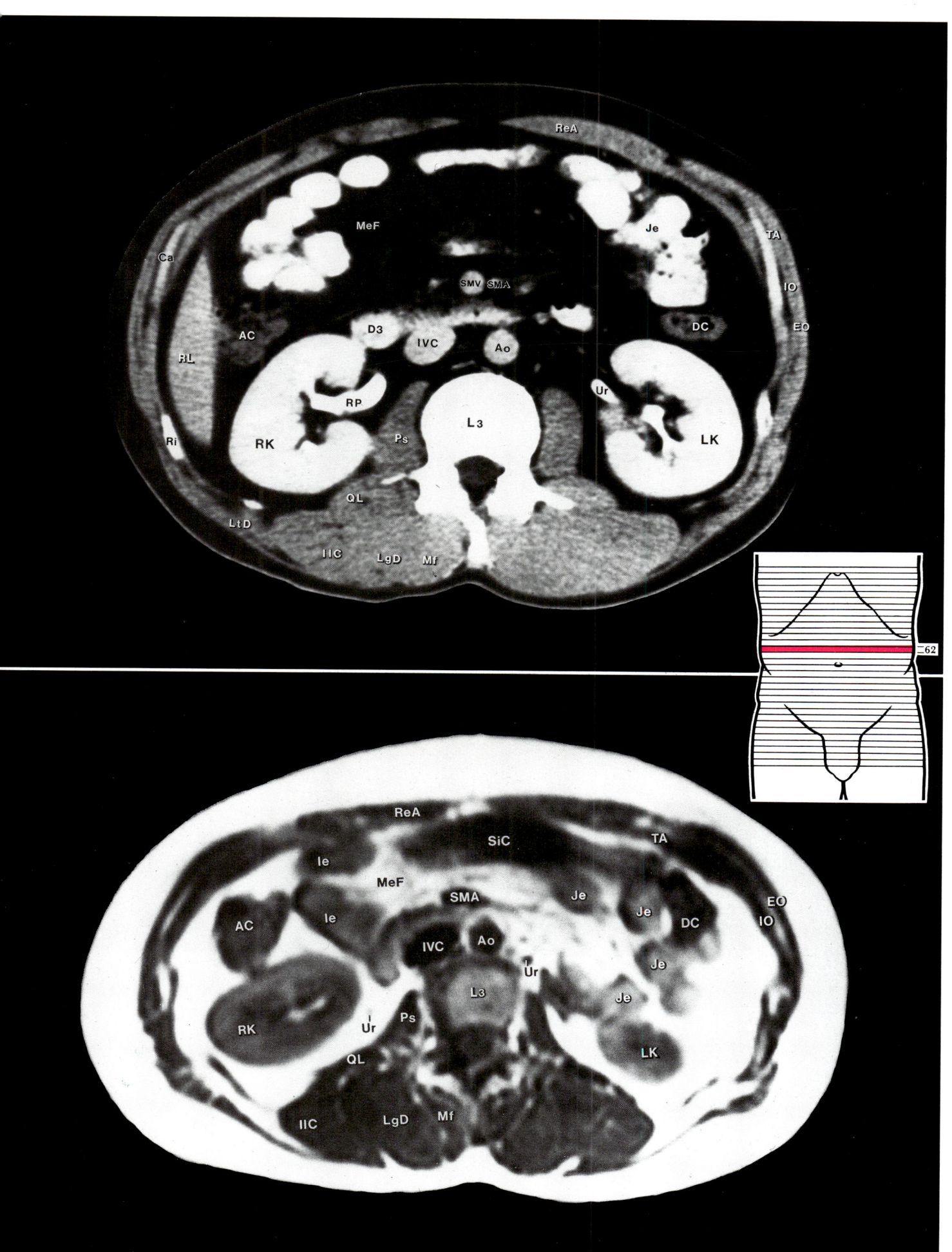

Plate 63. Transverse ABDOMEN

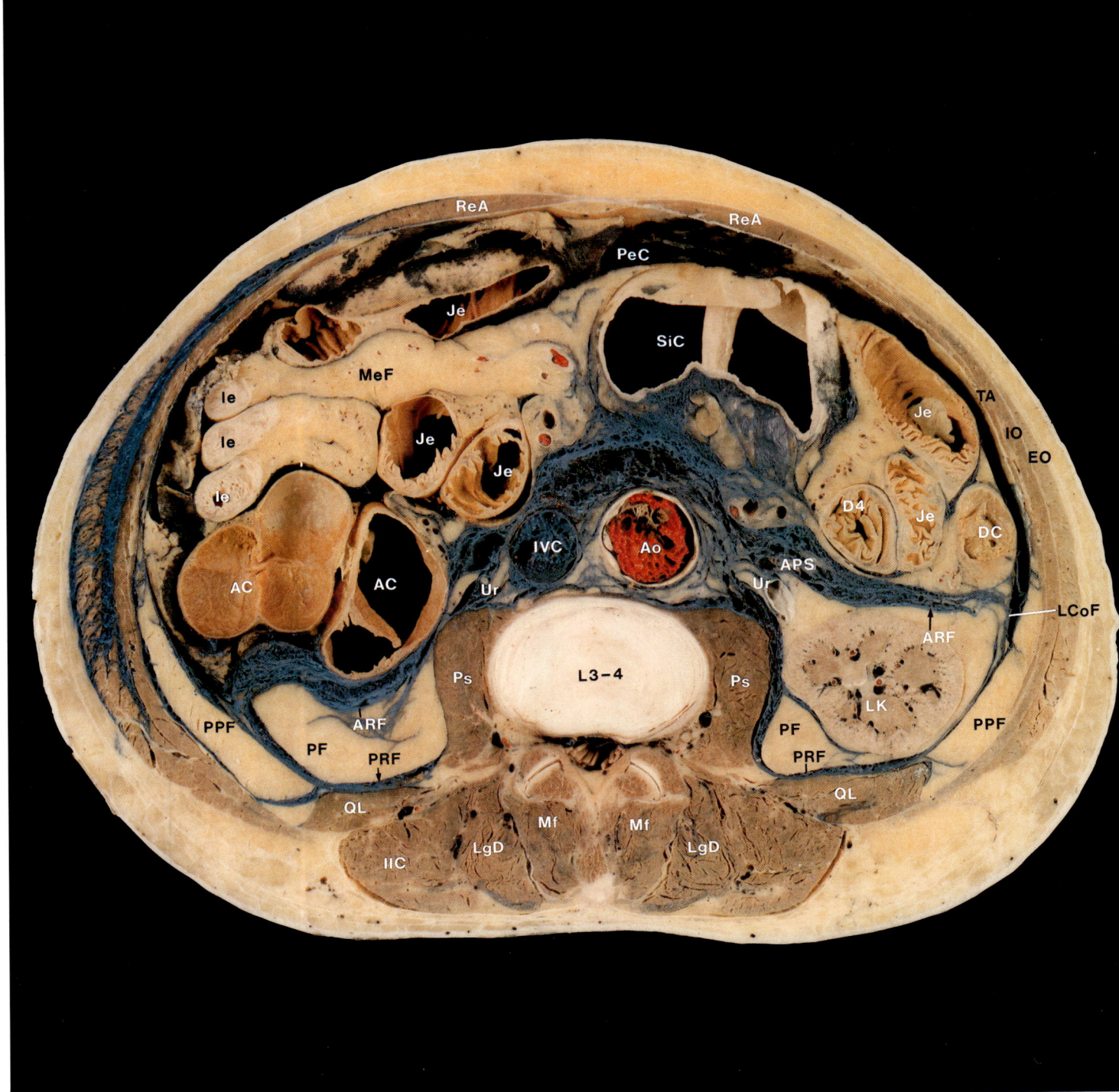

AC	Ascending colon	LtD	Latissimus dorsi muscle	TA	Transversus abdominis muscle
APS	Anterior pararenal space	MeF	Mesenteric fat	Ur	Ureter
ARF	Anterior renal fascia	Mf	Multifidus muscle		
Ao	Aorta	PF	Perirenal fat		
D3	Third portion of duodenum	PPF	Posterior pararenal fat		
D4	Fourth portion of duodenum	PRF	Posterior renal fascia		
DC	Descending colon	PeC	Peritoneal cavity		
EO	External oblique muscle	Ps	Psoas muscle		
IO	Internal oblique muscle	QL	Quadratus lumborum muscle		
IVC	Inferior vena cava	RC	Right diaphragmatic crus		
Ie	Ileum	RK	Right kidney		
IlC	Iliocostalis muscle	RL	Right lobe of liver		
Je	Jejunum	RP	Renal pelvis		
L3-4	L3-4 intervertebral disc	ReA	Rectus abdominis muscle		
LC	Left diaphragmatic crus	Ri	Rib		
LCoF	Lateroconal fascia	SMA	Superior mesenteric artery		
LK	Left kidney	SMV	Superior mesenteric vein		
LgD	Longissimus dorsi muscle	SiC	Sigmoid colon		

— 142 —

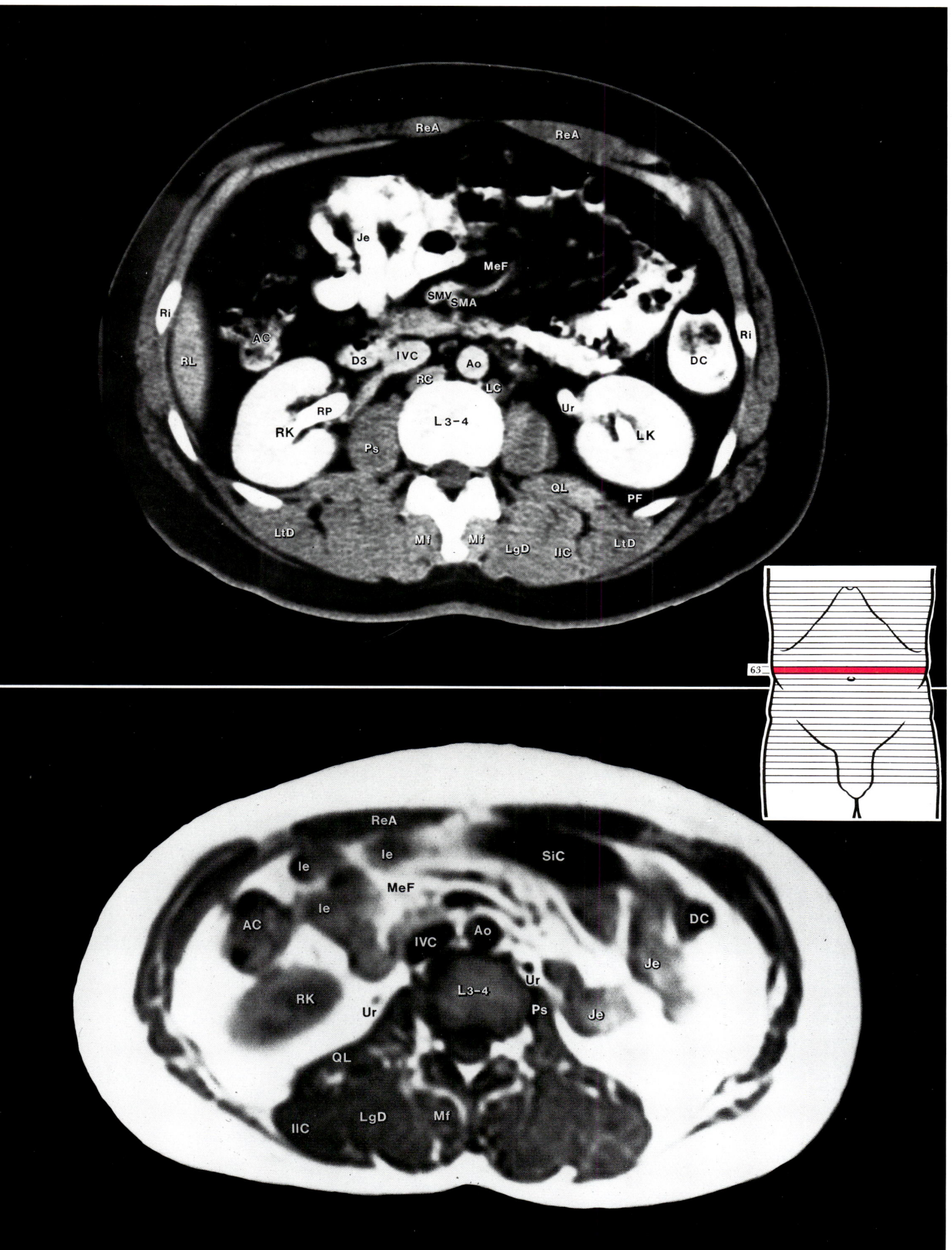

Plate 64. Transverse ABDOMEN

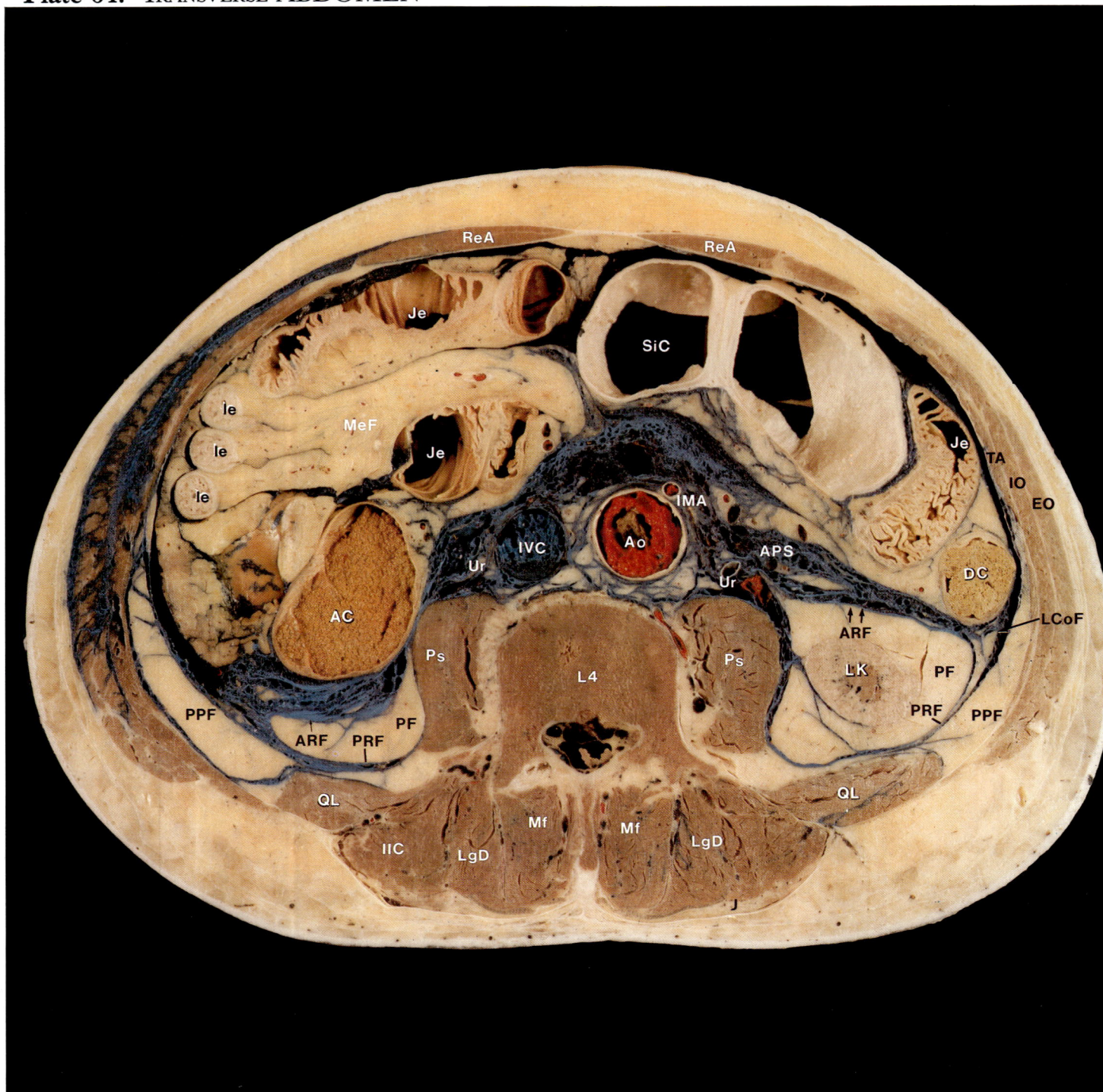

AC	Ascending colon	PF	Perirenal fat
APS	Anterior pararenal space	PPF	Posterior pararenal fat
ARF	Anterior renal fascia	PRF	Posterior renal fascia
Ao	Aorta	Ps	Psoas muscle
DC	Descending colon	QL	Quadratus lumborum muscle
EO	External oblique muscle	RK	Right kidney
IMA	Inferior mesenteric artery	RP	Renal pelvis
IO	Internal oblique muscle	ReA	Rectus abdominis muscle
IVC	Inferior vena cava	SMA	Superior mesenteric artery
Ie	Ileum	SMV	Superior mesenteric vein
IlC	Iliocostalis muscle	SiC	Sigmoid colon
Je	Jejunum	TA	Transversus abdominis muscle
L4	L4 vertebral body	Ur	Ureter
LCoF	Lateroconal fascia		
LK	Left kidney		
LgD	Longissimus dorsi muscle		
MeF	Mesenteric fat		
Mf	Multifidus muscle		

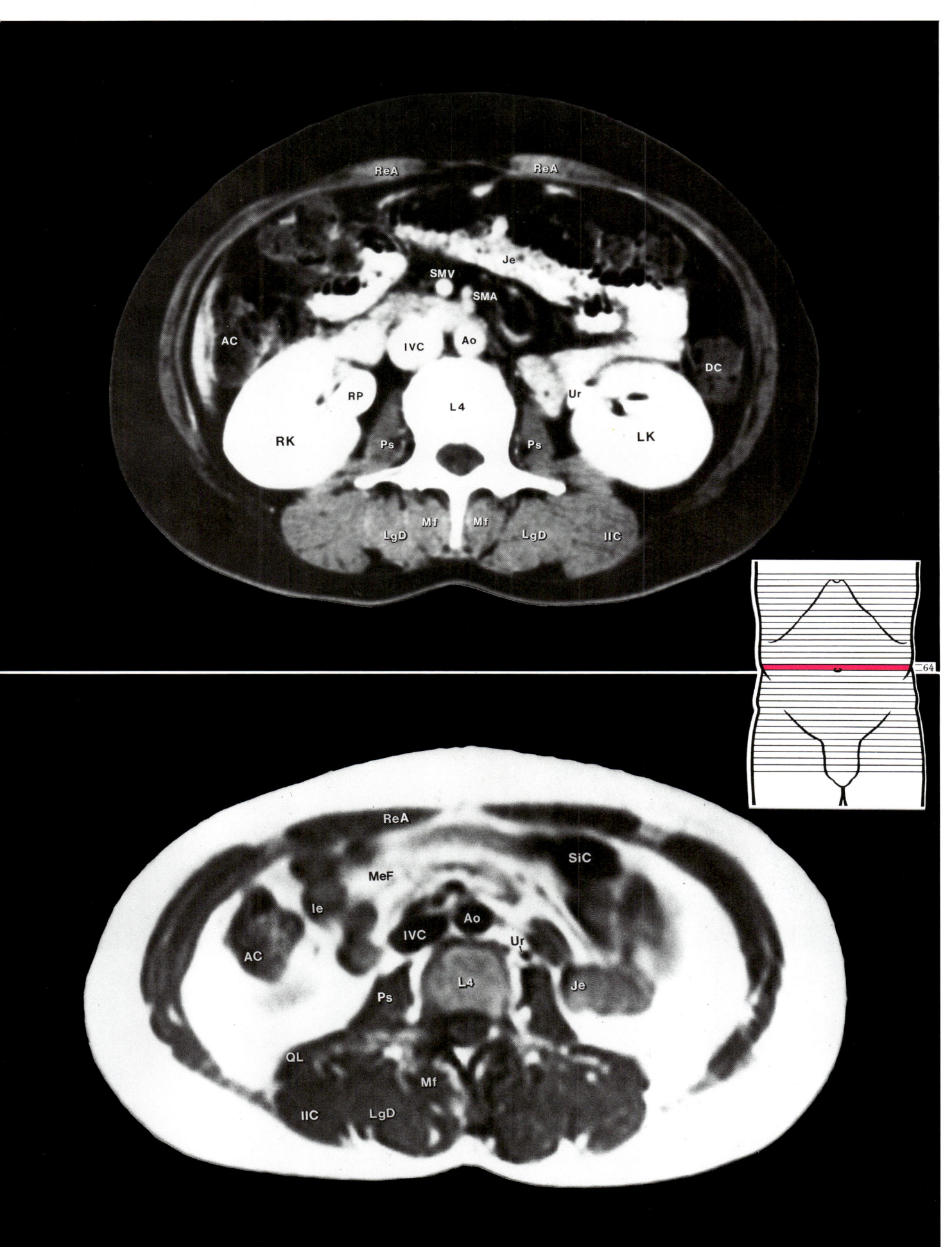

— 145 —

Plate 65. TRANSVERSE PELVIS-MALE

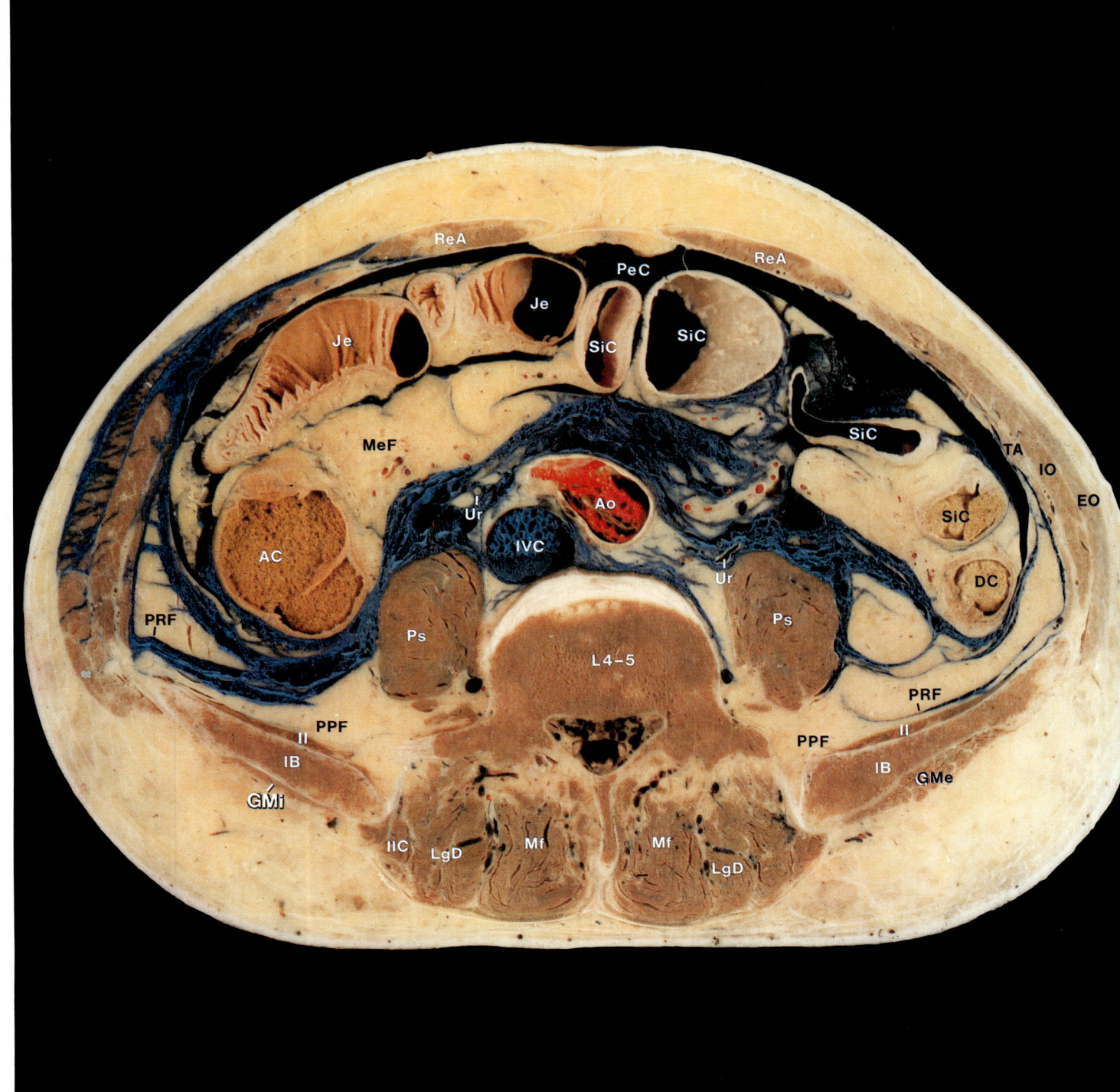

AC	Ascending colon	PPF	Posterior pararenal fat
Ao	Aorta	PRF	Posterior renal fascia
DC	Descending colon	PeC	Peritoneal cavity
EO	External oblique muscle	Ps	Psoas muscle
GMe	Gluteus medius muscle	QL	Quadratus lumborum muscle
GMi	Gluteus minimus muscle	ReA	Rectus abdominis muscle
IB	Iliac bone	SiC	Sigmoid colon
IMA	Inferior mesenteric artery	TA	Transversus abdominis muscle
IO	Internal oblique muscle	Ur	Ureter
IVC	Inferior vena cava		
IlC	Iliocostalis muscle		
Il	Iliacus muscle		
Je	Jejunum		
L4	L4 vertebral body		
L4-5	L4-5 intervertebral disc		
LgD	Longissimus dorsi muscle		
MeF	Mesenteric fat		
Mf	Multifidus muscle		

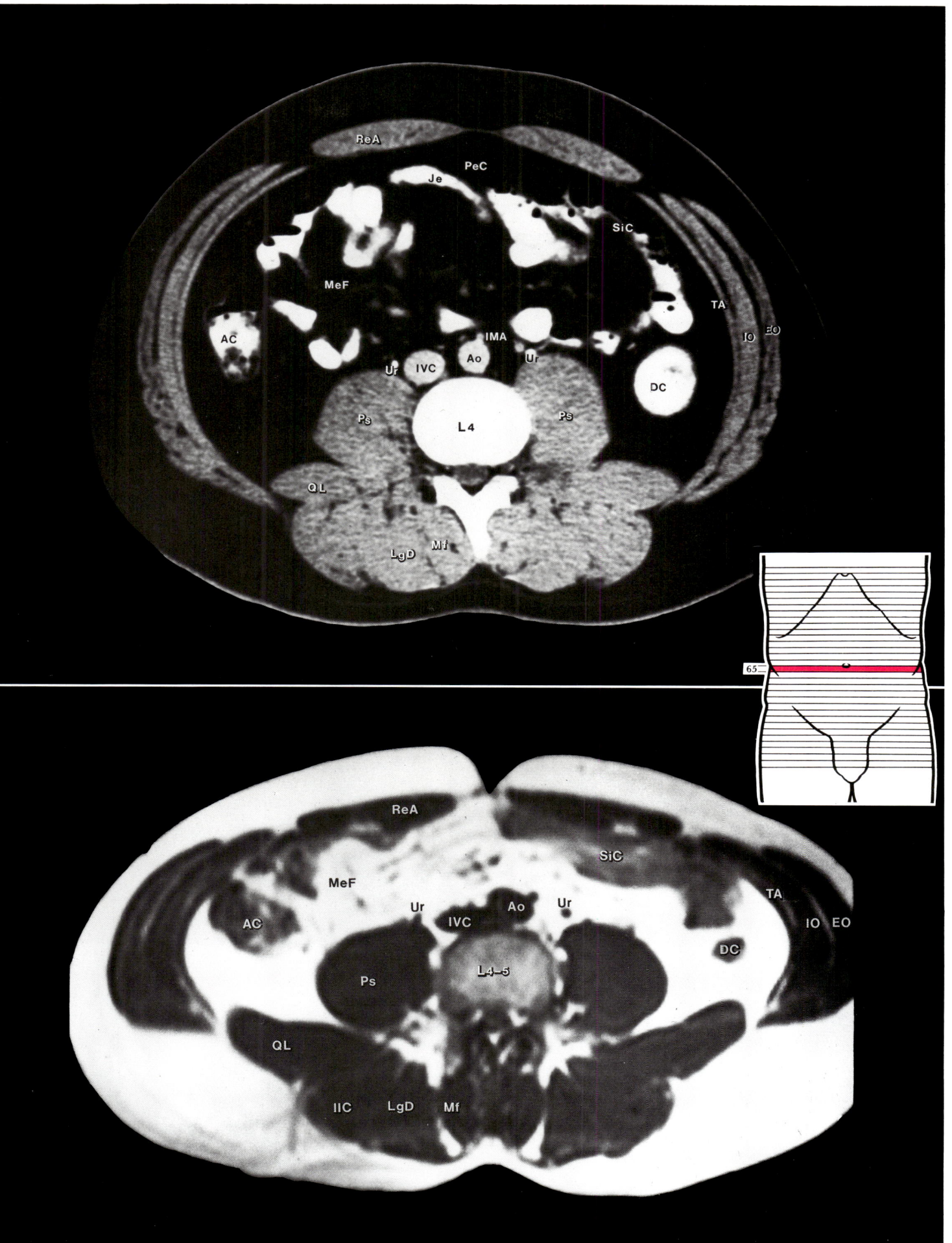

Plate 66. Transverse Pelvis–male

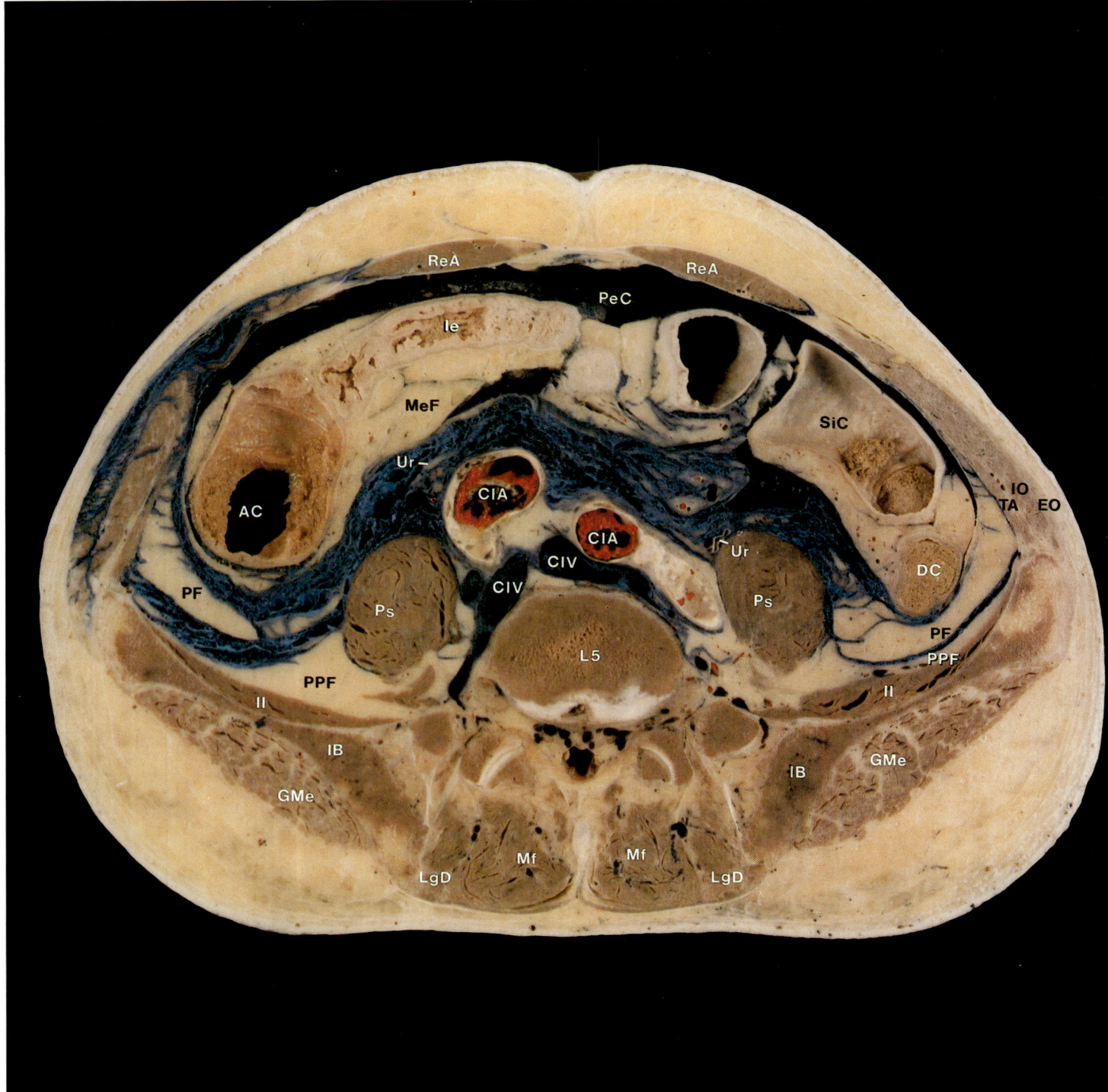

AC	Ascending colon	PeC	Peritoneal cavity
CIA	Common iliac artery	Ps	Psoas muscle
CIV	Common iliac vein	ReA	Rectus abdominis muscle
DC	Descending colon	SiC	Sigmoid colon
EO	External oblique muscle	TA	Transversus abdominis muscle
GMe	Gluteus medius muscle	Ur	Ureter
IB	Iliac bone		
IO	Internal oblique muscle		
IVC	Inferior vena cava		
Ie	Ileum		
Il	Iliacus muscle		
IlC	Iliocostalis muscle		
L5	L5 vertebral body		
LgD	Longissimus dorsi muscle		
MeF	Mesenteric fat		
Mf	Multifidus muscle		
PF	Perirenal fat		
PPF	Posterior pararenal fat		

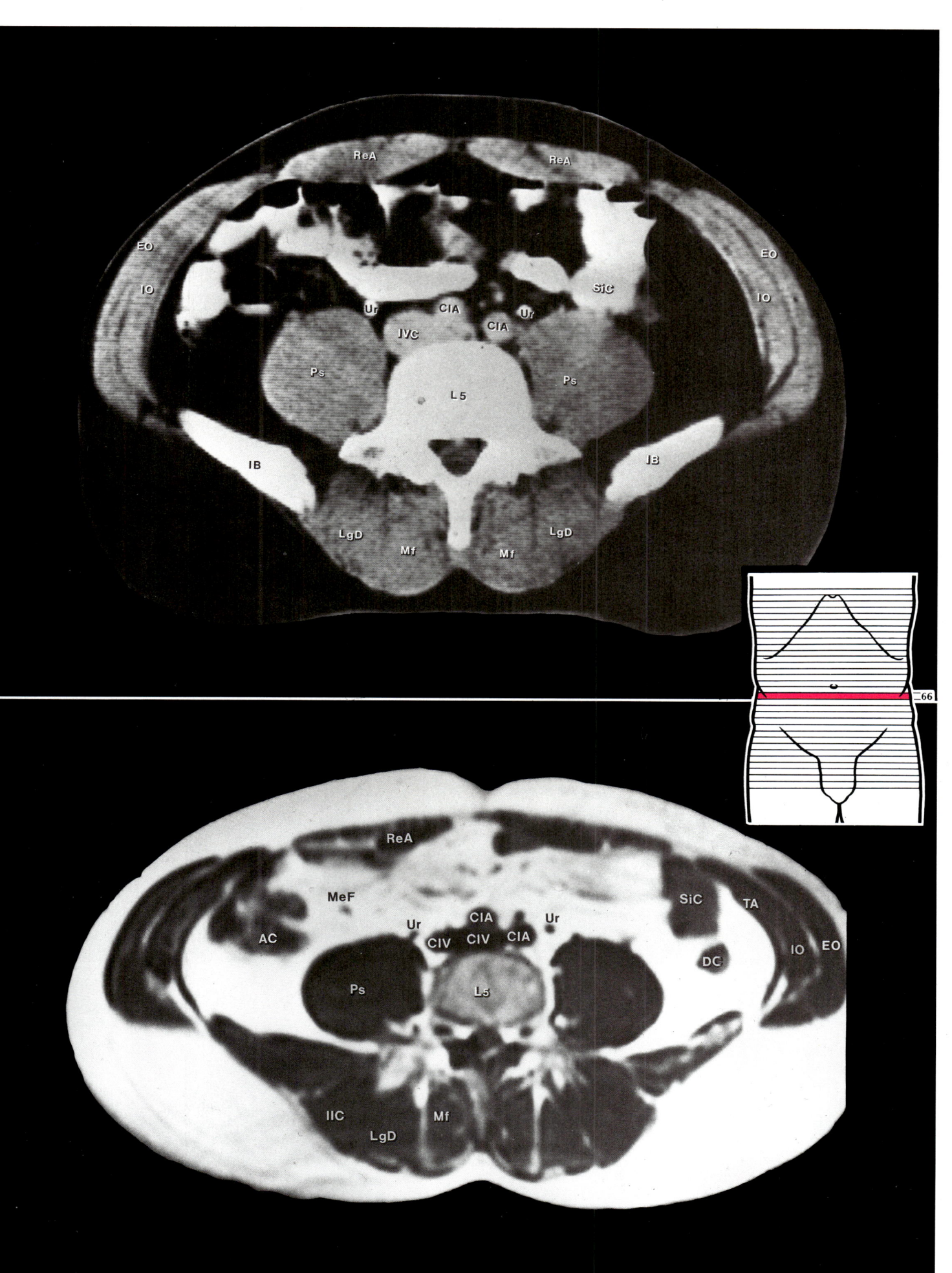

Plate 67. Transverse Pelvis—Male

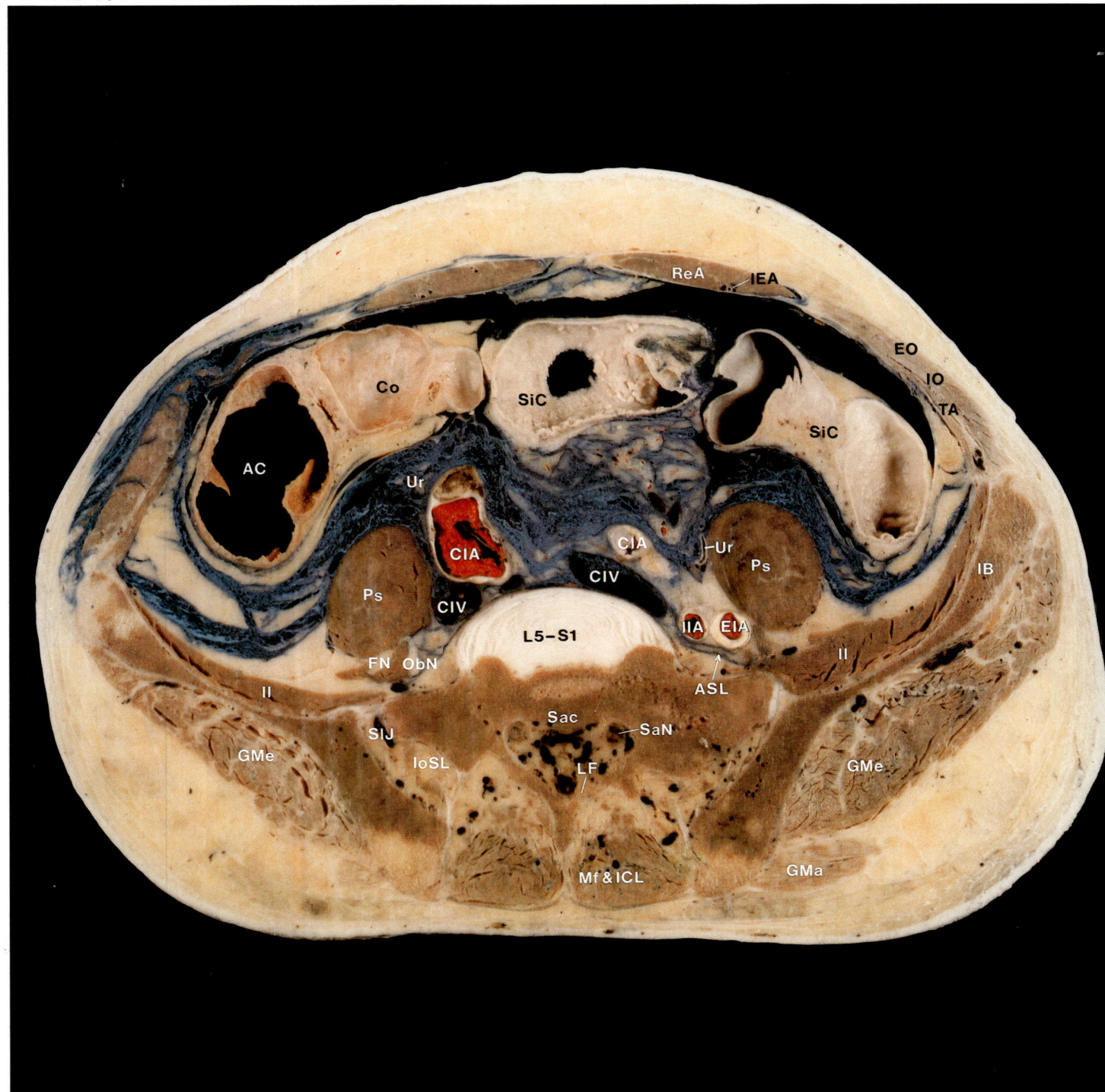

AC	Ascending colon	L5-Sl	L5-Sl intervertebral disc
ASL	Anterior sacroiliac ligament	LF	Ligamentum flavum
CIA	Common iliac artery	Mf	Multifidus muscle
CIV	Common iliac vein	ObN	Obturator nerve
Co	Colon	Ps	Psoas muscle
DC	Descending colon	ReA	Rectus abdominis muscle
EIA	External iliac artery	SIJ	Sacroiliac joint
EO	External oblique muscle	SaN	Sacral nerve
FN	Femoral nerve	Sac	Sacrum
GMa	Gluteus maximus muscle	SiC	Sigmoid colon
GMe	Gluteus medius muscle	TA	Transversus abdominis muscle
IB	Iliac bone	Ur	Ureter
ICL	Iliocostalis lumborum muscle		
IEA	Inferior epigastric artery		
IIA	Internal iliac artery		
IO	Internal oblique muscle		
Il	Iliacus muscle		
IoSL	Interosseous sacroiliac ligament		

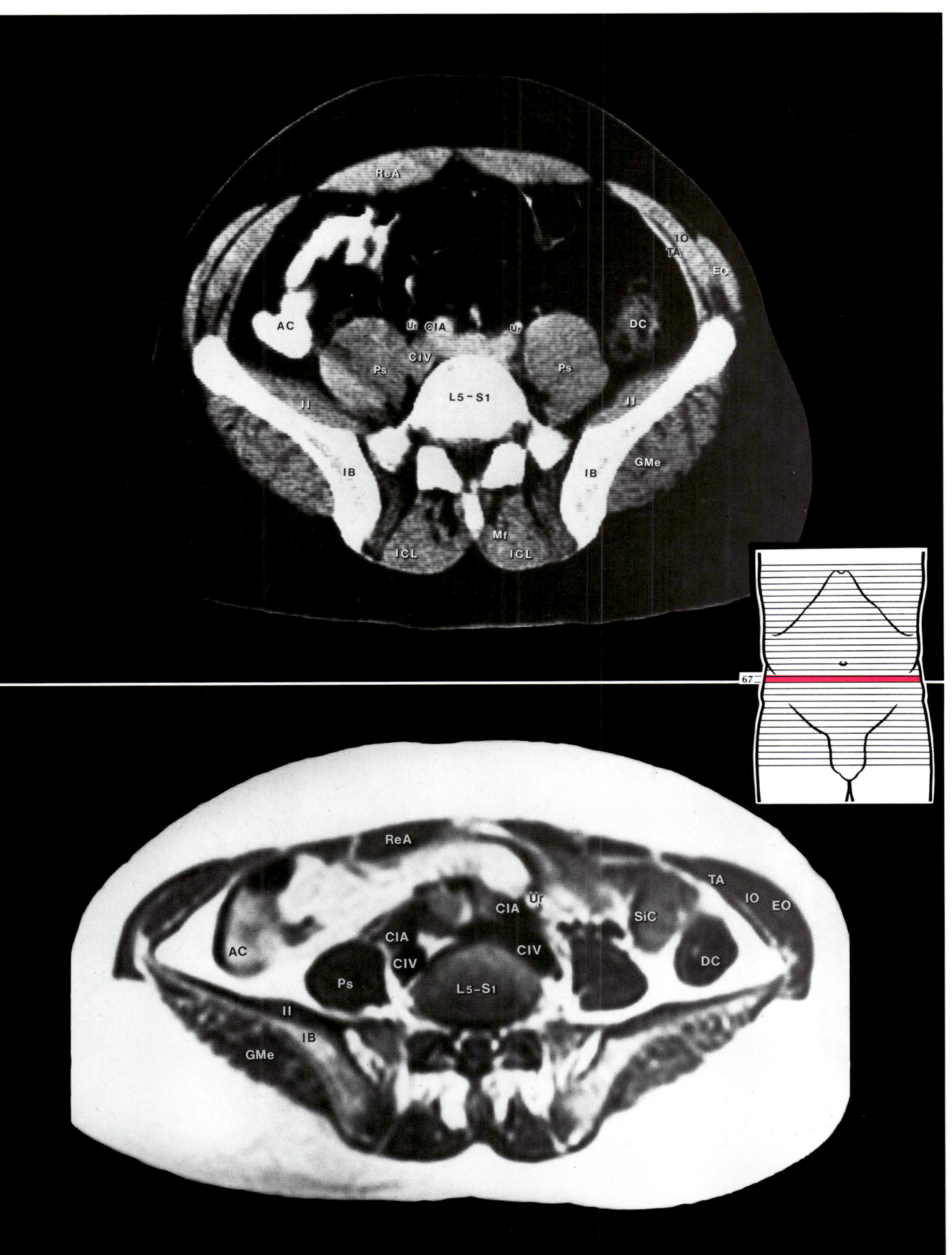

Plate 68. Transverse PELVIS-male

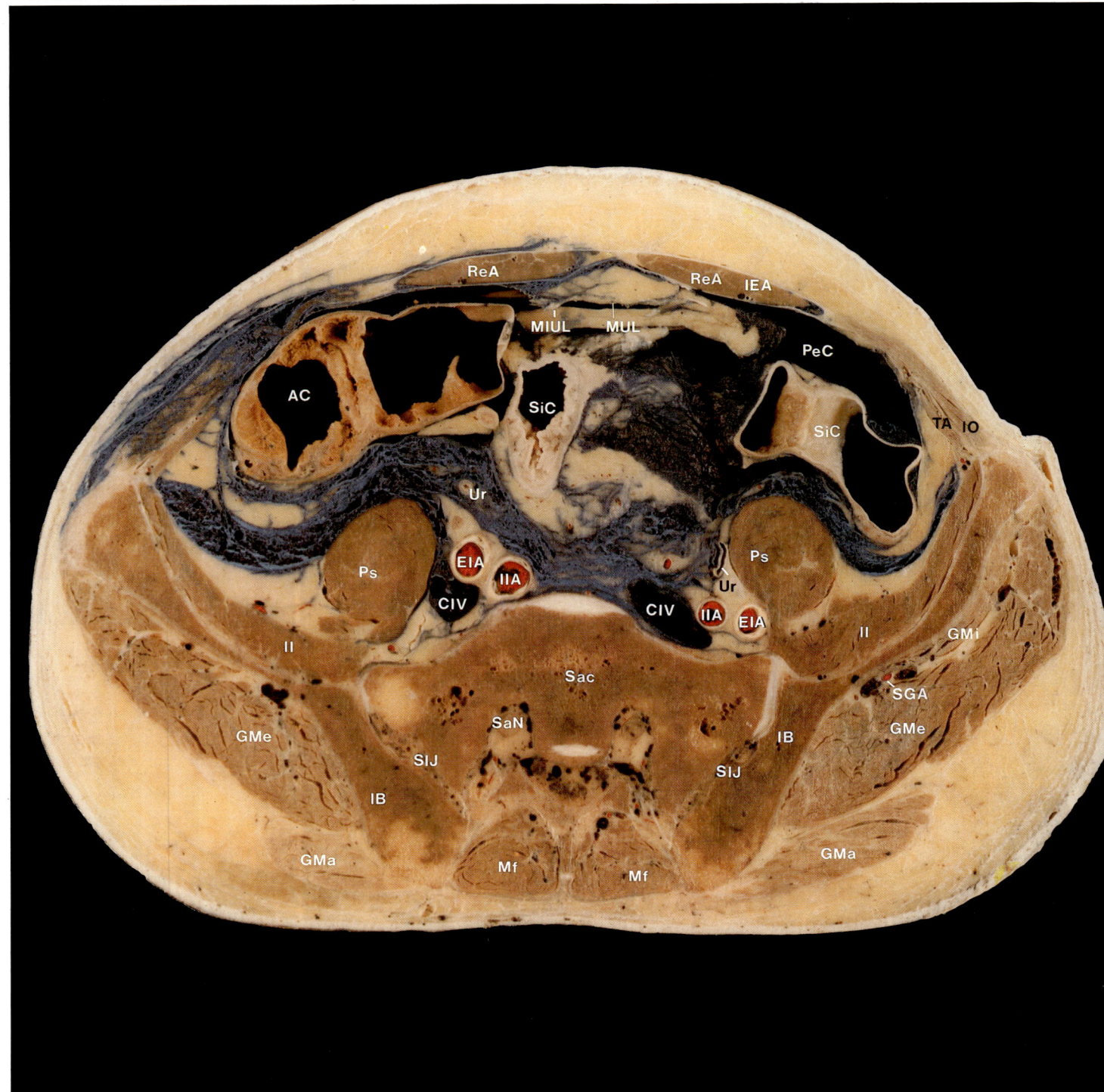

AC	Ascending colon	MlUL	Medial umbilical ligament
CIA	Common iliac artery	PeC	Peritoneal cavity
CIV	Common iliac vein	Ps	Psoas muscle
DC	Descending colon	ReA	Rectus abdominis muscle
EIA	External iliac artery	SGA	Superior gluteal artery
EO	External oblique muscle	SIJ	Sacroiliac joint
GMa	Gluteus maximus muscle	SaN	Sacral nerve
GMe	Gluteus medius muscle	Sac	Sacrum
GMi	Gluteus minimus muscle	SiC	Sigmoid colon
IB	Iliac bone	TA	Transversus abdominis muscle
ICL	Iliocostalis lumborum muscle	Ur	Ureter
IEA	Inferior epigastric artery		
IIA	Internal iliac artery		
IO	Internal oblique muscle		
Il	Iliacus muscle		
L5-Sl	L5-Sl intervertebral disc		
MUL	Median umbilical ligament		
Mf	Multifidus muscle		

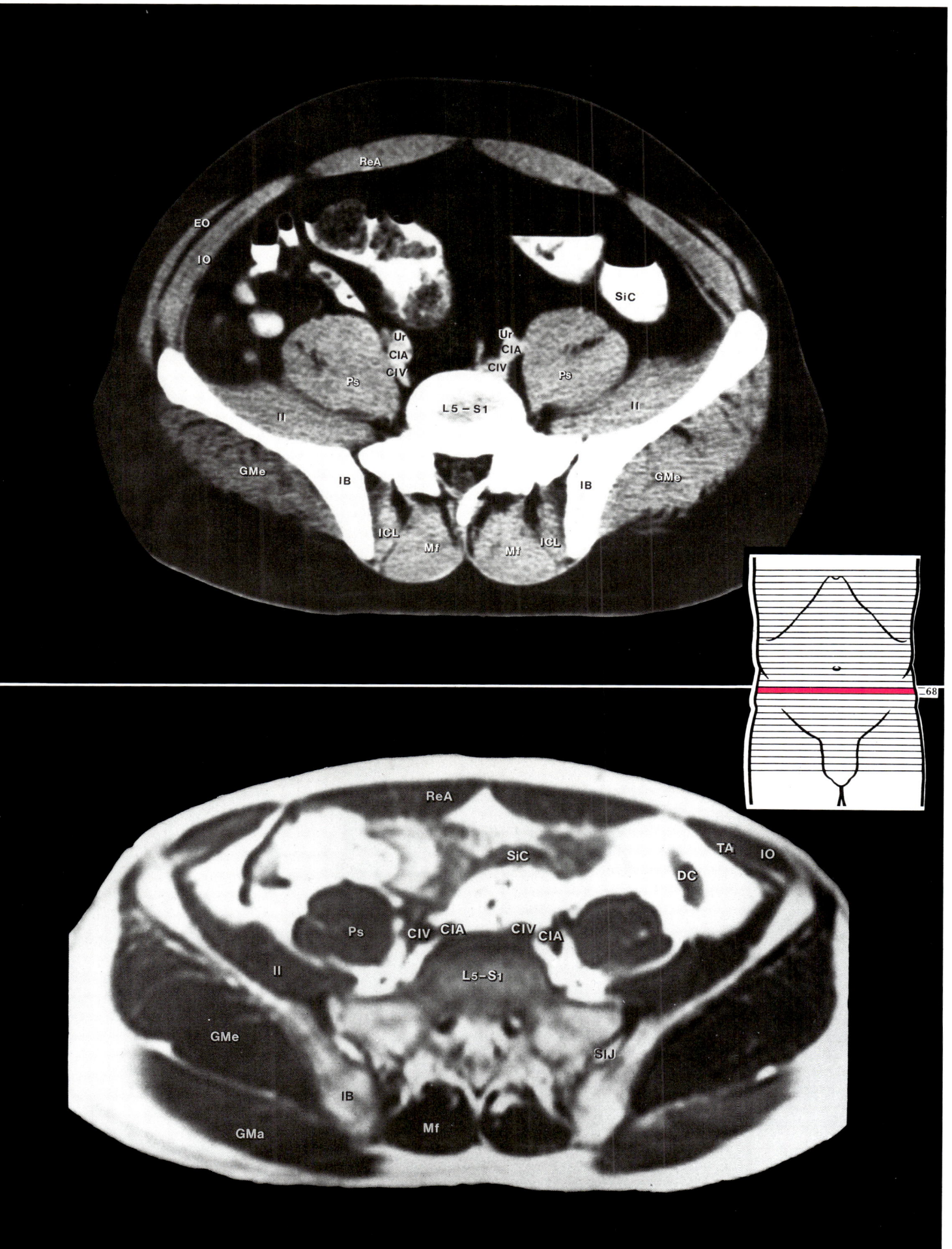

— 153 —

Plate 69. Transverse PELVIS-male

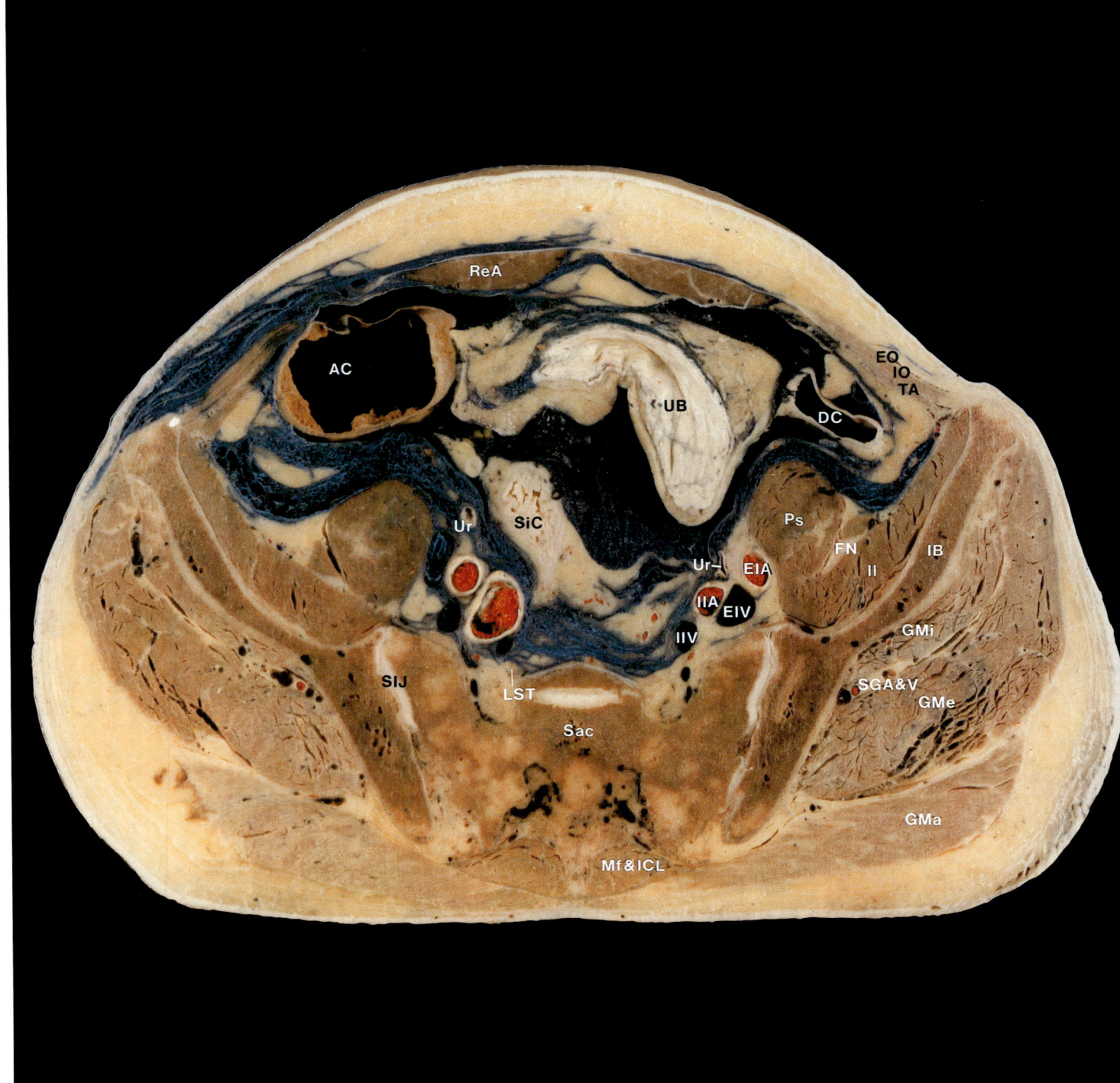

AC	Ascending colon	Mf	Multifidus muscle
Ce	Cecum	Ps	Psoas muscle
DC	Descending colon	ReA	Rectus abdominis muscle
EIA	External iliac artery	SGA	Superior gluteal artery
EIV	External iliac vein	SGV	Superior gluteal vein
EO	External oblique muscle	SIJ	Sacroiliac joint
FN	Femoral nerve	Sac	Sacrum
GMa	Gluteus maximus muscle	SiC	Sigmoid colon
GMe	Gluteus medius muscle	TA	Transversus abdominis muscle
GMi	Gluteus minimus muscle	UB	Urinary bladder
IB	Iliac bone	Ur	Ureter
ICL	Iliocostalis lumborum muscle		
IIA	Internal iliac artery		
IIV	Internal iliac vein		
IO	Internal oblique muscle		
Ie	Ileum		
Il	Iliacus muscle		
LST	Lumbosacral trunk		

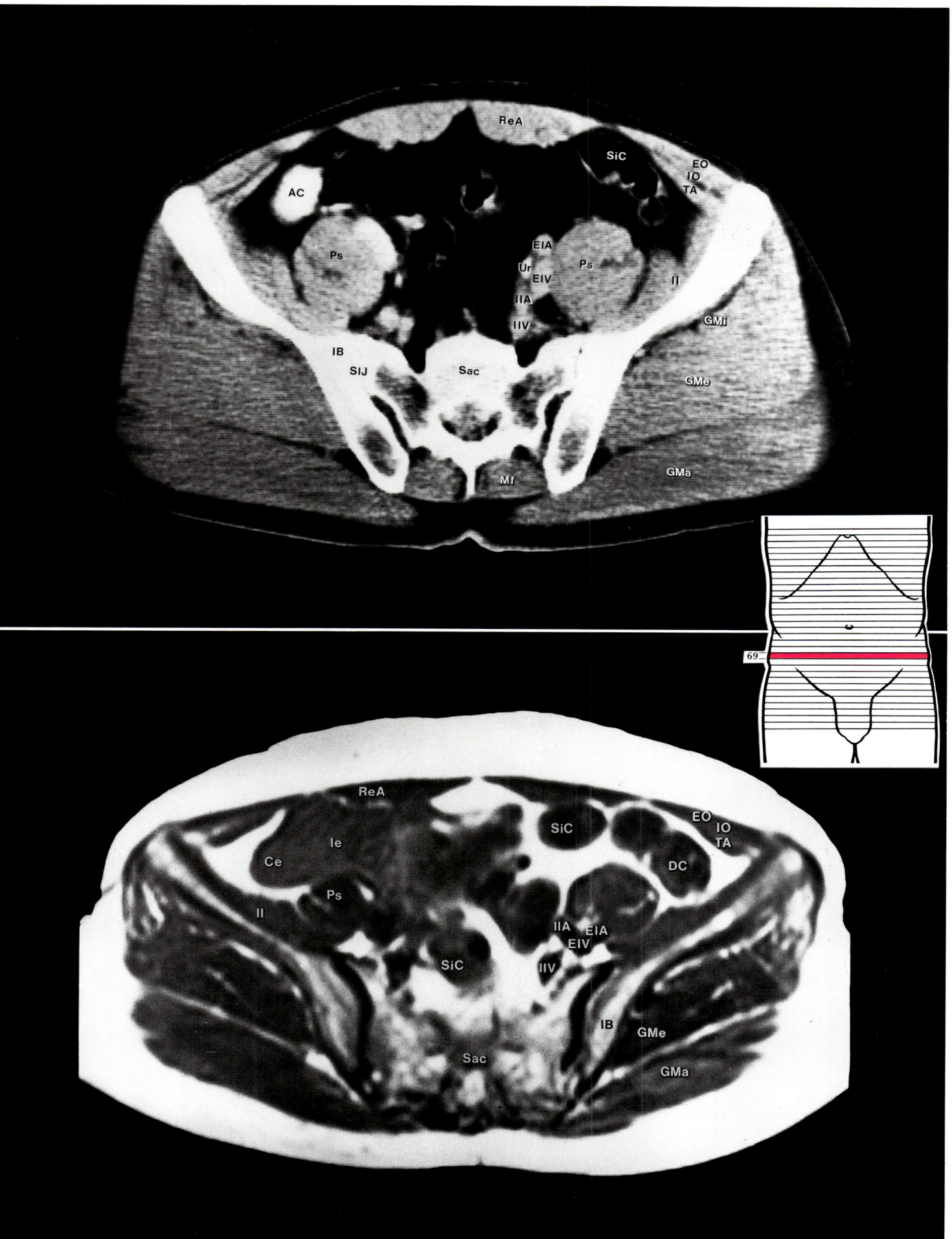

Plate 70. Transverse Pelvis-male

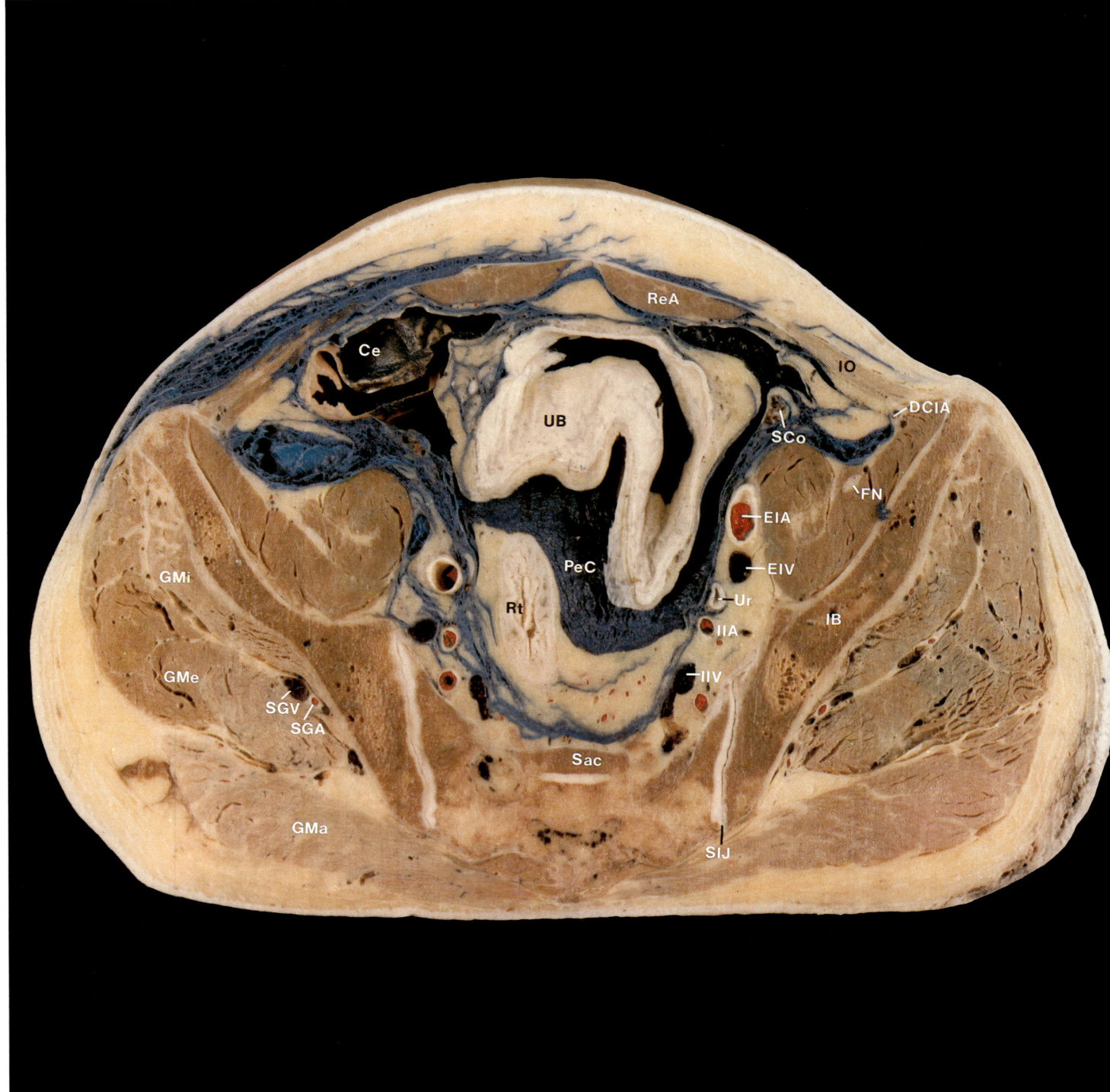

Ce	Cecum	Rt	Rectum
DCIA	Deep circumflex iliac artery	SCo	Spermatic cord
EIA	External iliac artery	SGA	Superior gluteal artery
EIV	External iliac vein	SGV	Superior gluteal vein
FN	Femoral nerve	SIJ	Sacroiliac joint
GMa	Gluteus maximus muscle	Sac	Sacrum
GMe	Gluteus medius muscle	SiC	Sigmoid colon
GMi	Gluteus minimus muscle	UB	Urinary bladder
IB	Iliac bone	Ur	Ureter
ICL	Iliocostalis lumborum muscle		
IIA	Internal iliac artery		
IIV	Internal iliac vein		
IO	Internal oblique muscle		
Il	Iliacus muscle		
Mf	Multifidus muscle		
PeC	Peritoneal cavity		
Ps	Psoas muscle		
ReA	Rectus abdominis muscle		

— 156 —

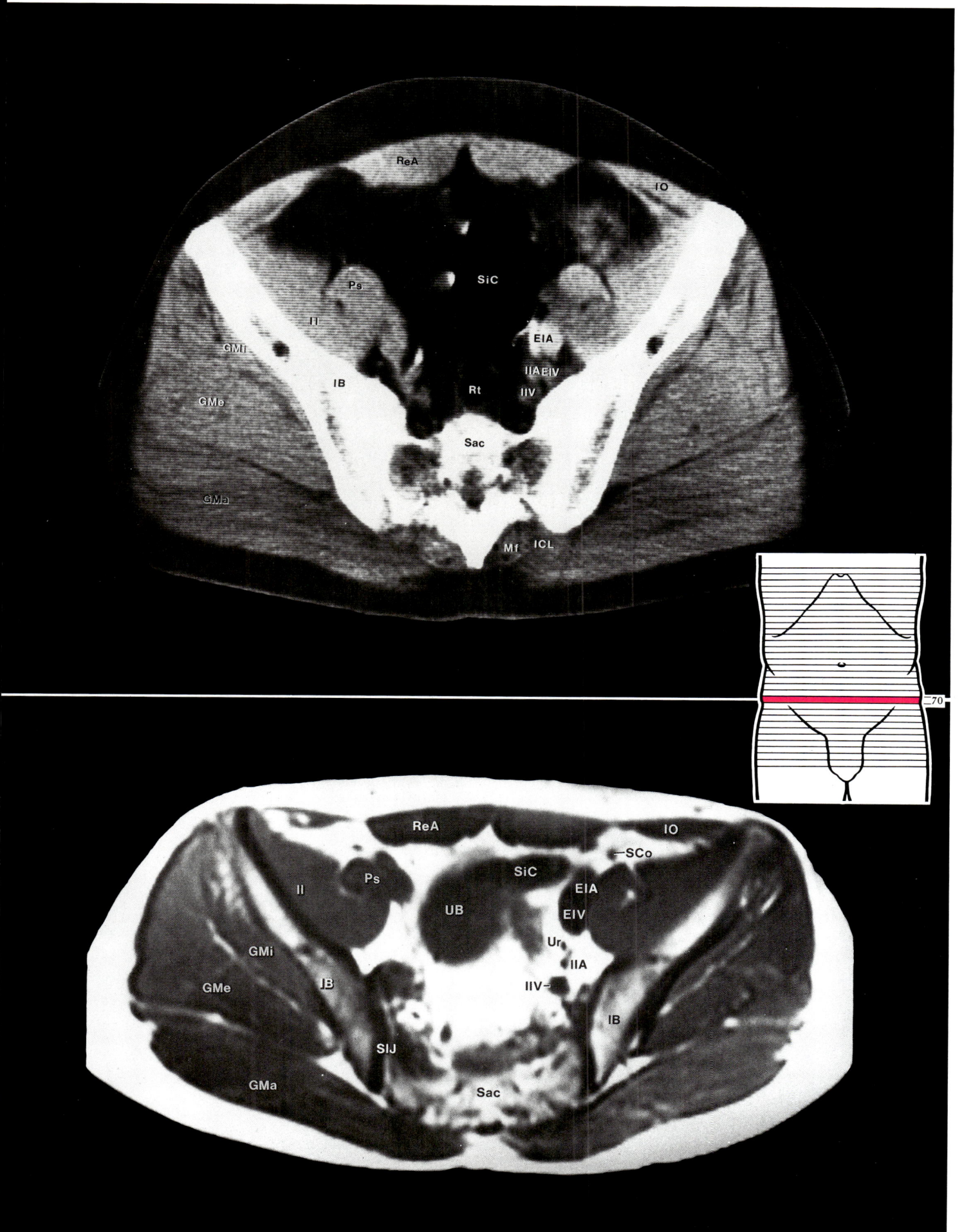

— 157 —

Plate 71. Transverse PELVIS-male

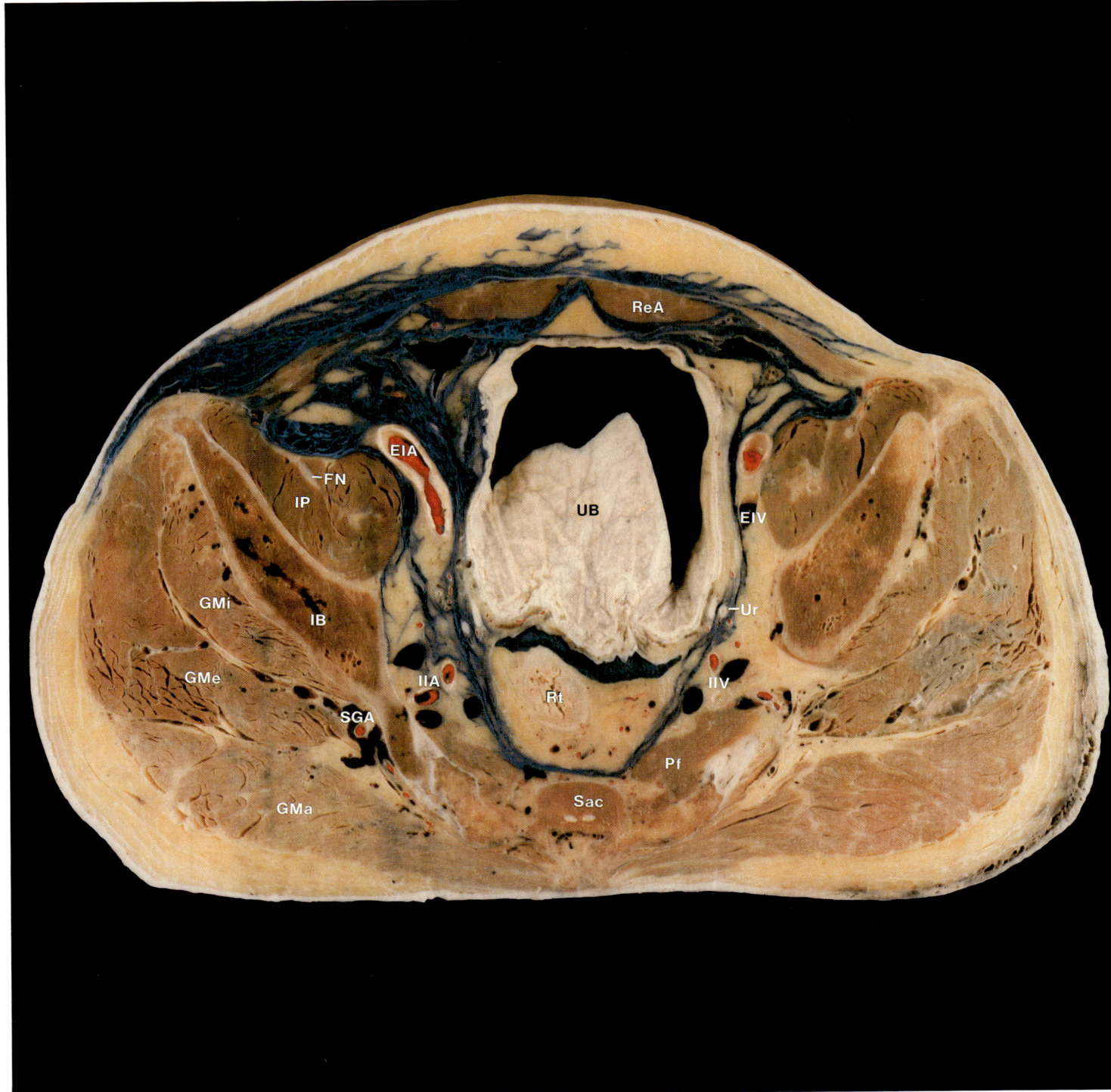

EIA	External iliac artery
EIV	External iliac vein
FN	Femoral nerve
GMa	Gluteus maximus muscle
GMe	Gluteus medius muscle
GMi	Gluteus minimus muscle
IB	Iliac bone
IIA	Internal iliac artery
IIV	Internal iliac vein
IP	Iliopsoas muscle
Pf	Piriformis muscle
ReA	Rectus abdominis muscle
Rt	Rectum
SGA	Superior gluteal artery
Sac	Sacrum
Sar	Sartorius muscle
UB	Urinary bladder
Ur	Ureter

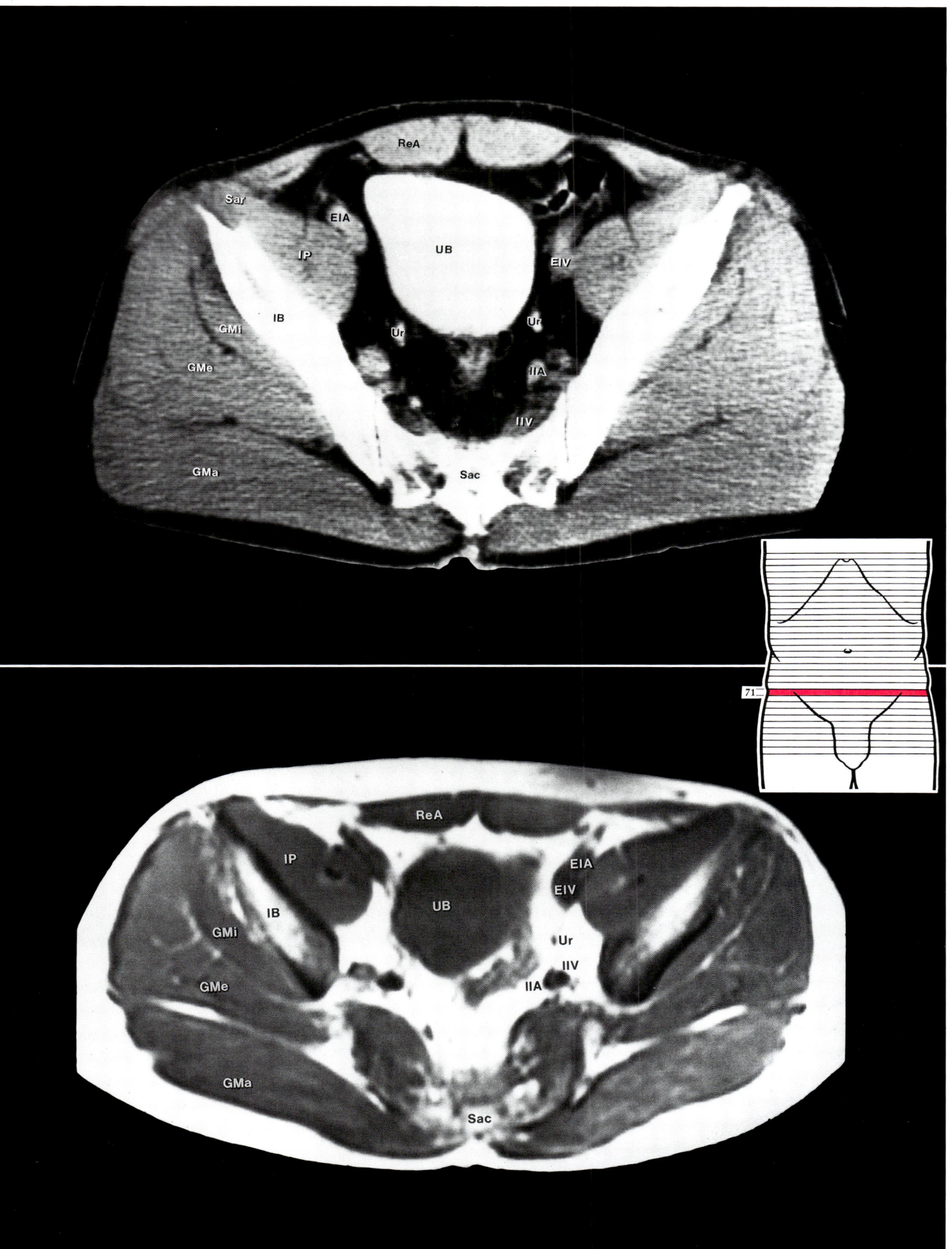

Plate 72. TRANSVERSE PELVIS-MALE

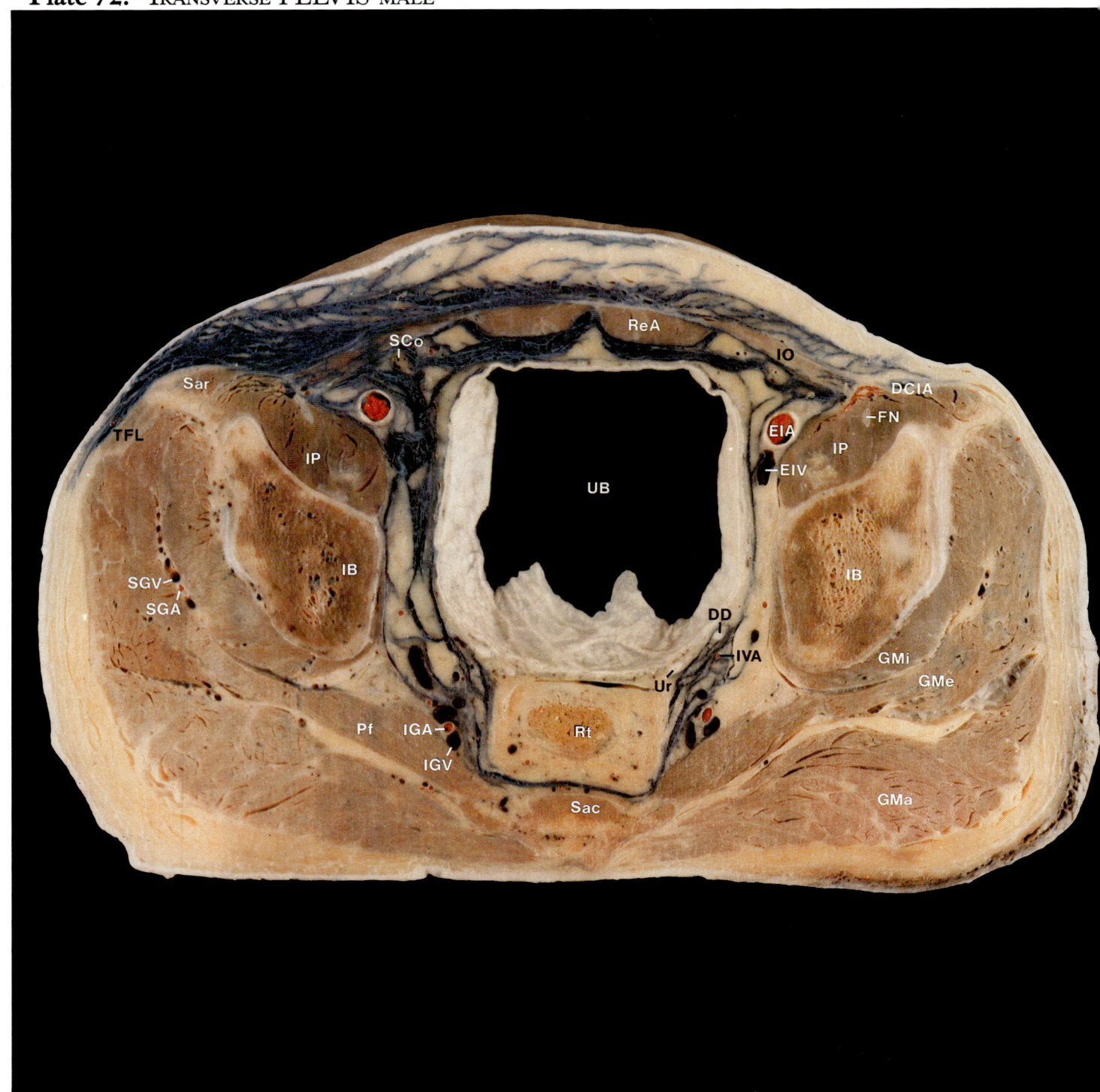

DCIA	Deep circumflex iliac artery	SGA	Superior gluteal artery
DD	Ductus deferens	SGV	Superior gluteal vein
EIA	External iliac artery	Sac	Sacrum
EIV	External iliac vein	Sar	Sartorius muscle
FN	Femoral nerve	TFL	Tensor fascia lata
GMa	Gluteus maximus muscle	UB	Urinary bladder
GMe	Gluteus medius muscle	Ur	Ureter
GMi	Gluteus minimus muscle		
IB	Iliac bone		
IGA	Inferior gluteal artery		
IGV	Inferoior gluteal vein		
IO	Internal oblique muscle		
IP	Iliopsoas muscle		
IVA	Inferior vesical artery		
Pf	Piriformis muscle		
ReA	Rectus abdominis muscle		
Rt	Rectum		
SCo	Spermatic cord		

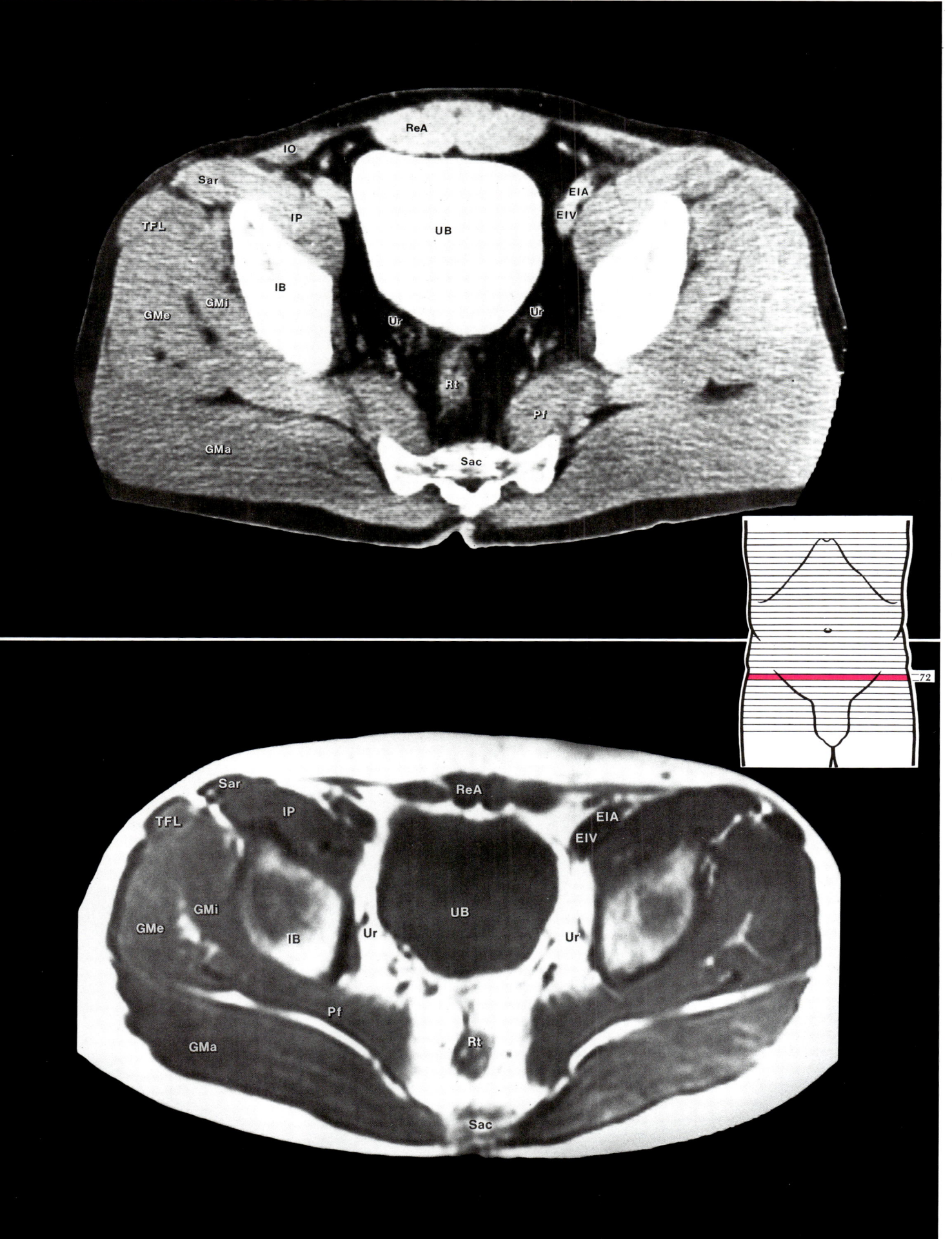

Plate 73. Transverse PELVIS-male

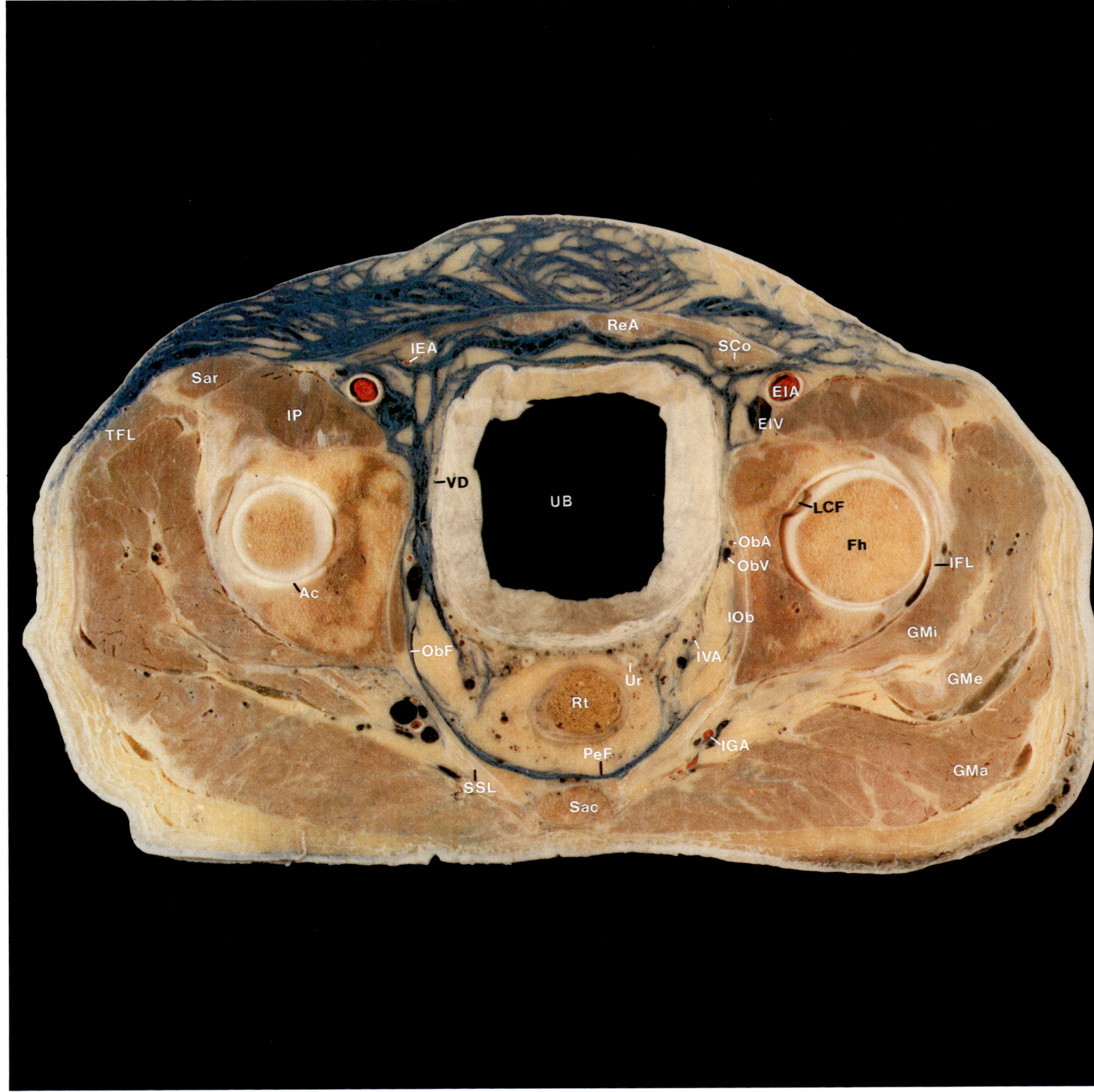

Ac	Acetabulum	PeF	Pelvic fascia
EIA	External iliac artery	ReA	Rectus abdominis muscle
EIV	External iliac vein	Rt	Rectum
Fh	Femur, head	SCo	Spermatic cord
GMa	Gluteus maximus muscle	SSL	Sacrospinous ligament
GMe	Gluteus medius muscle	Sac	Sacrum
GMi	Gluteus minimus muscle	Sar	Sartorius muscle
IEA	Inferior epigastric artery	TFL	Tensor fascia lata
IFL	Iliofemoral ligament	UB	Urinary bladder
IGA	Inferior gluteal artery	Ur	Ureter
IOb	Internal obturator muscle	VD	Vas deferens
IP	Iliopsoas muscle		
IVA	Inferior vesical artery		
LCF	Ligamentum capitis femoris		
Ob	Obtuator muscle		
ObA	Obturator artery		
ObF	Obturator fascia		
ObV	Obturator vein		

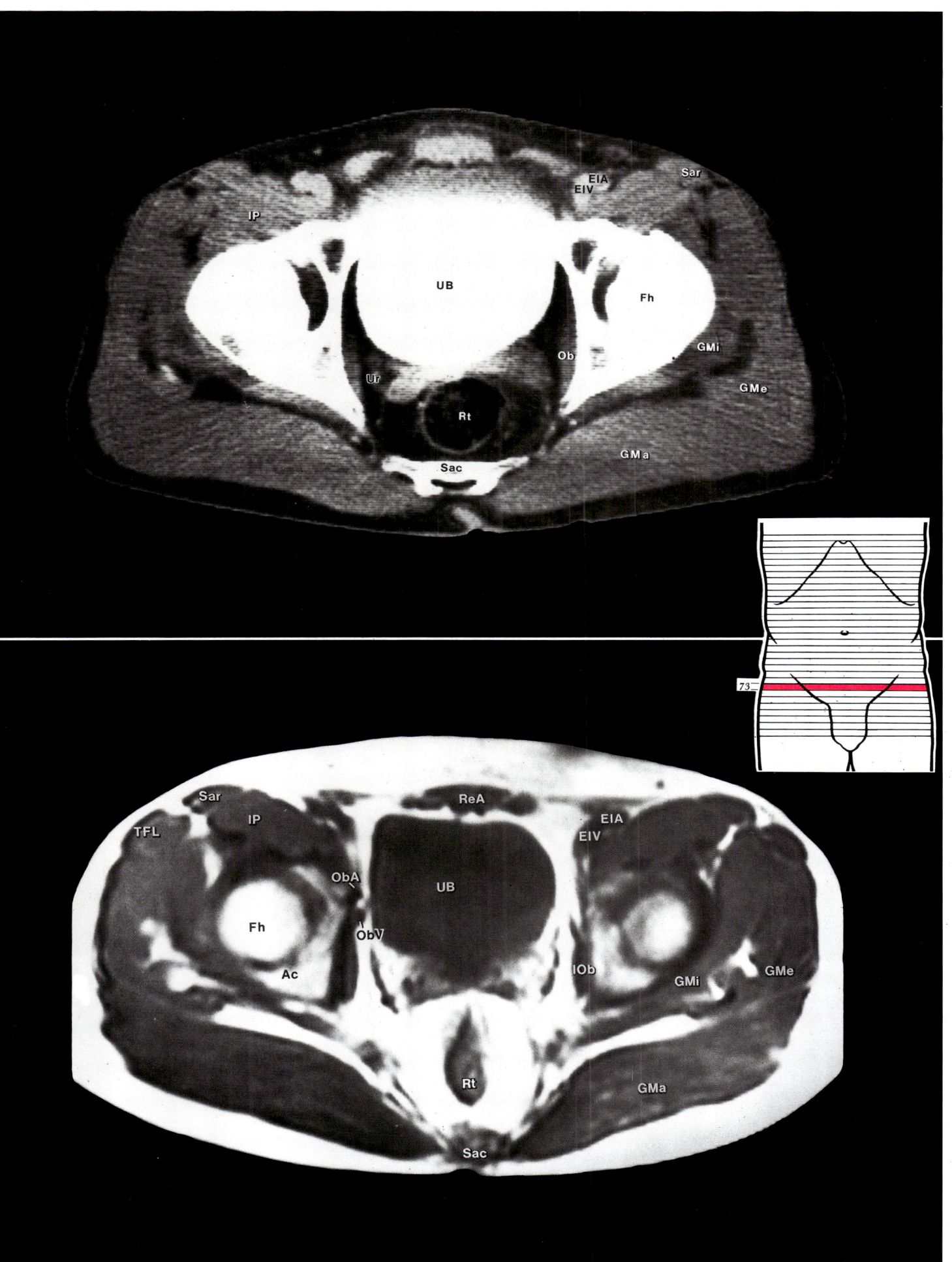

Plate 74. Transverse PELVIS-male

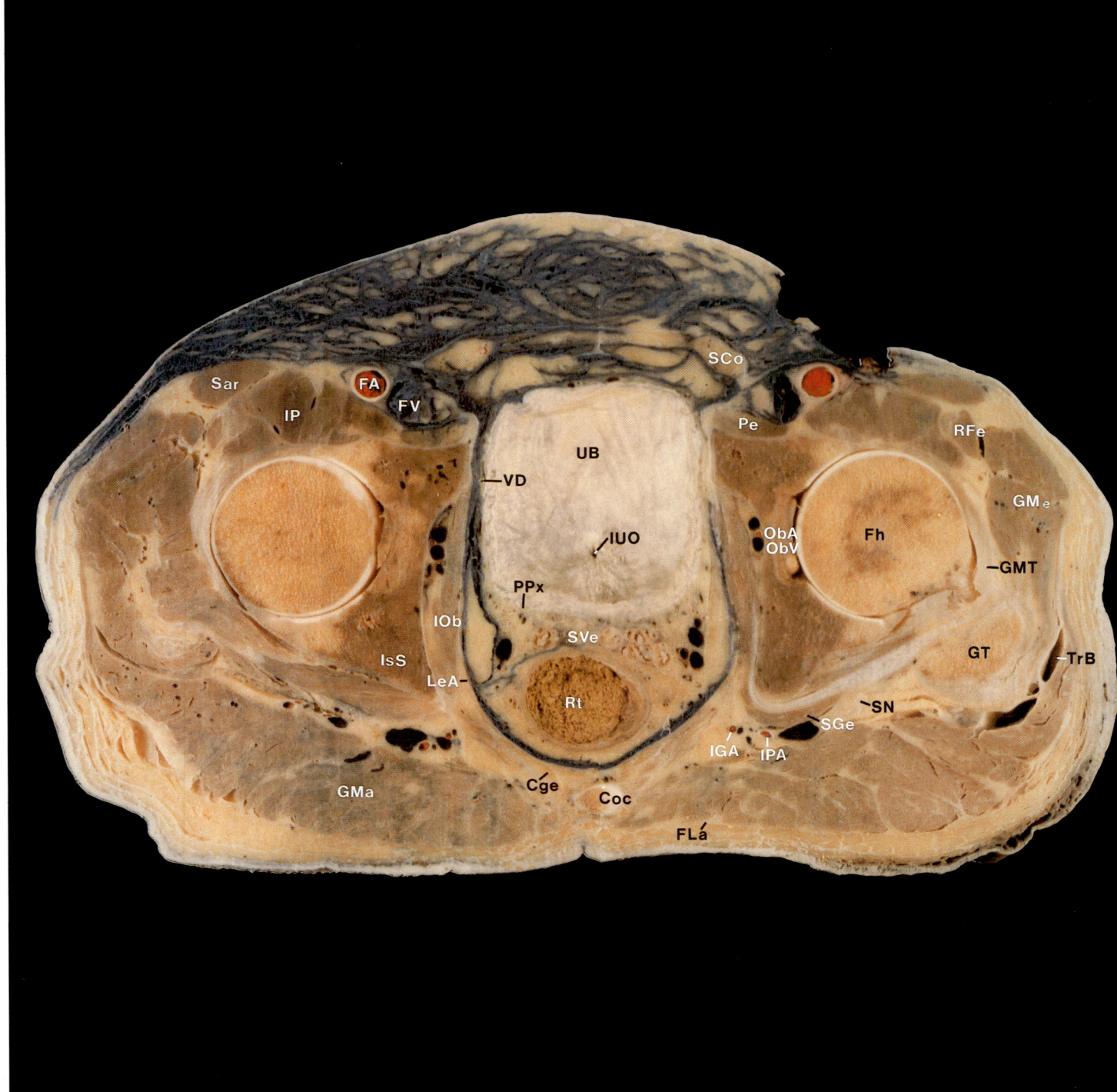

Cge	Coccygeus muscle	ObV	Obturator vein
Coc	Coccyx	PPx	Pudental plexus
FA	Femoral artery	Pe	Pectineus muscle
FLa	Fascia lata	RFe	Rectus femoris muscle
FV	Femoral vein	Rt	Rectum
Fh	Femur, head	SCo	Spermatic cord
GMT	Gluteus minimus tendon	SGe	Superior gemellus muscle
GMa	Gluteus maximus muscle	SN	Sciatic nerve
GMe	Gluteus medius muscle	Sar	Sartorius muscle
GT	Greater trochanter	SVe	Seminal vesicle
IGA	Inferior gluteal artery	TrB	Trochanteric bursa
IOb	Internal obturator muscle	UB	Urinary bladder
IP	Iliopsoas muscle	VD	Vas deferens
IPA	Internal pudendal artery		
IUO	Internal urethral opening		
IsS	Ischial spine		
LeA	Levator ani muscle		
ObA	Obturator artery		

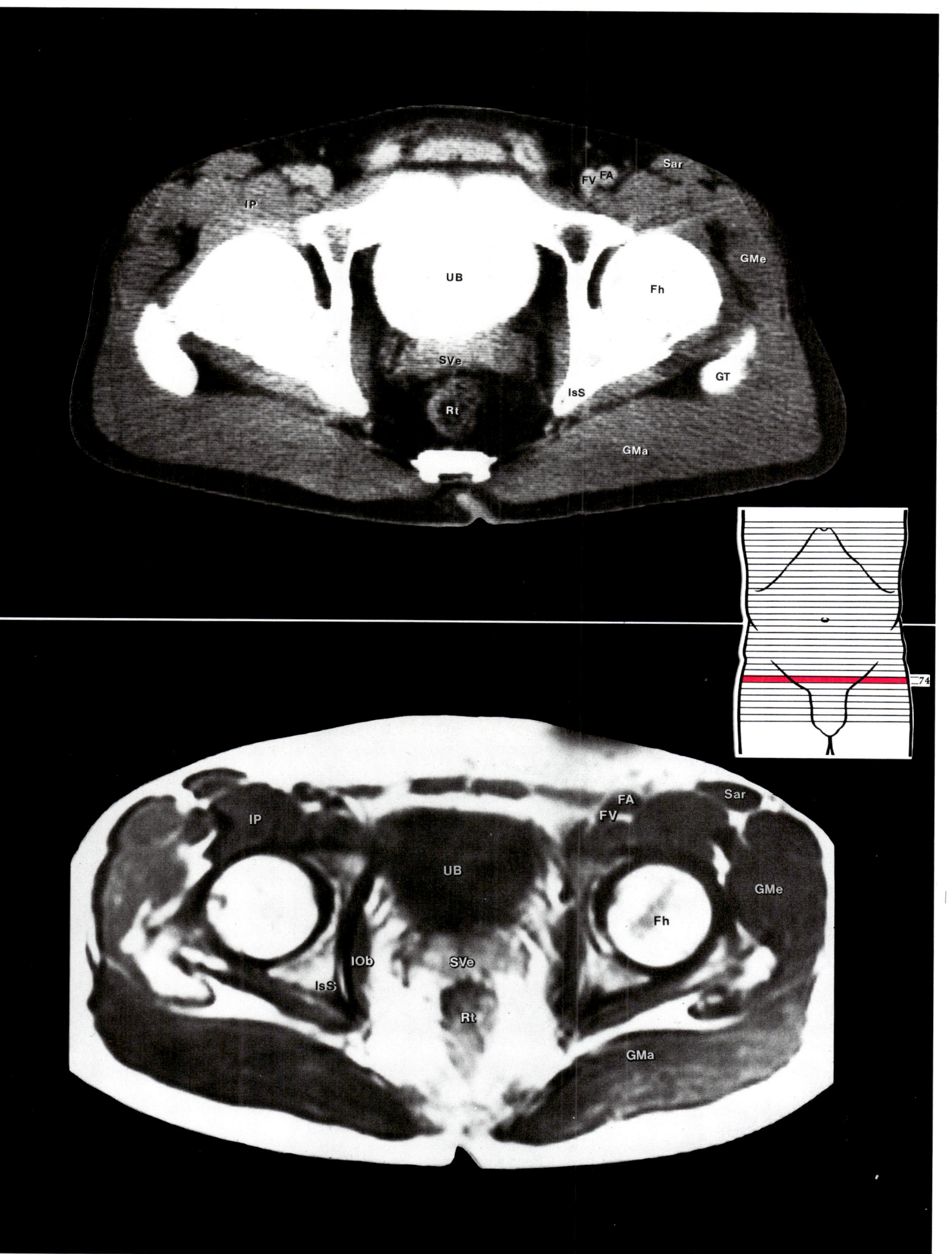

Plate 75. Transverse Pelvis-Male

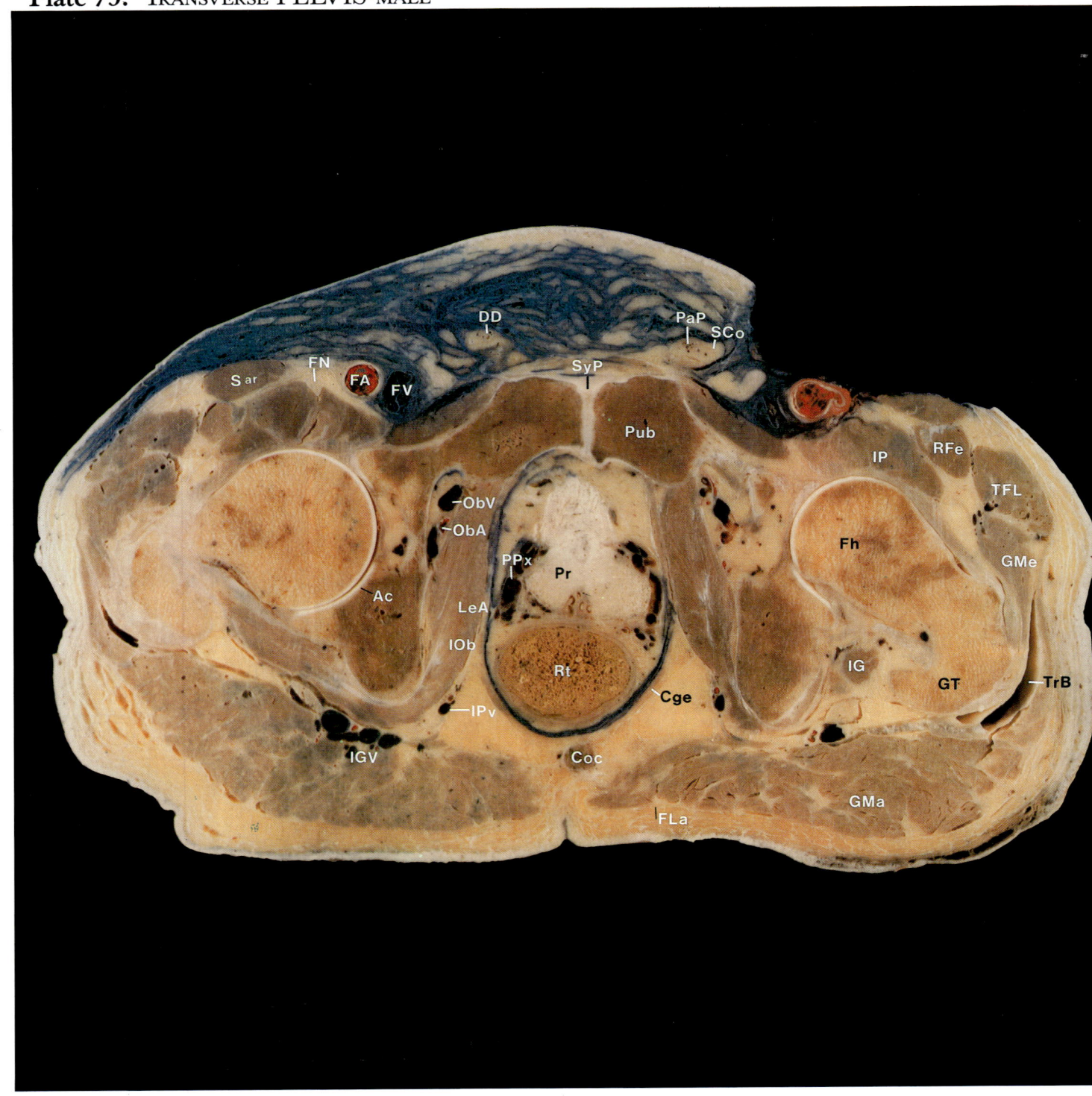

Ac	Acetabulum	ObA	Obturator artery
Cge	Coccygeus muscle	ObV	Obturator vein
Coc	Coccyx	PPx	Pudendal plexus
DD	Ductus deferens	PaP	Panpiniform plexus
FA	Femoral artery	Pr	Prostate
FLa	Fascia lata	Pub	Pubic bone
FN	Femoral nerve	RFe	Rectus femoris muscle
FV	Femoral vein	Rt	Rectum
Fh	Femur, head	SCo	Spermatic cord
GMa	Gluteus maximus muscle	Sar	Sartorius muscle
GMe	Gluteus medius muscle	SyP	Symphysis pubis
GT	Greater trochanter	TFL	Tensor fascia lata
IG	Inferior gemellus muscle	TrB	Trochanteric bursa
IGV	Inferior gluteal vein	UB	Urinary bladder
IOb	Internal obturator muscle		
IP	Iliopsoas muscle		
IPv	Internal pudendal vessel		
LeA	Levator ani muscle		

— 166 —

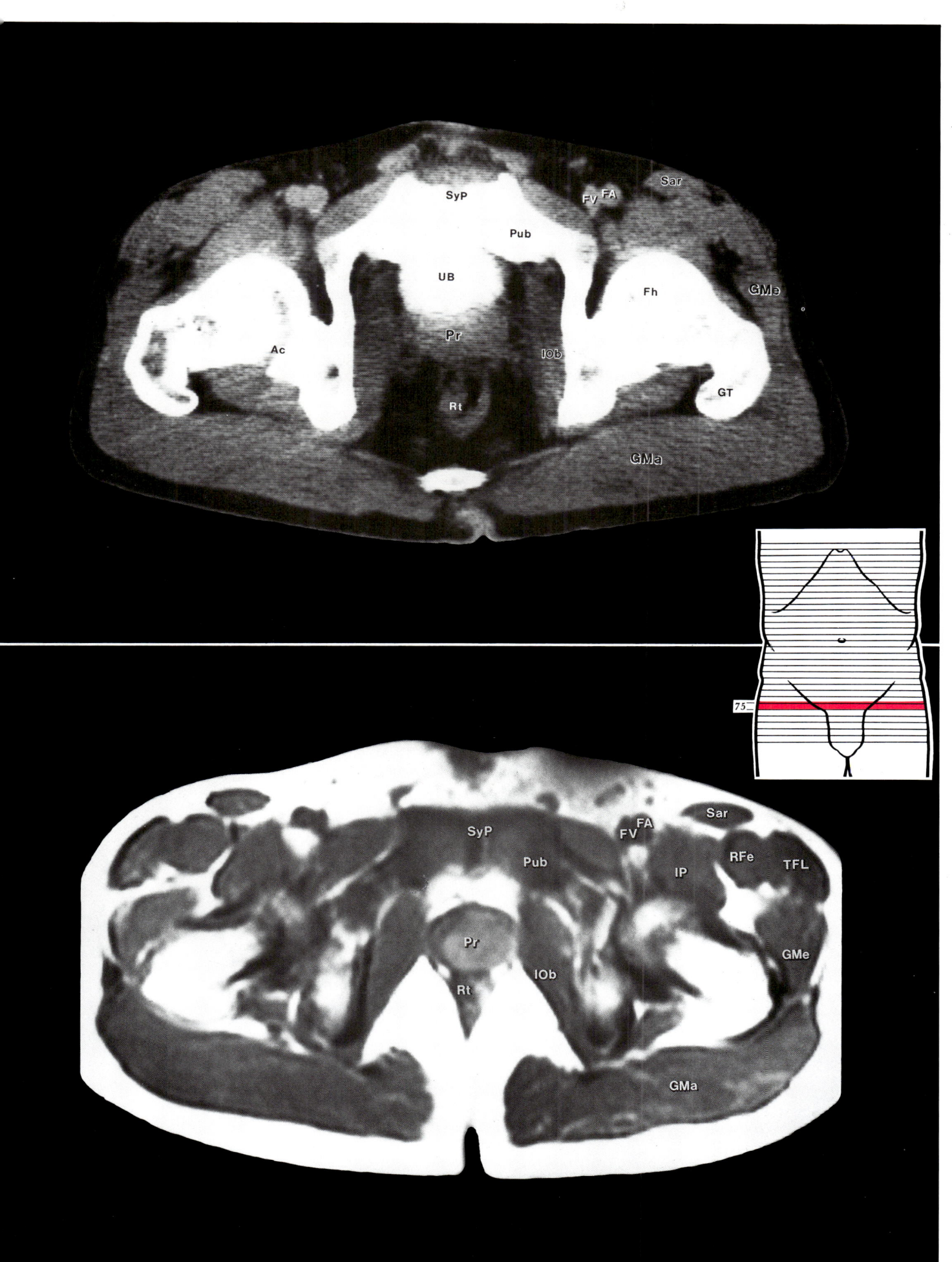

Plate 76. TRANSVERSE PELVIS-MALE

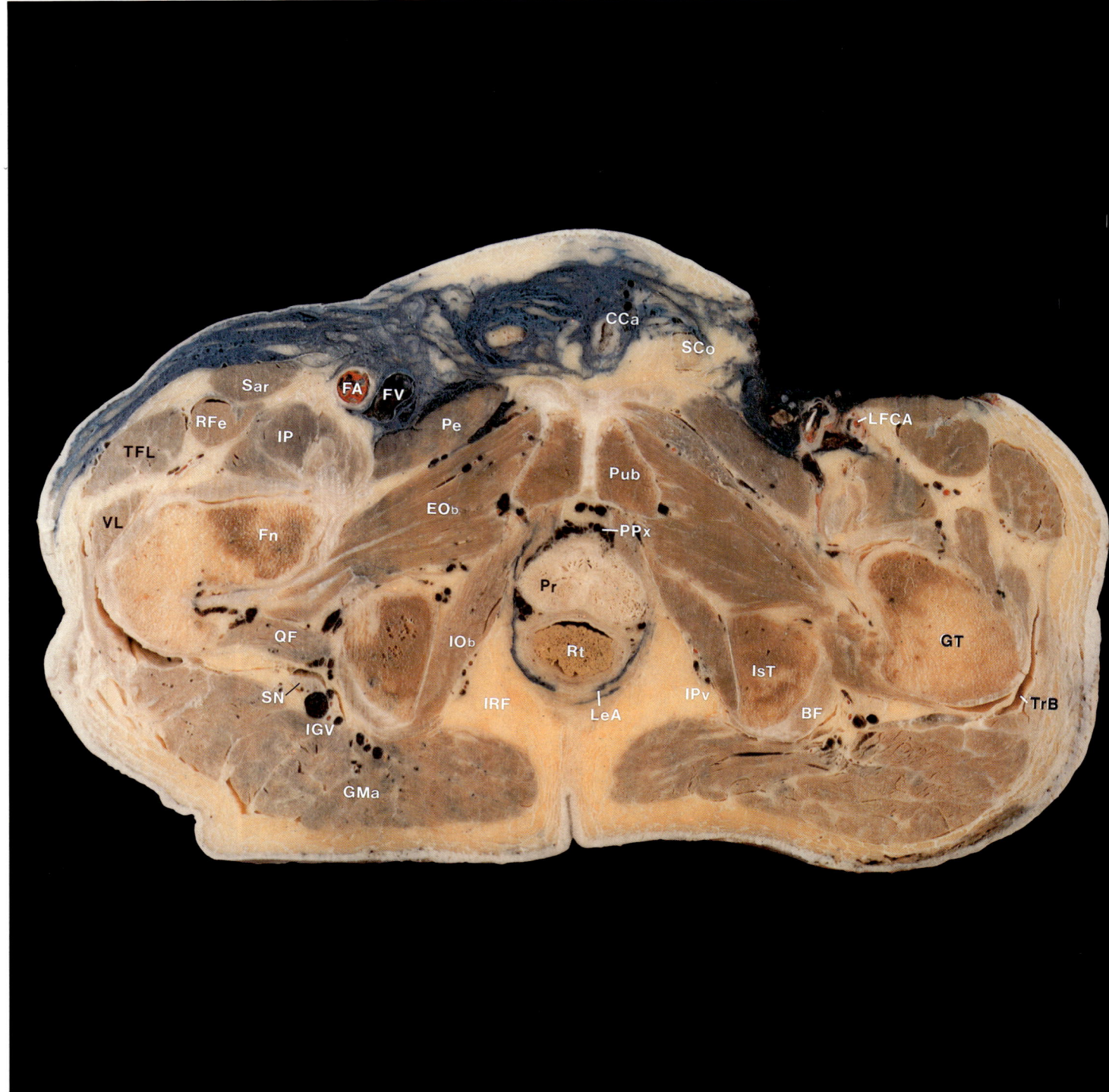

BF	Biceps femoris muscle	Pe	Pectineus muscle
CCa	Corpus cavernosum	Pr	Prostate
Coc	Coccyx	Pub	Pubic bone
EOb	External obturator muscle	QF	Quadratus femoris muscle
FA	Femoral artery	RFe	Rectus femoris muscle
FV	Femoral vein	RPe	Root of penis
Fn	Femur, neck	Rt	Rectum
GMa	Gluteus maximus muscle	SCo	Spermatic cord
GT	Greater trochanter	SN	Sciatic nerve
IGV	Inferior gluteal vein	Sar	Satorius muscle
IOb	Internal obturator muscle	TFL	Tensor fascia lata
IP	Iliopsoas muscle	TrB	Trochanteric bursa
IPv	Internal pudental vessel	VL	Vastus lateralis muscle
IRF	Ischiorectal fossa		
IsT	Ischial tuberosity		
LFCA	Lateral femoral circumflex artery		
LeA	Levator ani muscle		
PPx	Pudental plexus		

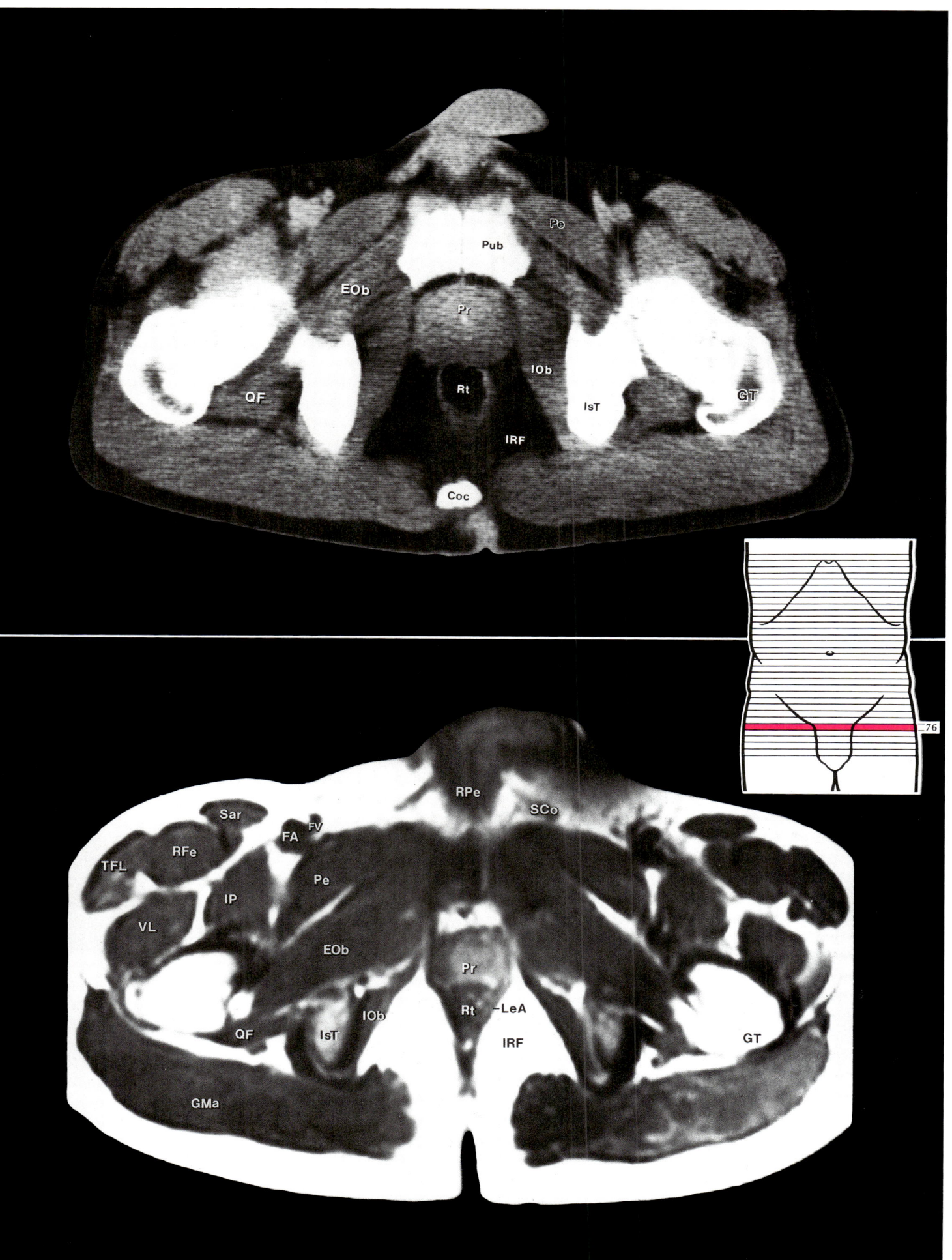

Plate 77. TRANSVERSE PELVIS-MALE

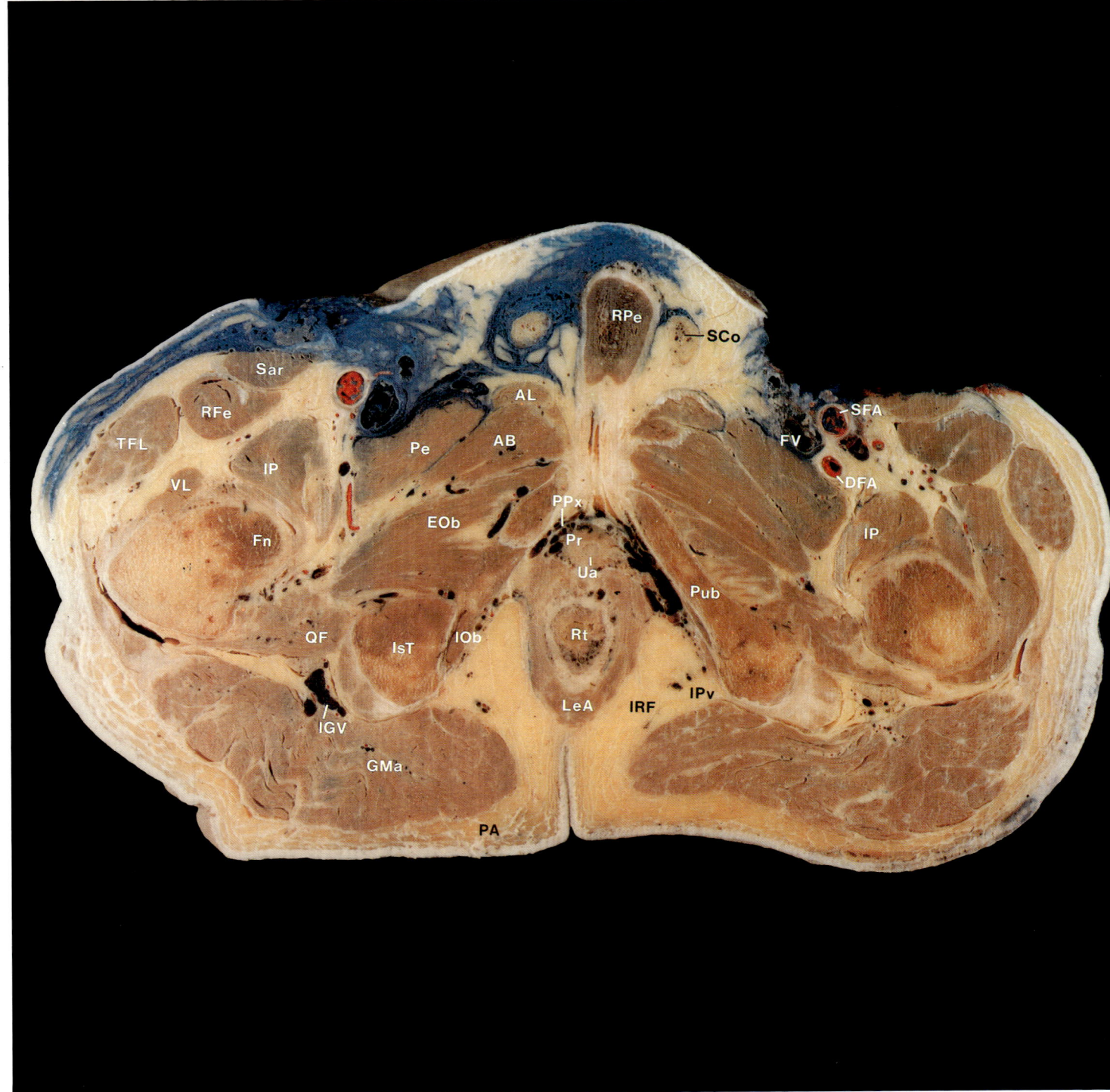

AB	Adductor brevis muscle	Pe	Pectineus muscle
AL	Adductor longus muscle	Pr	Prostate
Coc	Coccyx	Pub	Pubic bone
DFA	Deep femoral artery	QF	Quadratus femoris muscle
EOb	External obturator muscle	RFe	Rectus femoris muscle
FV	Femoral vein	RPe	Root of penis
Fn	Femur, neck	Rt	Rectum
GMa	Gluteus maximus muscle	SCo	Spermatic cord
GT	Greater trochanter	SFA	Superficial femoral artery
IGV	Inferior gluteal vein	Sar	Sartorius muscle
IOb	Internal obturator muscle	TFL	Tensor fascia lata
IP	Iliopsoas muscle	Ua	Urethra
IPv	Internal pudental vessel	VL	Vastus lateralis muscle
IRF	Ischiorectal fossa		
IsT	Ischial tuberosity		
LeA	Levator ani muscle		
PA	Panniculus adiposus		
PPx	Pudental plexus		

— 170 —

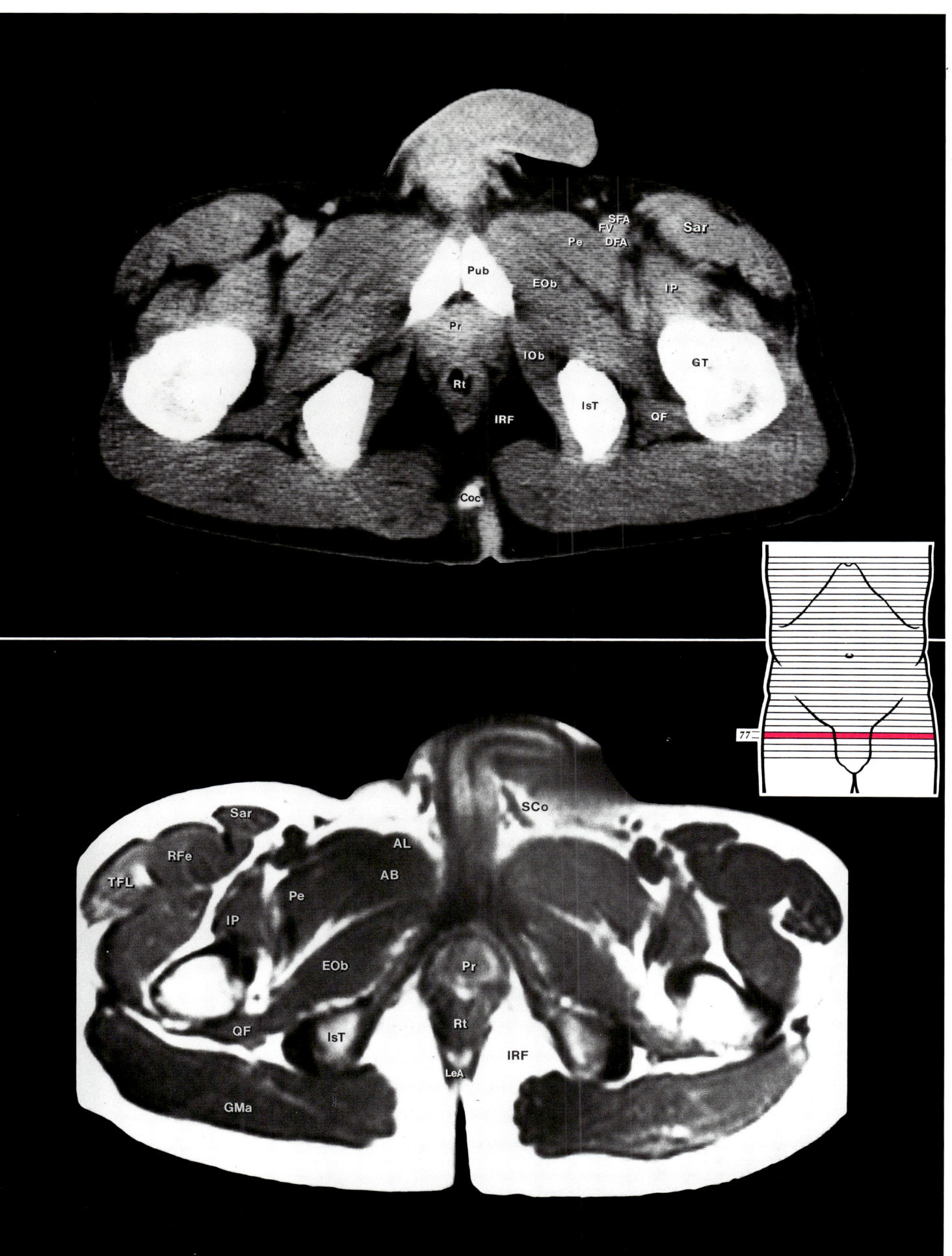

— 171 —

Plate 78. Transverse Pelvis-male

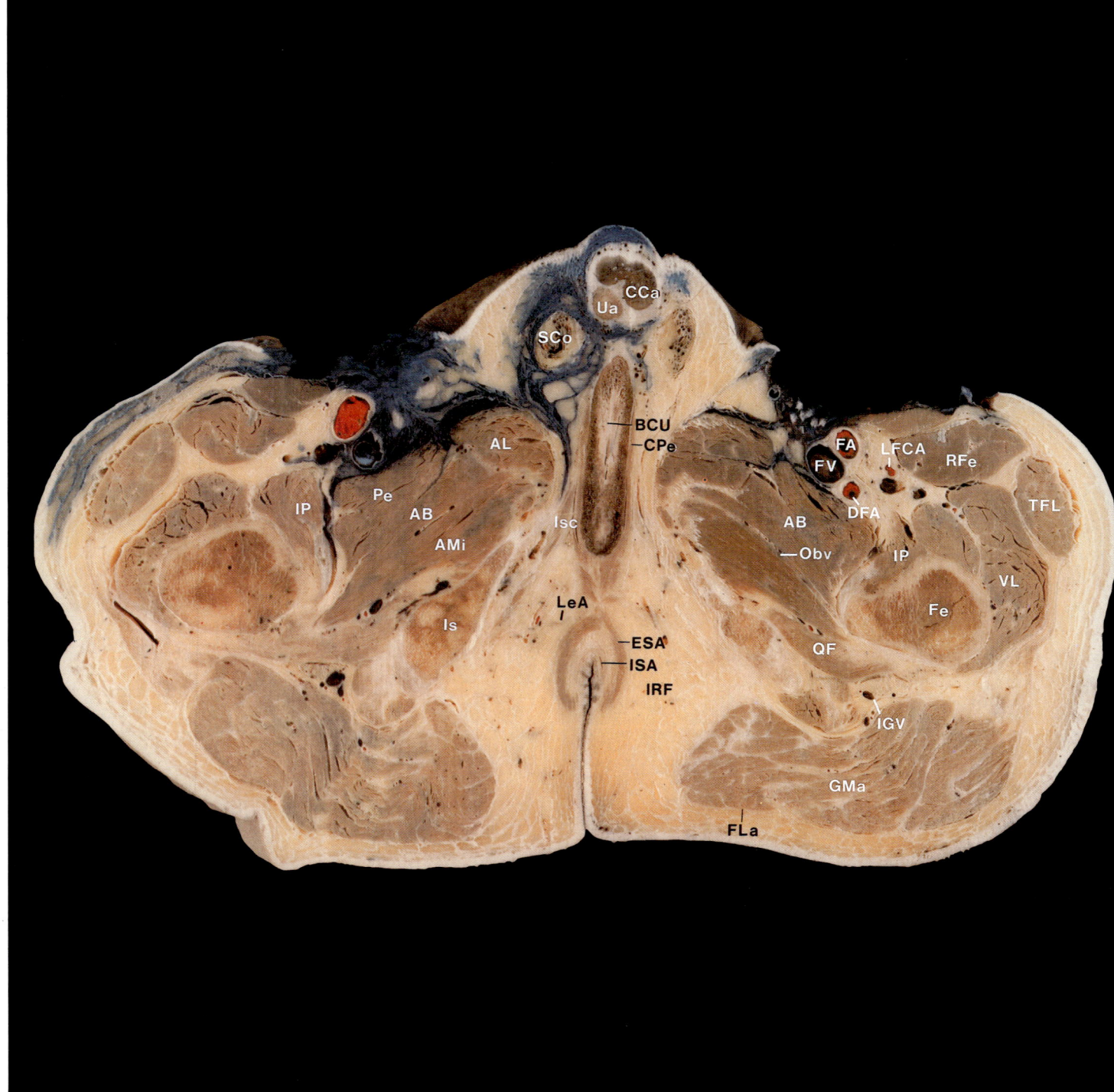

AB	Adductor brevis muscle	IsT	Ischial tuberosity
AL	Adductor longus muscle	Isc	Ischiocavernous muscle
AMi	Adductor minimus muscle	LFCA	Lateral femoral circumflex artery
BCU	Bulbocavernous urethra	LeA	Levator ani muscle
CCa	Corpus cavernosum	Obv	Obturator vessel
CPe	Crus penis	Pe	Pectineus muscle
DFA	Deep femoral artery	Pr	Prostate
ESA	External sphincter ani	QF	Quadratus femoris muscle
FA	Femoral artery	RFe	Rectus femoris muscle
FLa	Fascia lata	RPe	Root of penis
FV	Femoral vein	SCo	Spermatic cord
Fe	Femur	SFA	Superficial femoral artery
GMa	Gluteus maximus muscle	Sar	Sartorius muscle
IGV	Inferior gluteal vein	TFL	Tensor fascia lata
IP	Iliopsoas muscle	Tes	Testis
IRF	Ischiorectal fossa	Ua	Urethra
ISA	Internal sphincter ani	VL	Vastus lateralis muscle
Is	Ischium		

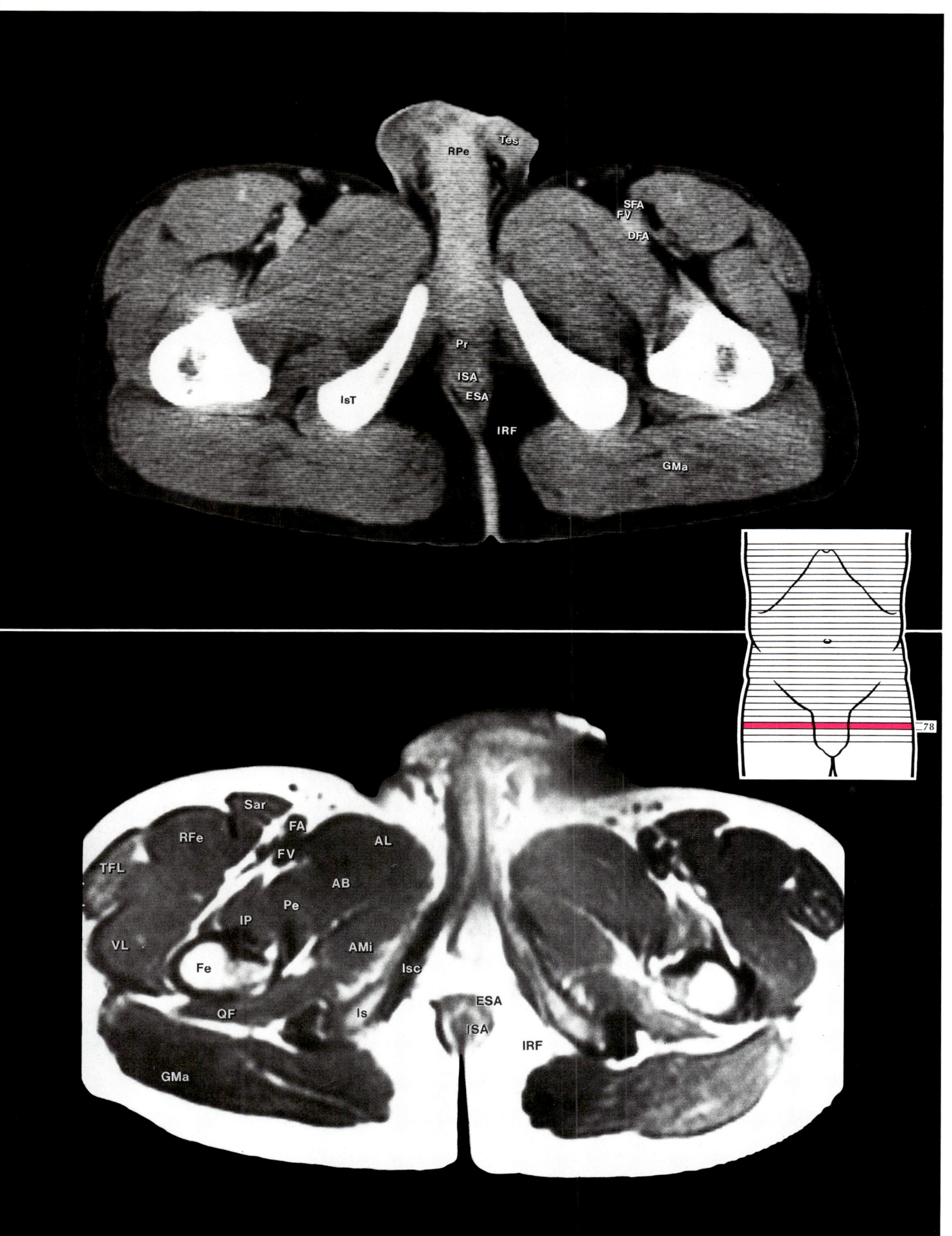

Plate 79. TRANSVERSE PELVIS-MALE

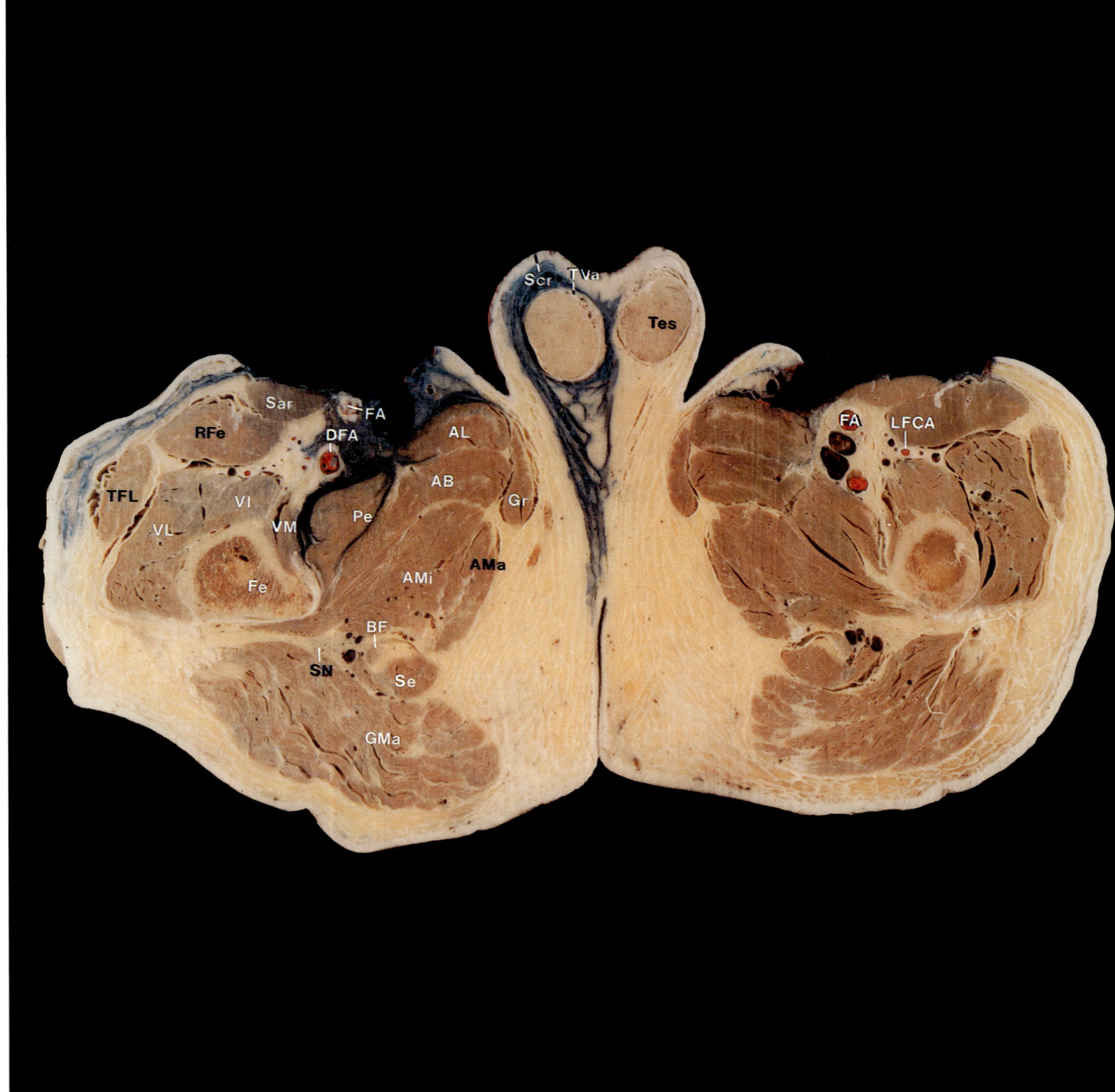

AB	Adductor brevis muscle	TVa	Tunica vaginalis
AL	Adductor longus muscle	Tes	Testis
AMa	Adductor magnus muscle	VI	Vastus intermedius muscle
AMi	Adductor minimus muscle	VL	Vastus lateralis muscle
BF	Biceps femoris muscle	VM	Vastus medialis muscle
DFA	Deep femoral artery		
FA	Femoral artery		
Fe	Femur		
GMa	Gluteus maximus muscle		
Gr	Gracilis muscle		
LFCA	Lateral femoral circumflex artery		
Pe	Pectineus muscle		
RFe	Rectus femoris muscle		
SN	Sciatic nerve		
Sar	Sartorius muscle		
Scr	Scrotum		
Se	Semitendinosus muscle		
TFL	Tensor fascia lata		

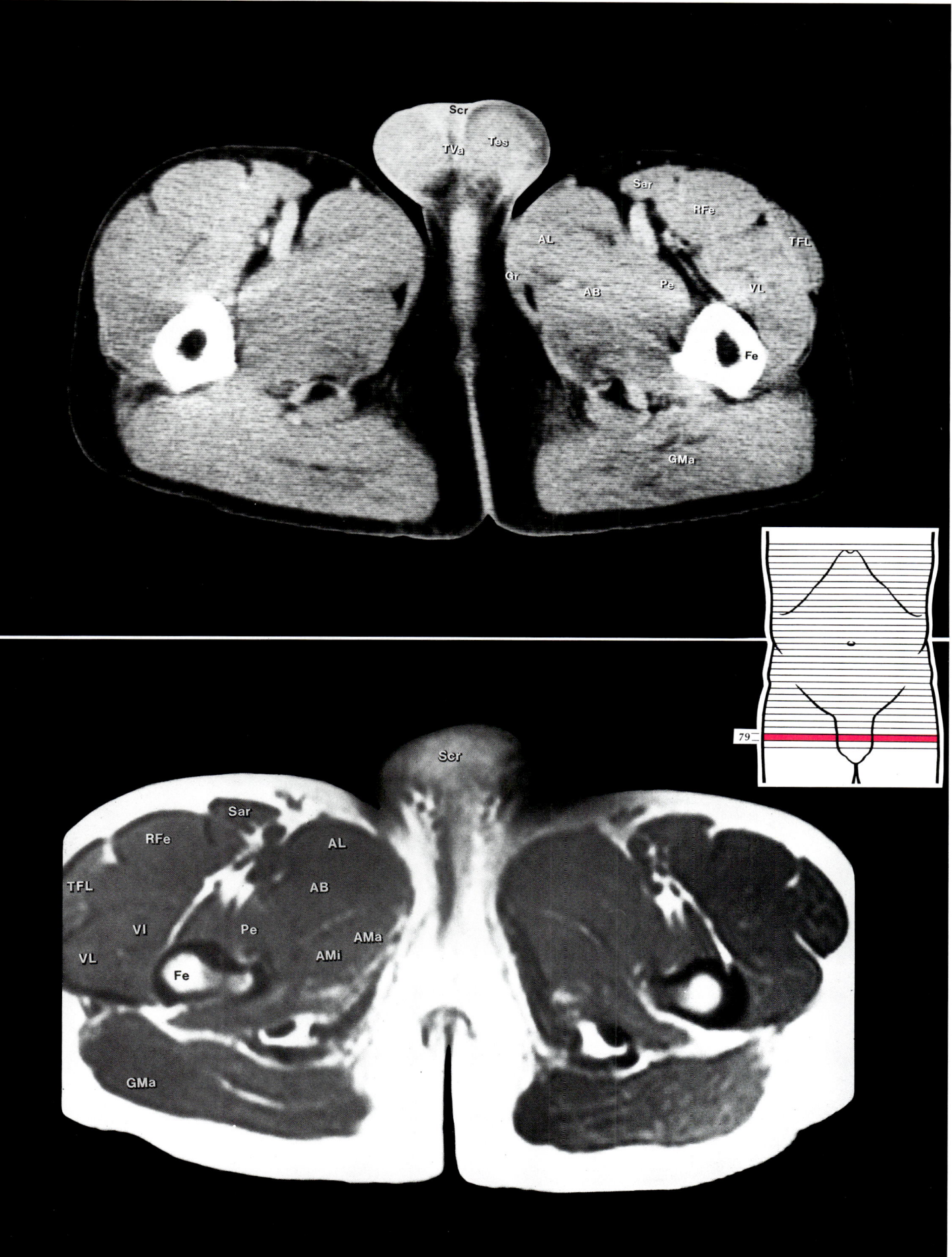

Plate 80. Transverse Pelvis-male

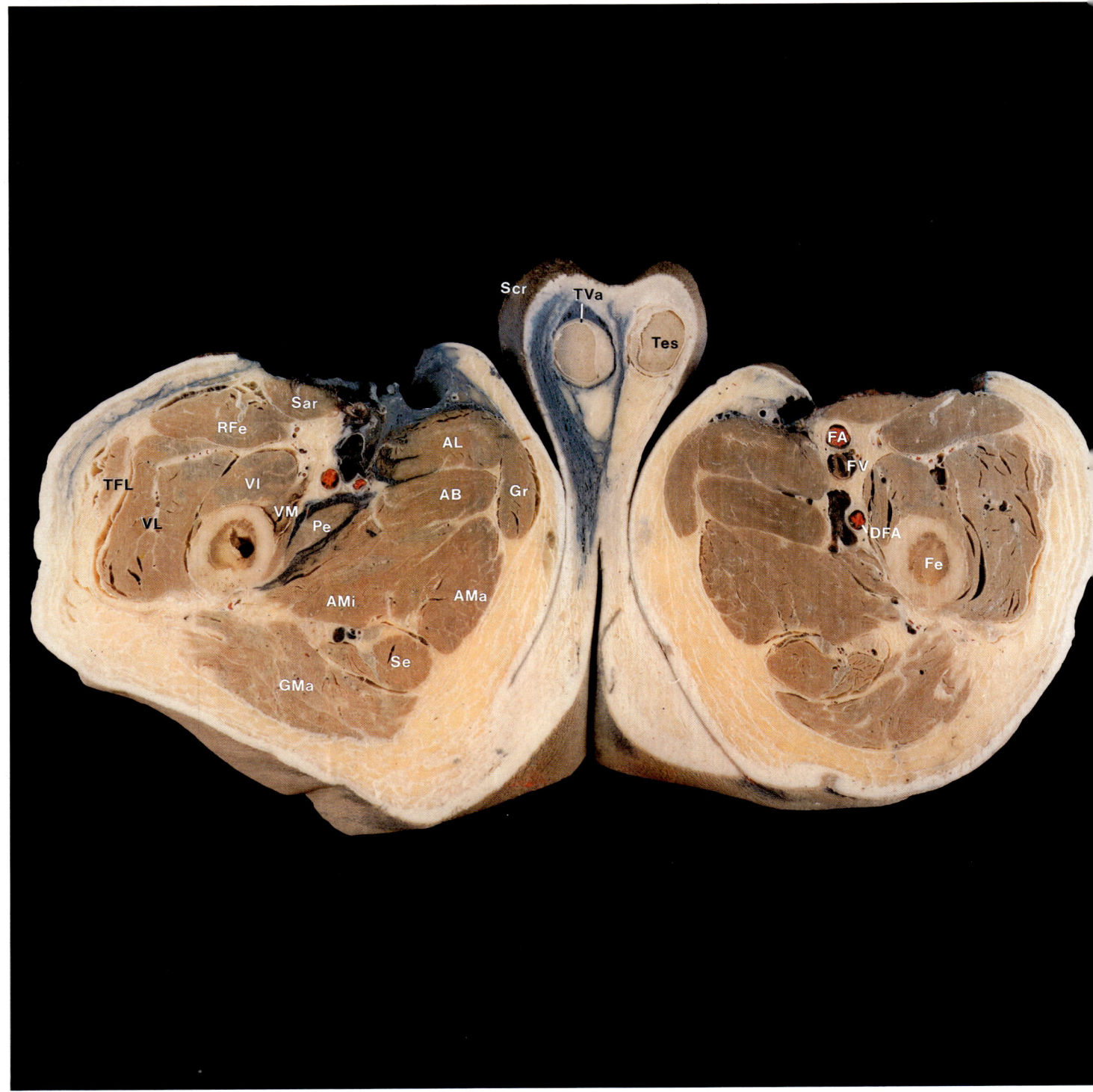

AB	Adductor brevis muscle	VI	Vastus intermedius muscle
AL	Adductor longus muscle	VL	Vastus lateralis muscle
AMa	Adductor magnus muscle	VM	Vastus medialis muscle
AMi	Adductor minimus muscle		
DFA	Deep femoral artery		
FA	Femoral artery		
FV	Femoral vein		
Fe	Femur		
GMa	Gluteus maximus muscle		
Gr	Gracilis muscle		
Pe	Pectineus muscle		
RFe	Rectus femoris muscle		
Sar	Sartorius muscle		
Scr	Scrotum		
Se	Semitendinosus muscle		
TFL	Tensor fascia lata		
TVa	Tunica vaginalis		
Tes	Testis		

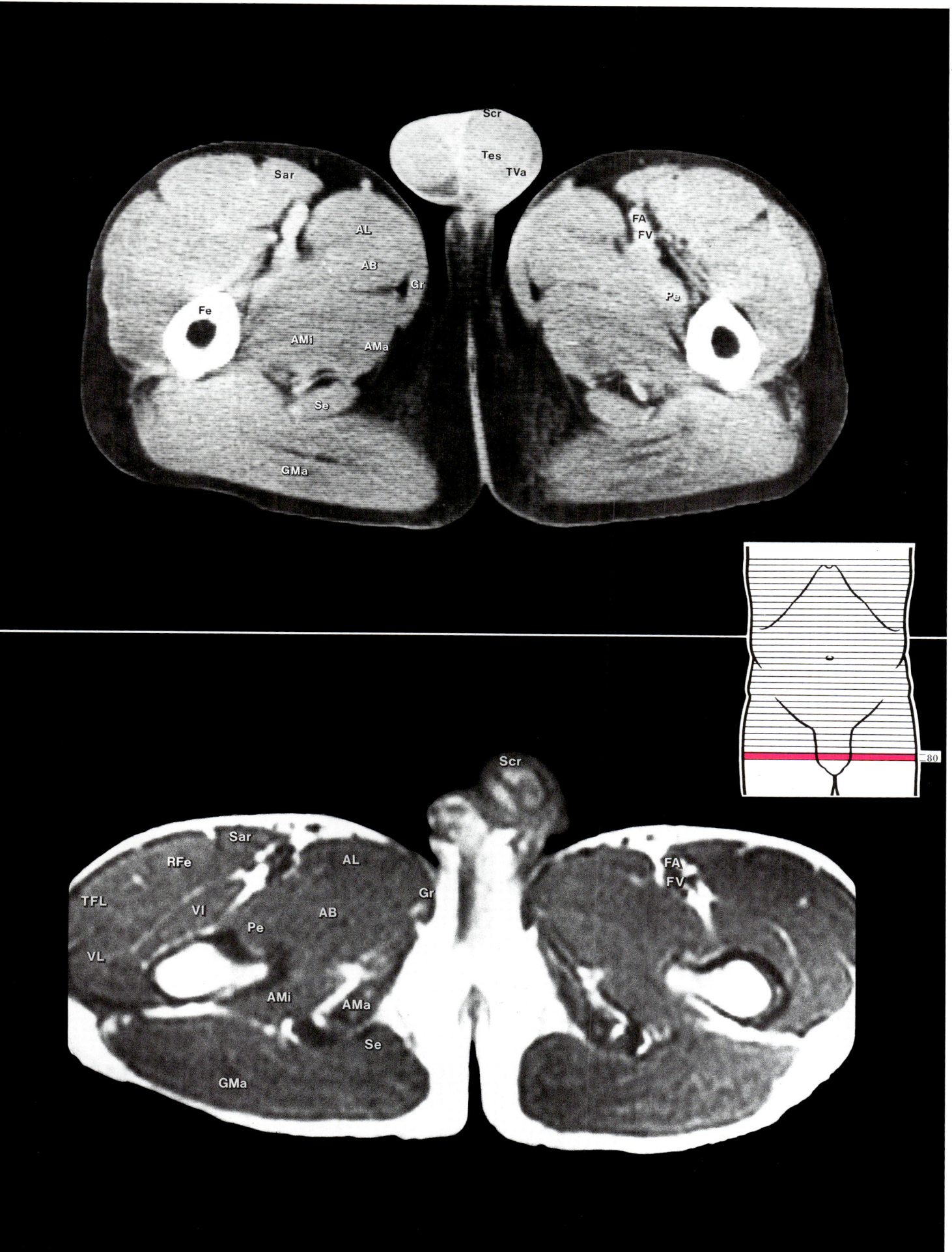

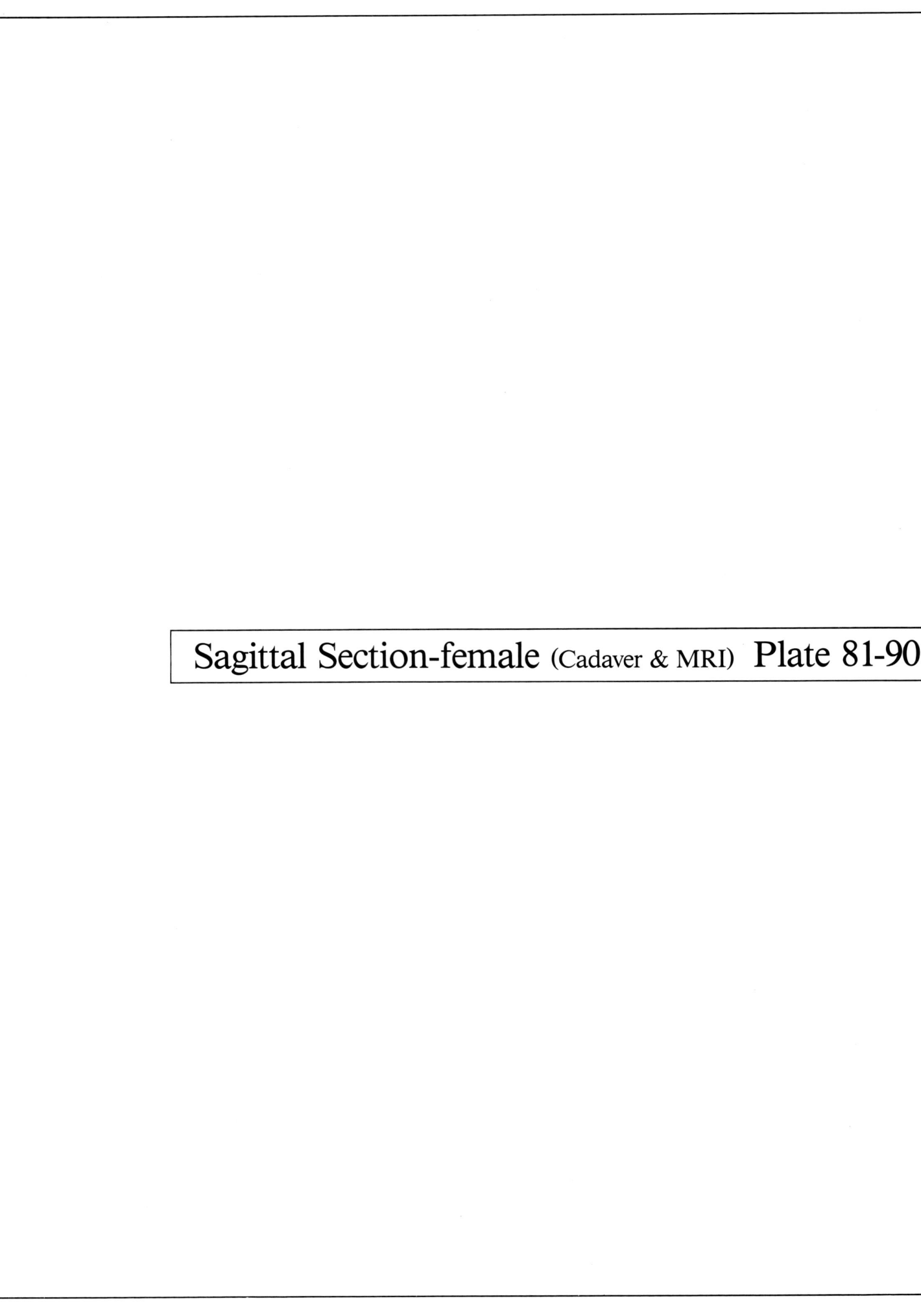

Sagittal Section-female (Cadaver & MRI) Plate 81-90

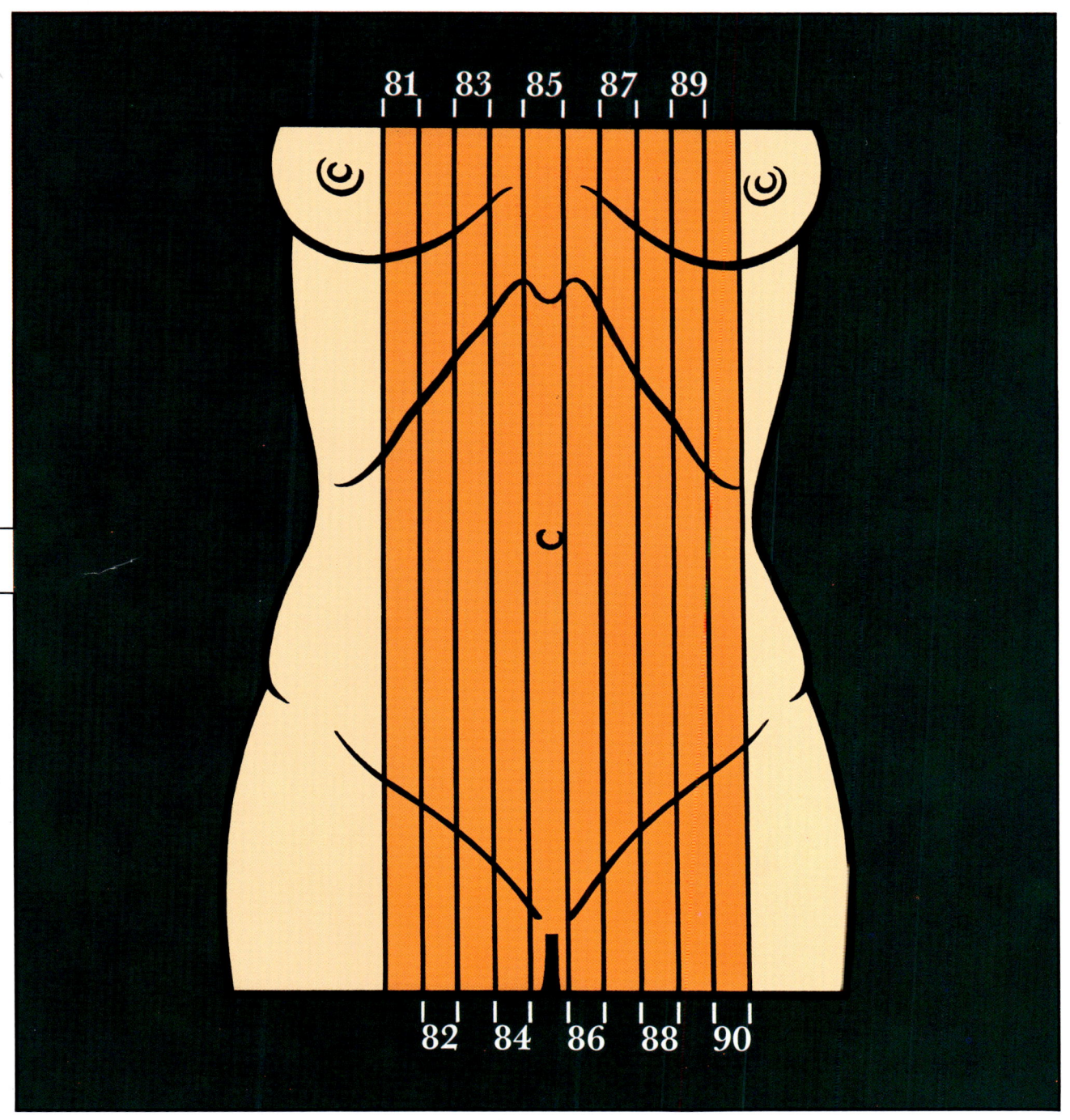

Plate 81. SAGITTAL ABDOMEN AND PELVIS-FEMALE

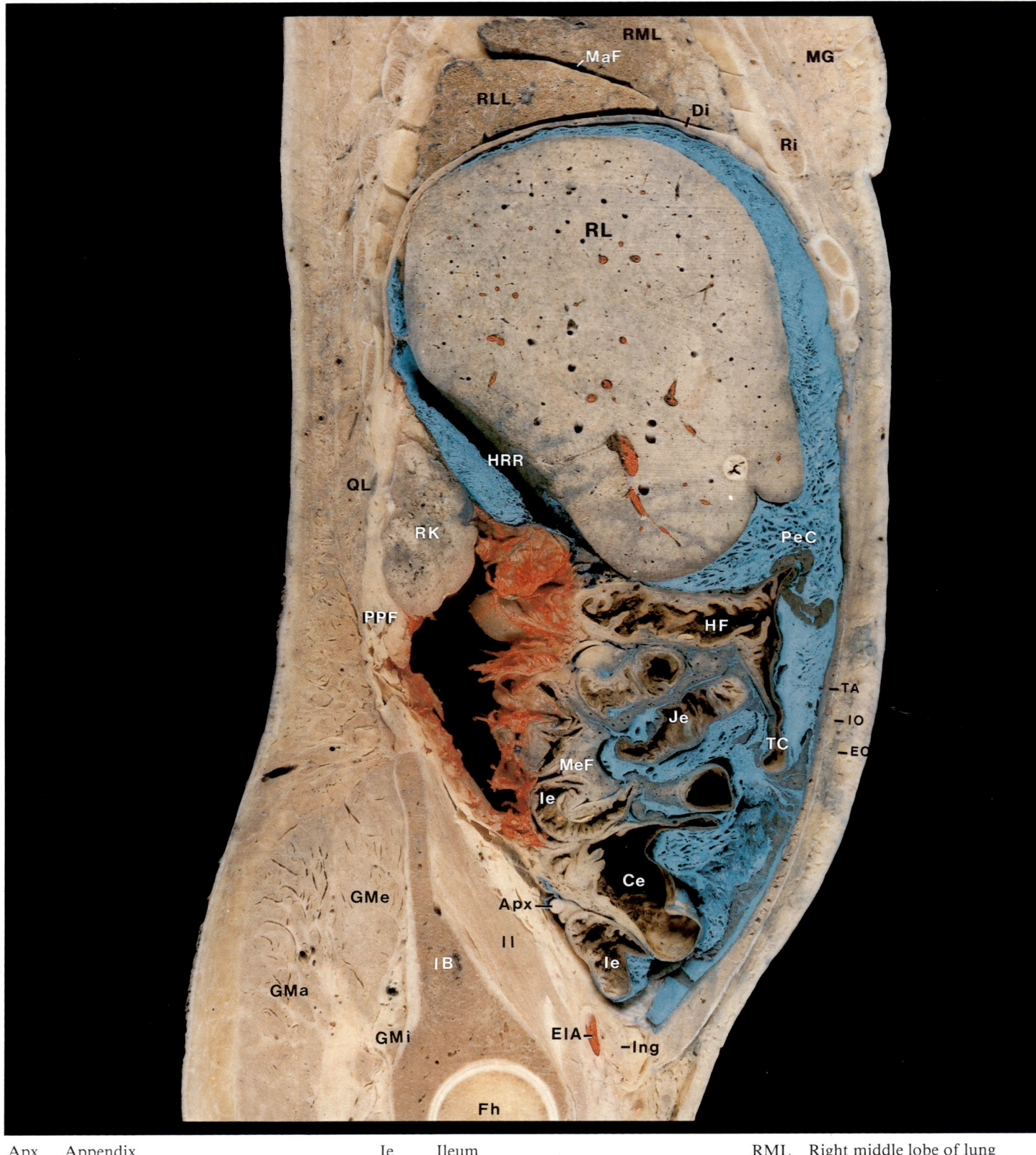

Apx	Appendix	Ie	Ileum	RML	Right middle lobe of lung
Ce	Cecum	Il	Iliacus muscle	Ri	Rib
Di	Diaphragm	Ing	Inguinal ligament	TA	Transversus abdominis muscle
EIA	External iliac artery	Je	Jejunum	TC	Transverse colon
EO	External oblique muscle	MG	Mammary gland		
Fh	Femur, head	MaF	Major fissure		
GMa	Gluteus maximus muscle	MeF	Mesenteric fat		
GMe	Gluteus medius muscle	PPF	Posterior pararenal fat		
GMi	Gluteus minimus muscle	PeC	Peritoneal cavity		
HF	Hepatic flexure of colon	QL	Quadratus lumborum muscle		
HRR	Hepatorenal recess	RK	Right kidney		
IB	Iliac bone	RL	Right lobe of liver		
IO	Internal oblique muscle	RLL	Right lower lobe of lung		

— 180 —

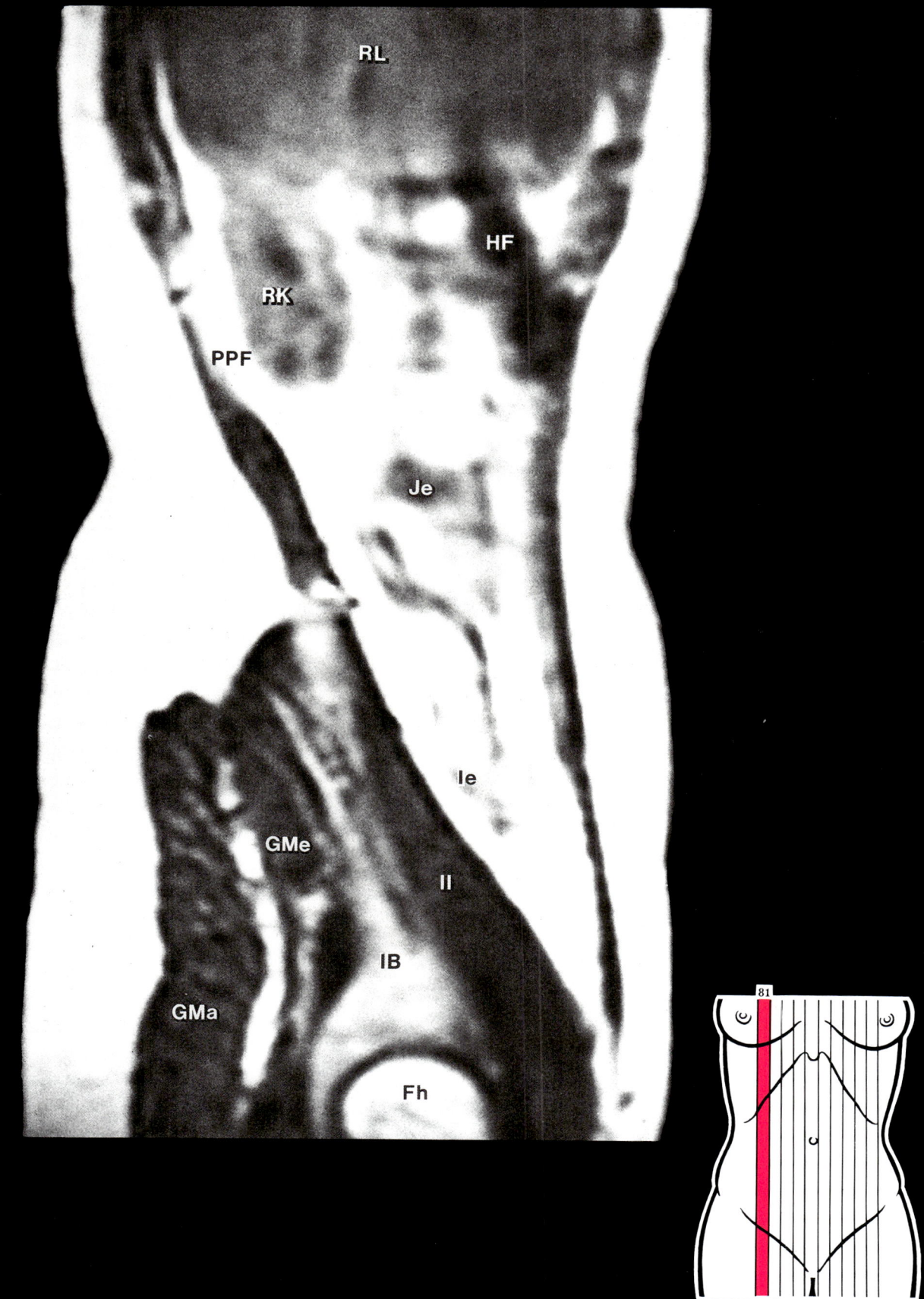

Plate 82. Sagittal ABDOMEN AND PELVIS–female

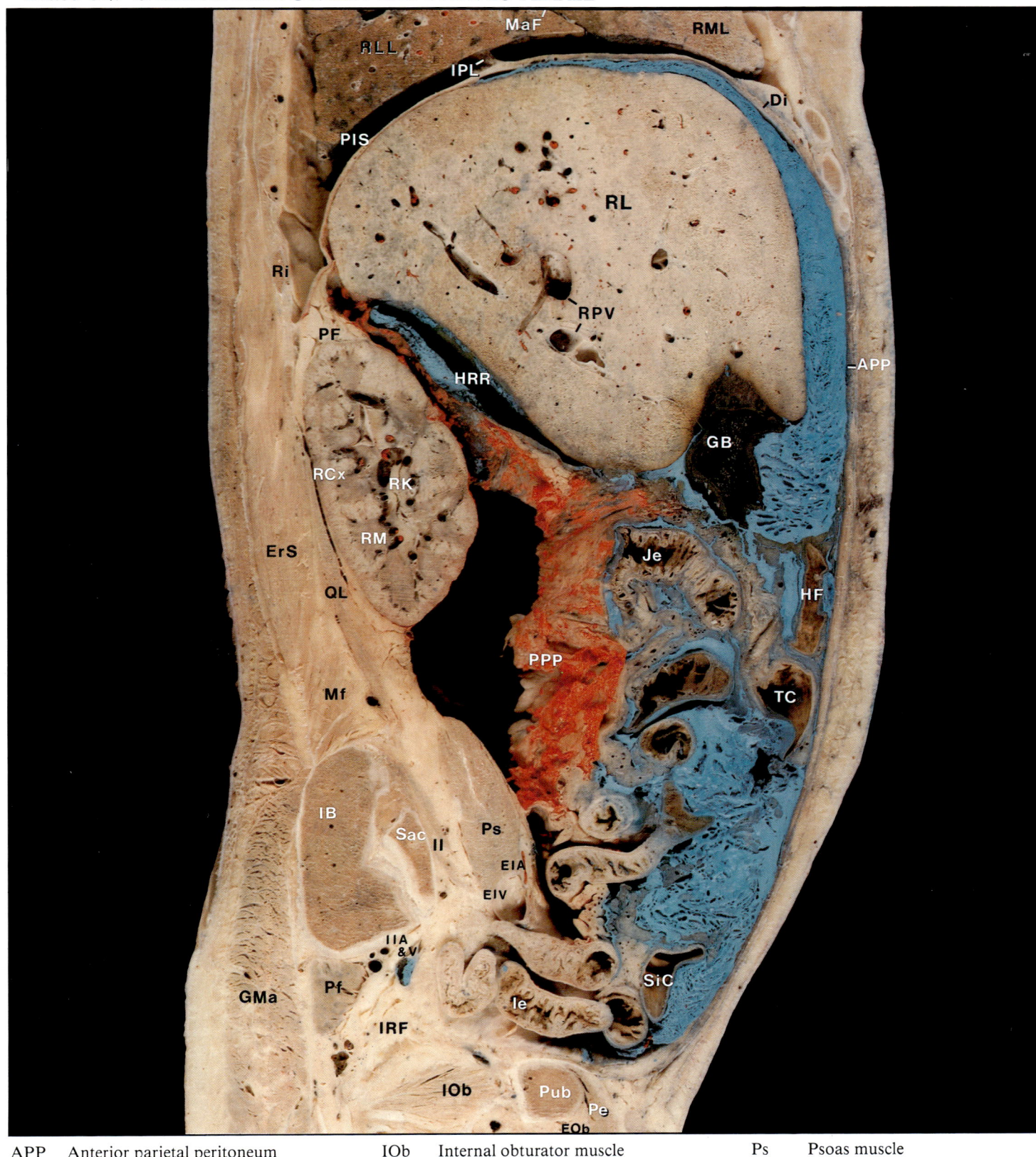

APP	Anterior parietal peritoneum	IOb	Internal obturator muscle	Ps	Psoas muscle
Di	Diaphragm	IPL	Inferior pulmonary ligament	Pub	Pubic bone
EIA	External iliac artery	IRF	Ischiorectal fossa	QL	Quadratus lumborum muscle
EIV	External iliac vein	Ie	Ileum	RCx	Renal cortex
EOb	External obturator muscle	Il	Iliacus muscle	RK	Right kidney
ErS	Erector spinae muscle	Je	Jejunum	RLL	Right lower lobe of lung
GB	Gall bladder	MaF	Major fissure	RM	Renal medulla
GMa	Gluteus maximus muscle	Mf	Multifidus muscle	RML	Right middle lobe of lung
HF	Hepatic flexure of colon	PF	Perirenal fat	RPV	Right portal vein
HRR	Hepatorenal recess	PPP	Posterior parietal peritoneum	Ri	Rib
IB	Iliac bone	Pe	Pectineus muscle	Sac	Sacrum
IIA	Internal iliac artery	Pf	Piriformis muscle	SiC	Sigmoid colon
IIV	Internal iliac vein	PlS	Pleural space	TC	Transverse colon

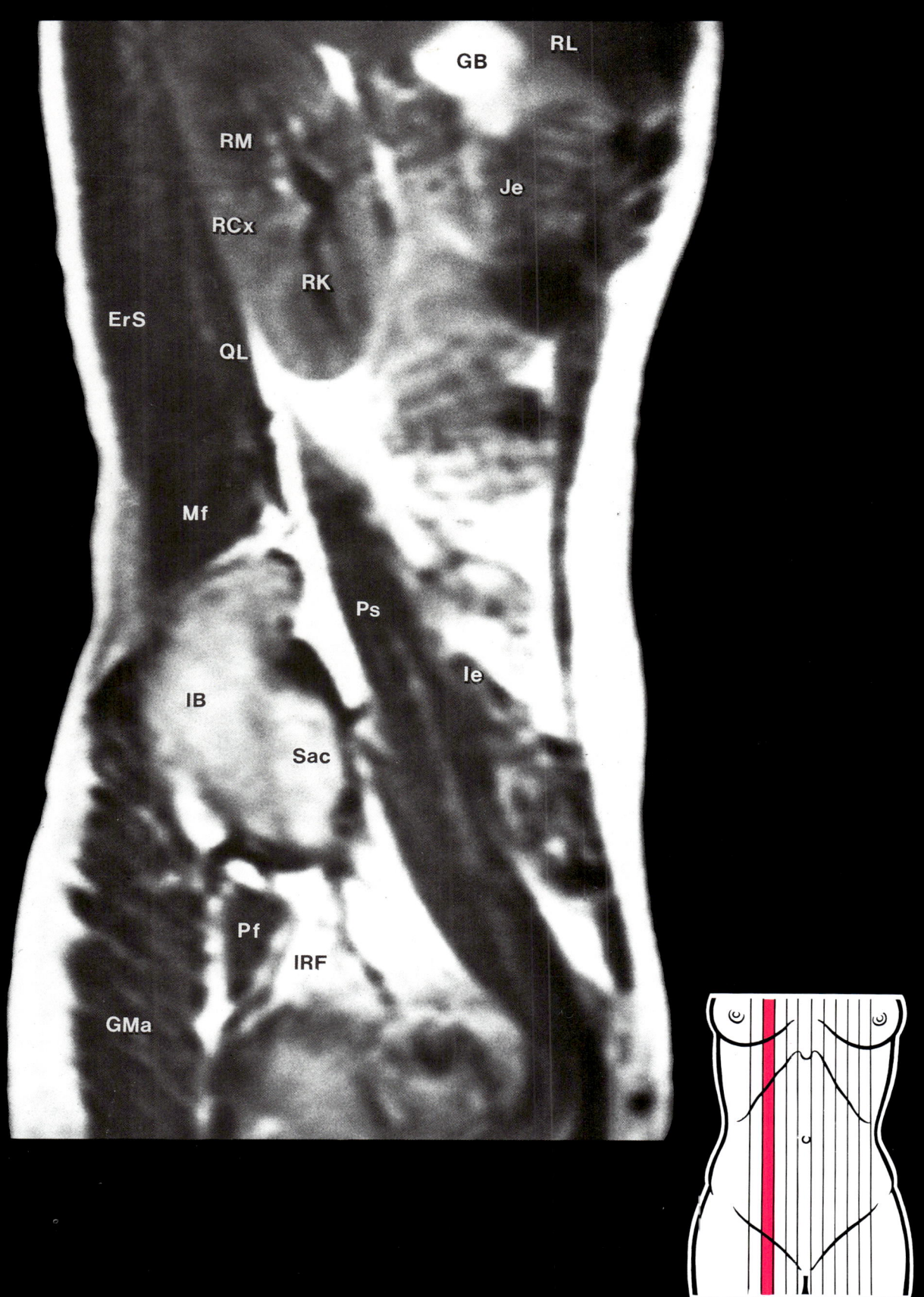

Plate 83. SAGITTAL ABDOMEN AND PELVIS-FEMALE

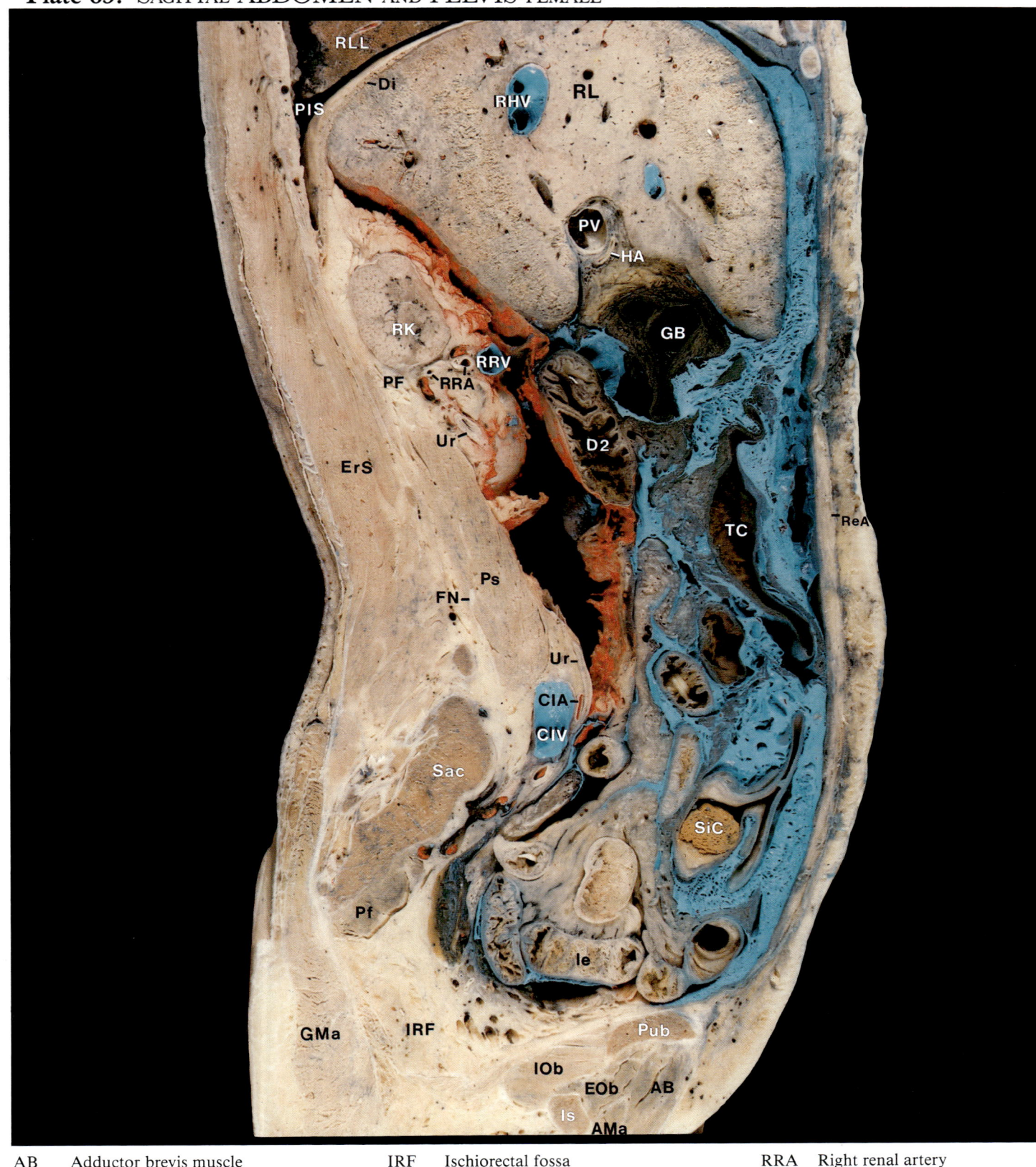

AB	Adductor brevis muscle	IRF	Ischiorectal fossa	RRA	Right renal artery
AMa	Adductor magnus muscle	Ie	Ileum	RRV	Right renal vein
CIA	Common iliac artery	Is	Ischium	ReA	Rectus abdominis muscle
CIV	Common iliac vein	PF	Perirenal fat	Sac	Sacrum
D2	Second portion of duodenum	PV	Portal vein	SiC	Sigmoid colon
Di	Diaphragm	Pf	Piriformis muscle	TC	Transverse colon
EOb	External obturator muscle	PlS	Pleural space	Ur	Ureter
ErS	Erector spinae muscle	Ps	Psoas muscle		
FN	Femoral nerve	Pub	Pubic bone		
GB	Gall bladder	RHV	Right hepatic vein		
GMa	Gluteus maximus muscle	RK	Right kidney		
HA	Hepatic artery	RL	Right lobe of liver		
IOb	Internal obturator muscle	RLL	Right lower lobe of lung		

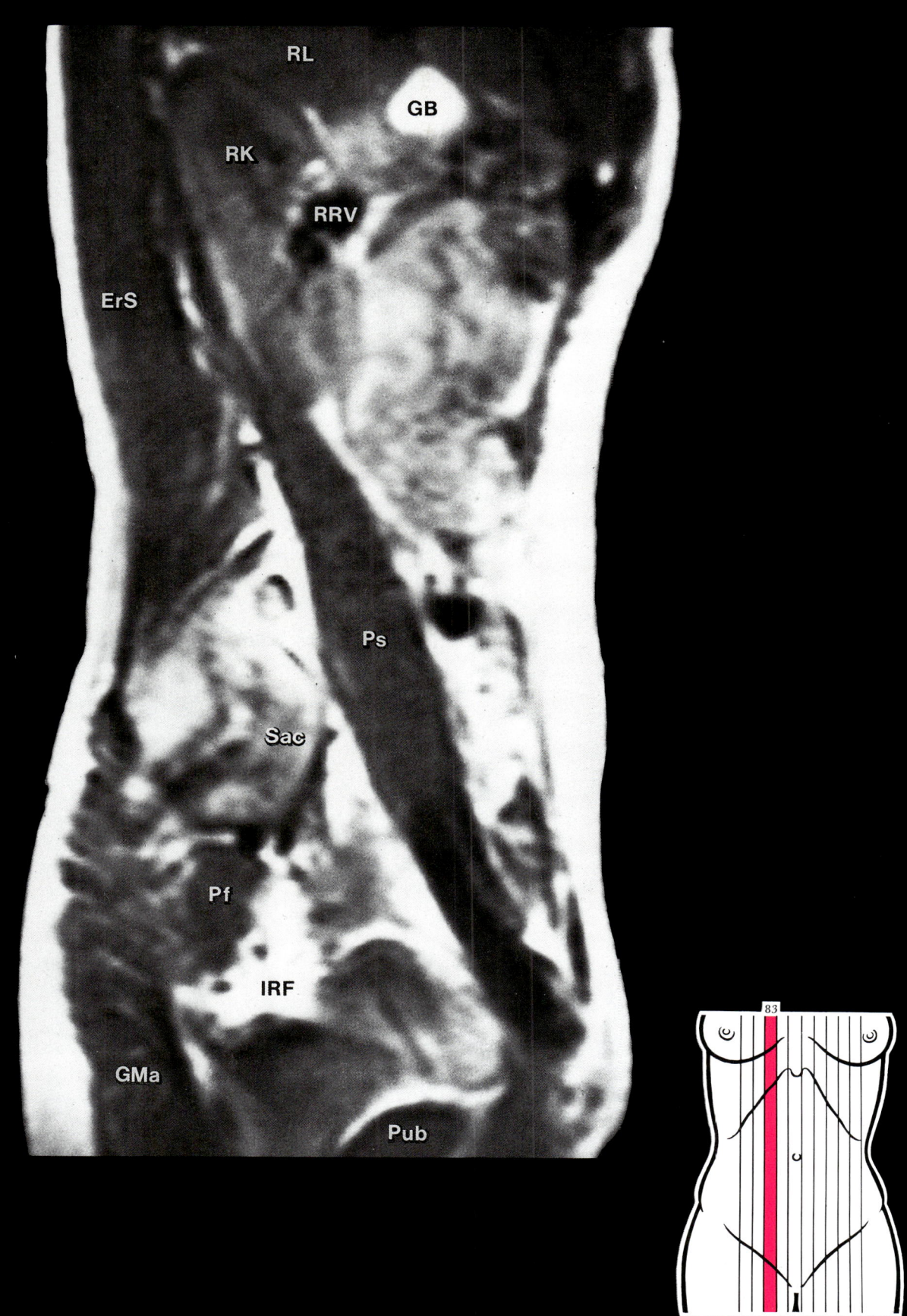

Plate 84. SAGITTAL ABDOMEN AND PELVIS-FEMALE

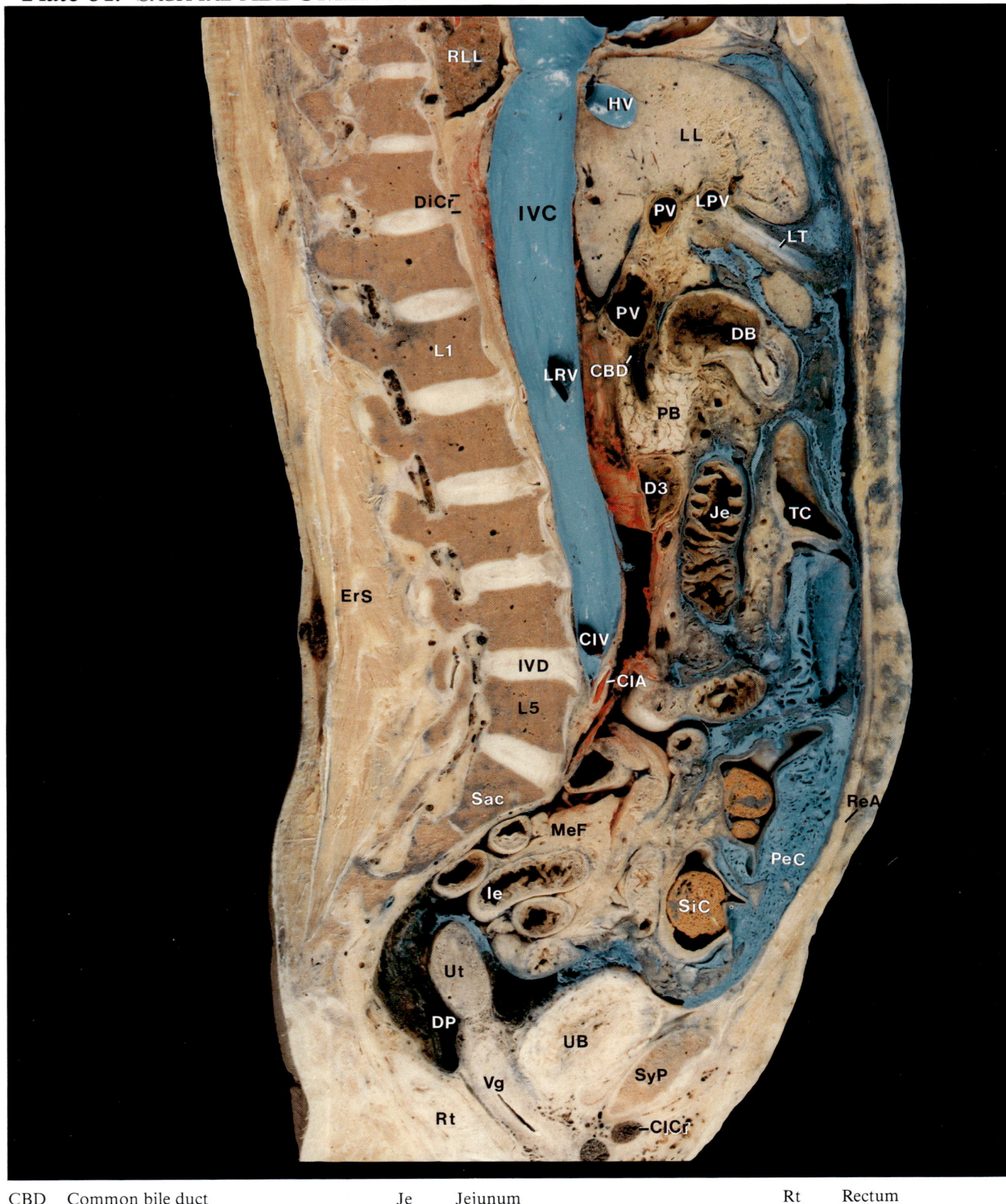

CBD	Common bile duct	Je	Jejunum	Rt	Rectum
CIA	Common iliac artery	L1	L1 vertebral body	Sac	Sacrum
CIV	Common iliac vein	L5	L5 vertebral body	SiC	Sigmoid colon
ClCr	Clitoris, crus	LL	Left lobe of liver	SyP	Symphysis pubis
D3	Third portion of duodenum	LPV	Left portal vein	TC	Transverse colon
DB	Duodenal bulb	LRV	Left renal vein	UB	Urinary bladder
DP	Douglas pouch	LT	Ligamentum teres	Ut	Uterus
DiCr	Diaphragmatic crus	MeF	Mesenteric fat	Vg	Vagina
ErS	Erector spinae muscle	PB	Pancreas, body		
HV	Hepatic vein	PV	Portal vein		
IVC	Inferior vena cava	PeC	Peritoneal cavity		
IVD	Intervertebral disc	RLL	Right lower lobe of lung		
Ie	Ileum	ReA	Rectus abdominis muscle		

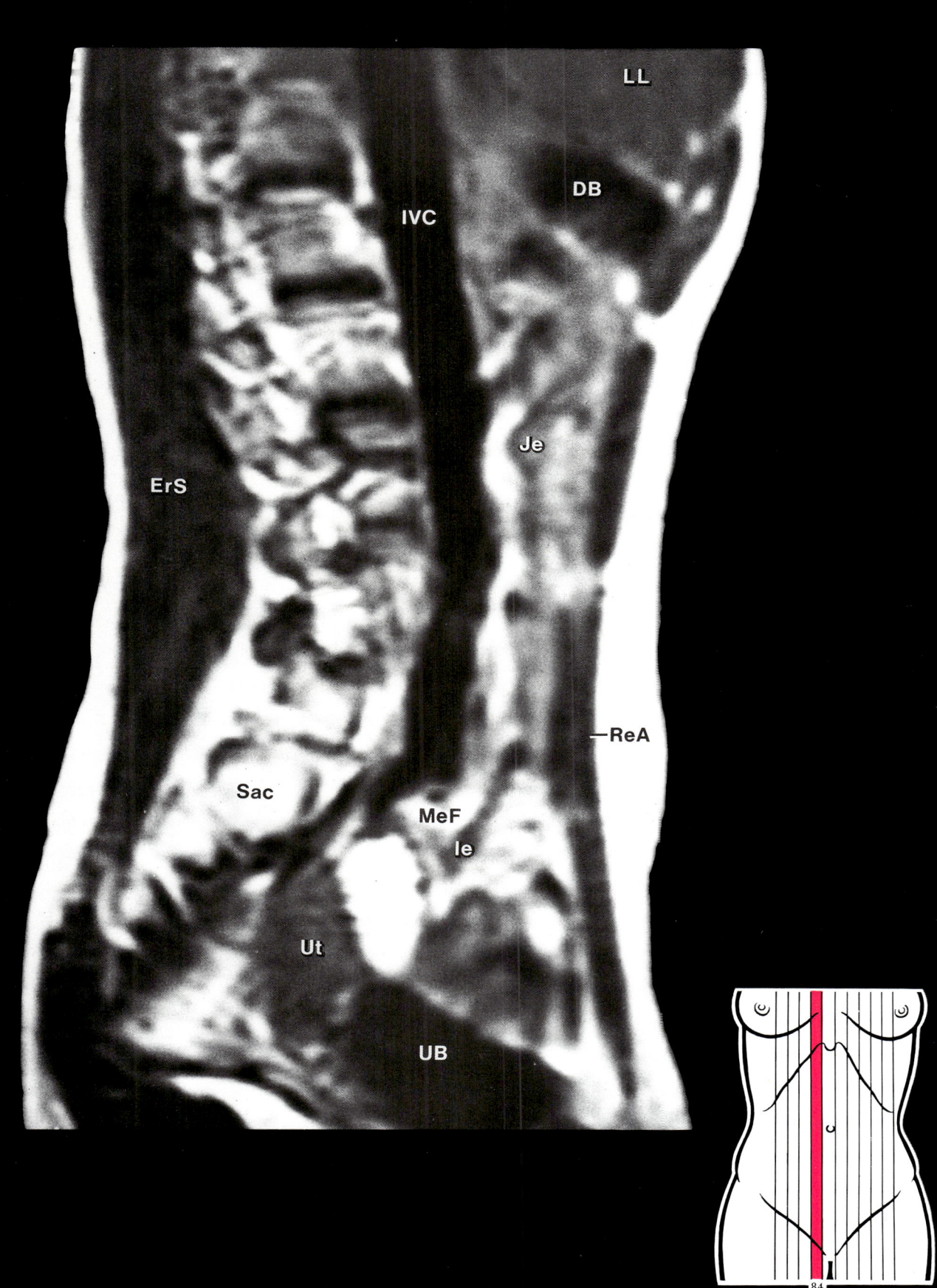

Plate 85. SAGITTAL ABDOMEN AND PELVIS-FEMALE

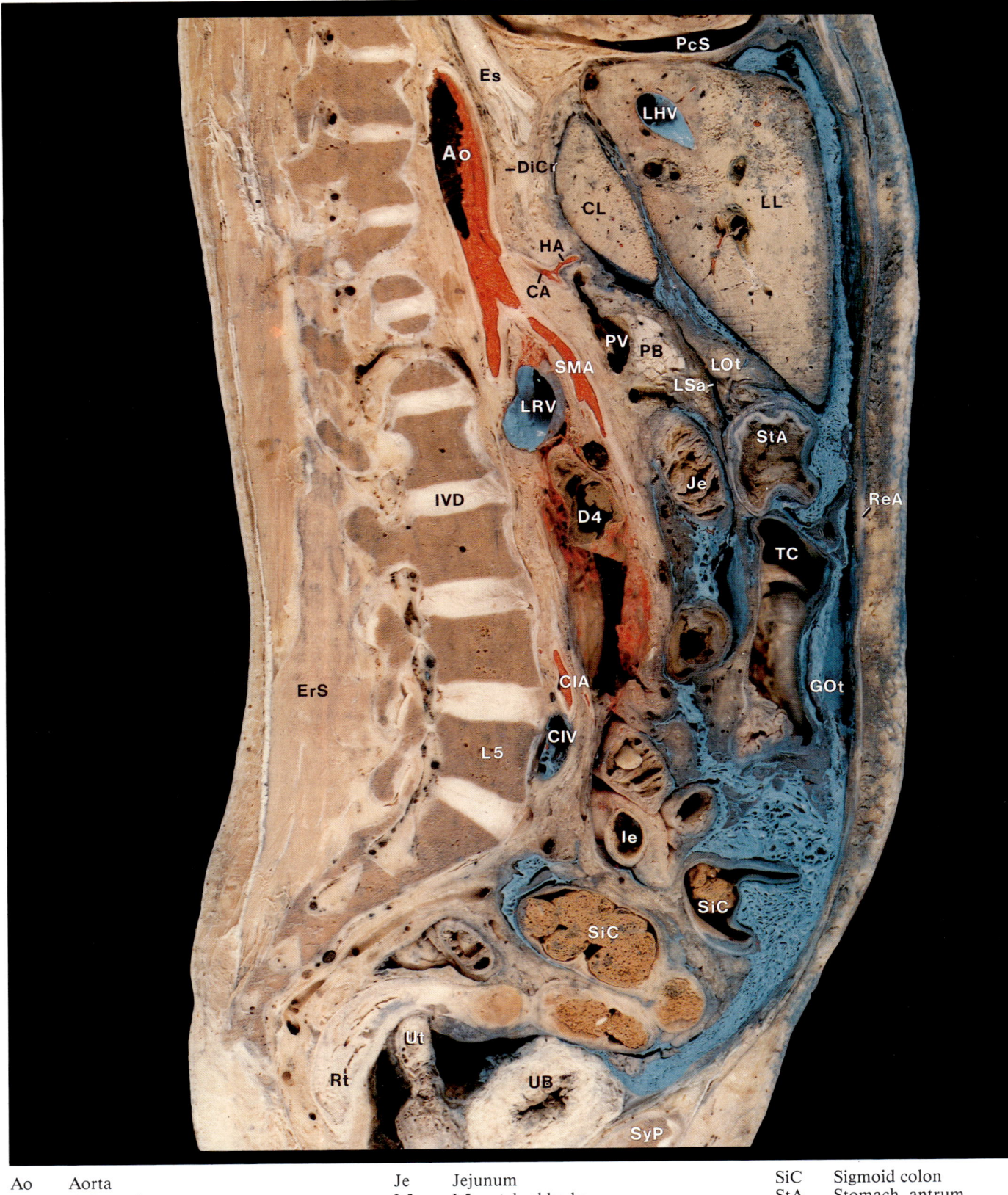

Ao	Aorta	Je	Jejunum	SiC	Sigmoid colon
CA	Celiac axis	L5	L5 vertebral body	StA	Stomach, antrum
CIA	Common iliac artery	LHV	Left hepatic vein	SyP	Symphysis pubis
CIV	Common iliac vein	LL	Left lobe of liver	TC	Transverse colon
CL	Caudate lobe of liver	LOt	Lesser omentum	UB	Urinary bladder
D4	Fourth portion of duodenum	LRV	Left renal vein	Ut	Uterus
DiCr	Diaphragmatic crus	LSa	Lesser sac		
ErS	Erector spinae muscle	PB	Pancreas, body		
Es	Esophagus	PV	Portal vein		
GOt	Greater omentum	PcS	Pericardial space		
HA	Hepatic artery	ReA	Rectus abdominis muscle		
IVD	Intervertebral disc	Rt	Rectum		
Ie	Ileum	SMA	Superior mesenteric artery		

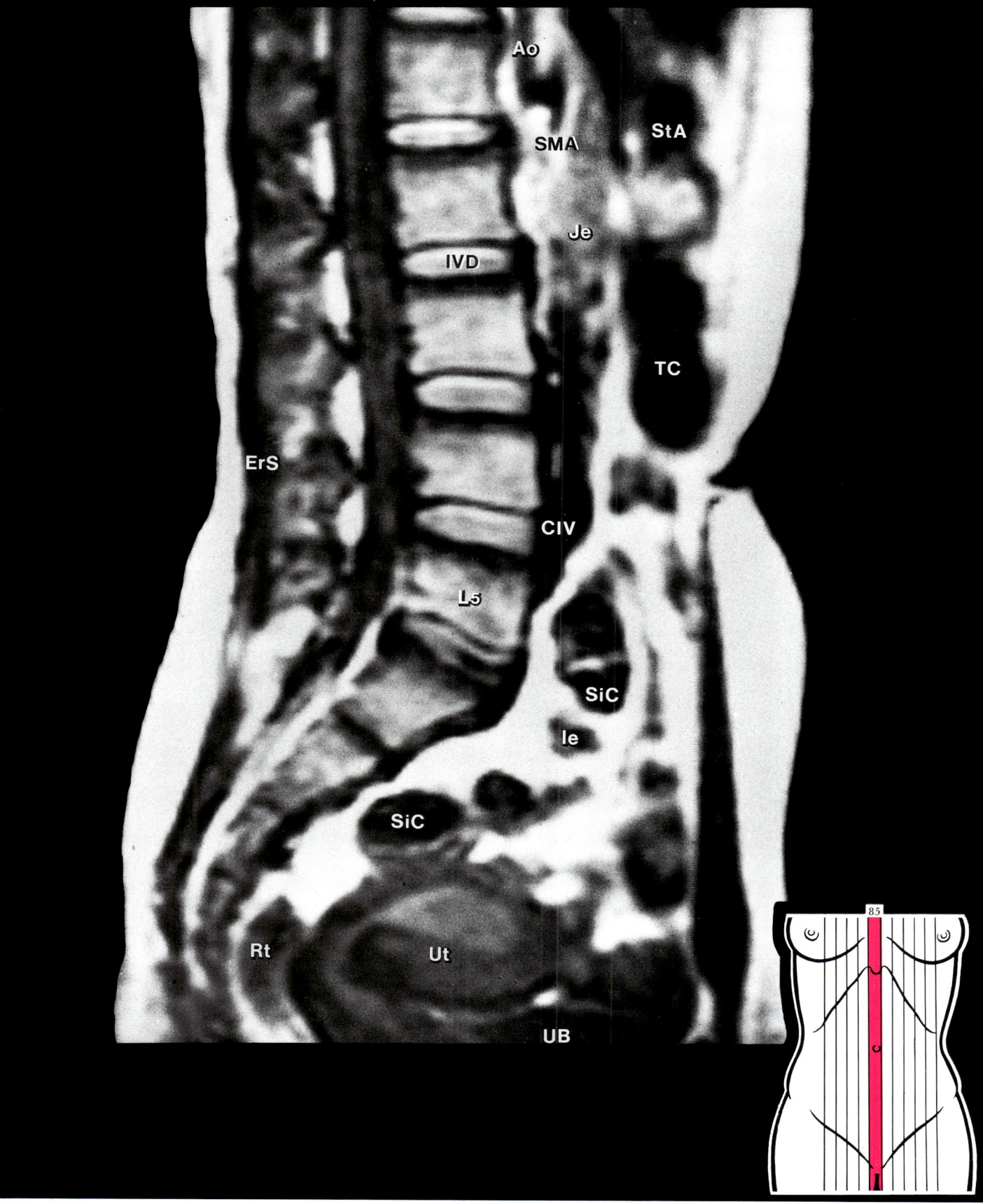

Plate 86. SAGITTAL ABDOMEN AND PELVIS-FEMALE

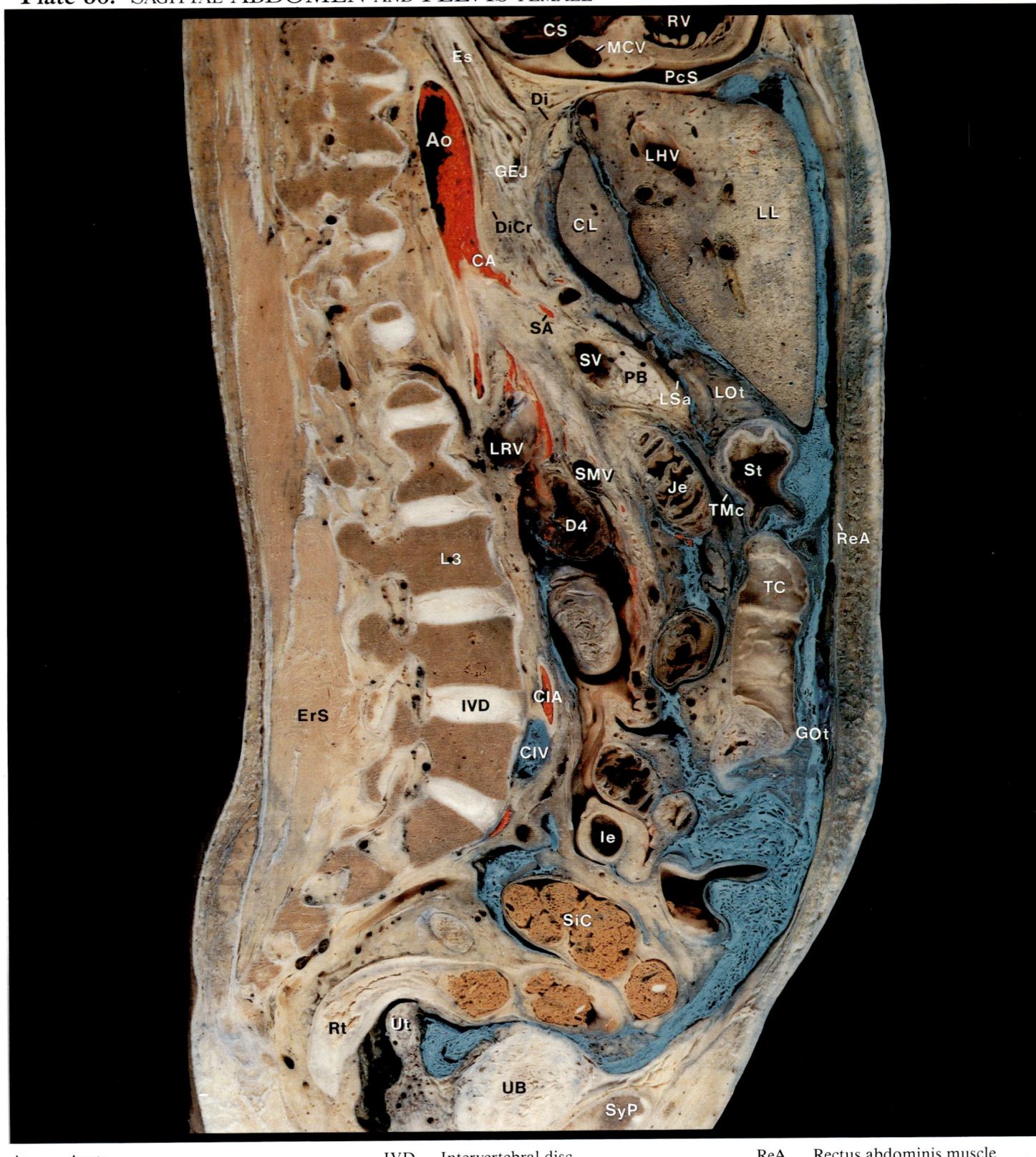

Ao	Aorta	IVD	Intervertebral disc	ReA	Rectus abdominis muscle
CA	Celiac axis	Ie	Ileum	Rt	Rectum
CIA	Common iliac artery	Je	Jejunum	SA	Splenic artery
CIV	Common iliac vein	L3	L3 vertebral body	SMV	Superior mesenteric vein
CL	Caudate lobe of liver	LHV	Left hepatic vein	SV	Splenic vein
CS	Coronary sinus	LL	Left lobe of liver	SiC	Sigmoid colon
D4	Fourth portion of duodenum	LOt	Lesser omentum	St	Stomach
Di	Diaphragm	LRV	Left renal vein	SyP	Symphysis pubis
DiCr	Diaphragmatic crus	LSa	Lesser sac	TC	Transverse colon
ErS	Erector spinae muscle	MCV	Middle cardiac vein	TMc	Transverse mesocolon
Es	Esophagus	PB	Pancreas, body	UB	Urinary bladder
GEJ	Gastroesophageal junction	PcS	Pericardial space	Ut	Uterus
GOt	Greater omentum	RV	Right ventricle of heart		

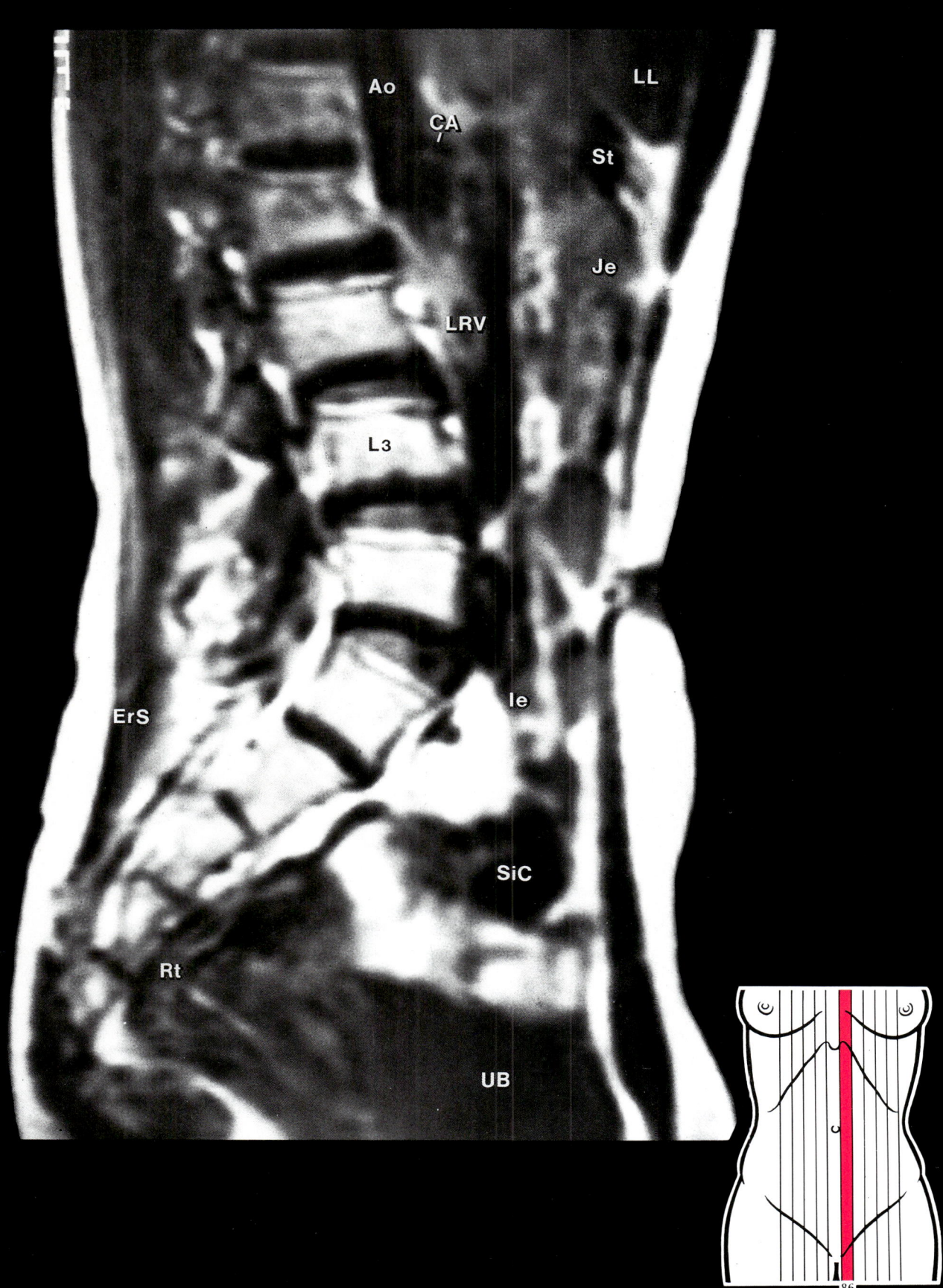

Plate 87. SAGITTAL ABDOMEN AND PELVIS-FEMALE

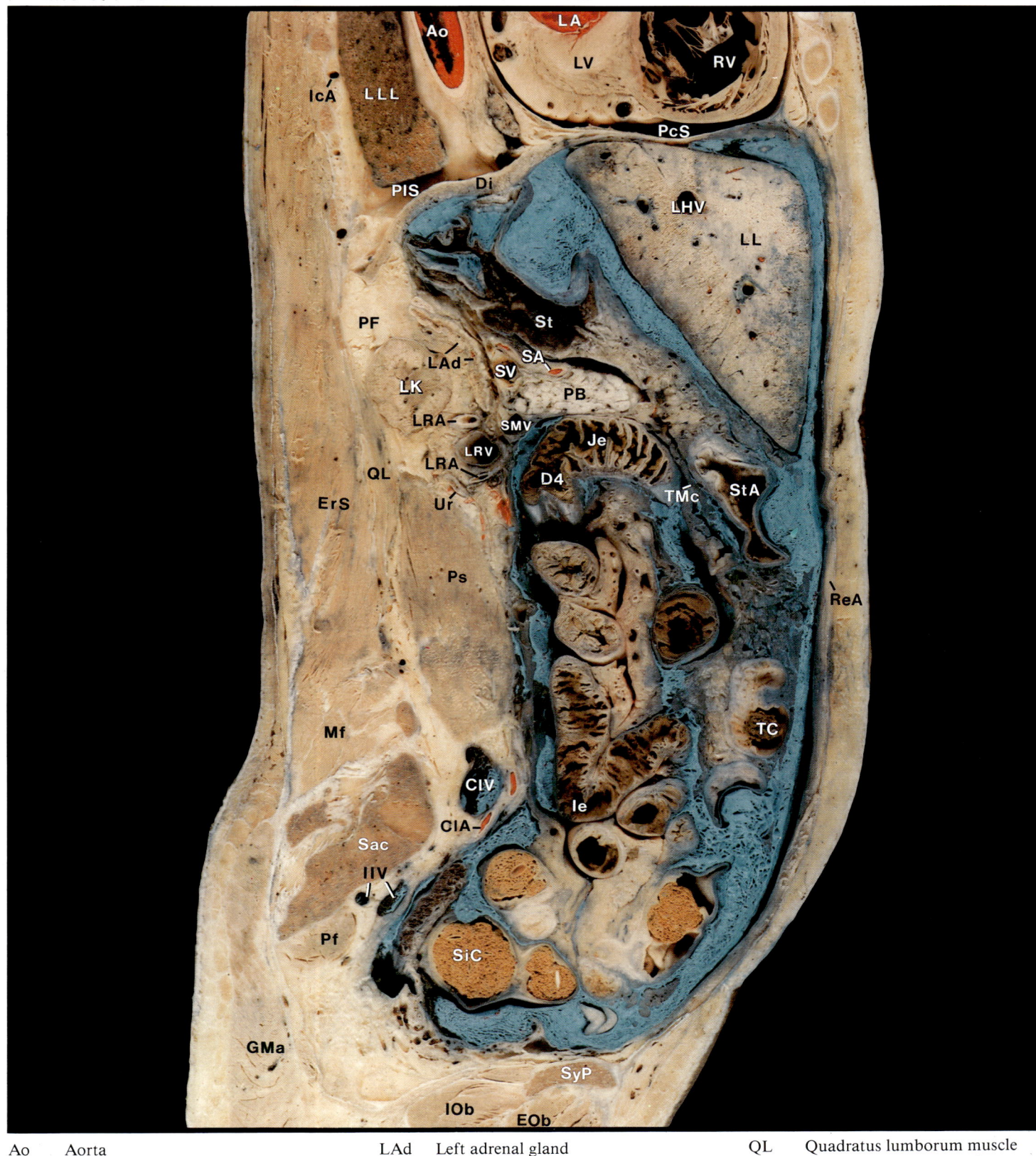

Ao	Aorta	LAd	Left adrenal gland	QL	Quadratus lumborum muscle
CIA	Common iliac artery	LHV	Left hepatic vein	ReA	Rectus abdominis muscle
CIV	Common iliac vein	LK	Left kidney	SA	Splenic artery
D4	Fourth portion of duodenum	LL	Left lobe of liver	SMV	Superior mesenteric vein
Di	Diaphragm	LRA	Left renal artery	SV	Splenic vein
EOb	External obturator muscle	LRV	Left renal vein	Sac	Sacrum
ErS	Erector spinae muscle	LV	Left ventricle of heart	SiC	Sigmoid colon
GMa	Gluteus maximus muscle	Mf	Multifidus muscle	StA	Stomach, antrum
IIV	Internal iliac vein	PB	Pancreas, body	SyP	Symphysis pubis
IOb	Internal obturator muscle	PF	Perirenal fat	TC	Transverse colon
IcA	Intercostal artery	Pf	Piriformis muscle	TMc	Transverse mesocolon
Ie	Ileum	PlS	Pleural space	UB	Urinary bladder
LA	Left atrium of heart	Ps	Psoas muscle	Ur	Ureter

— 192 —

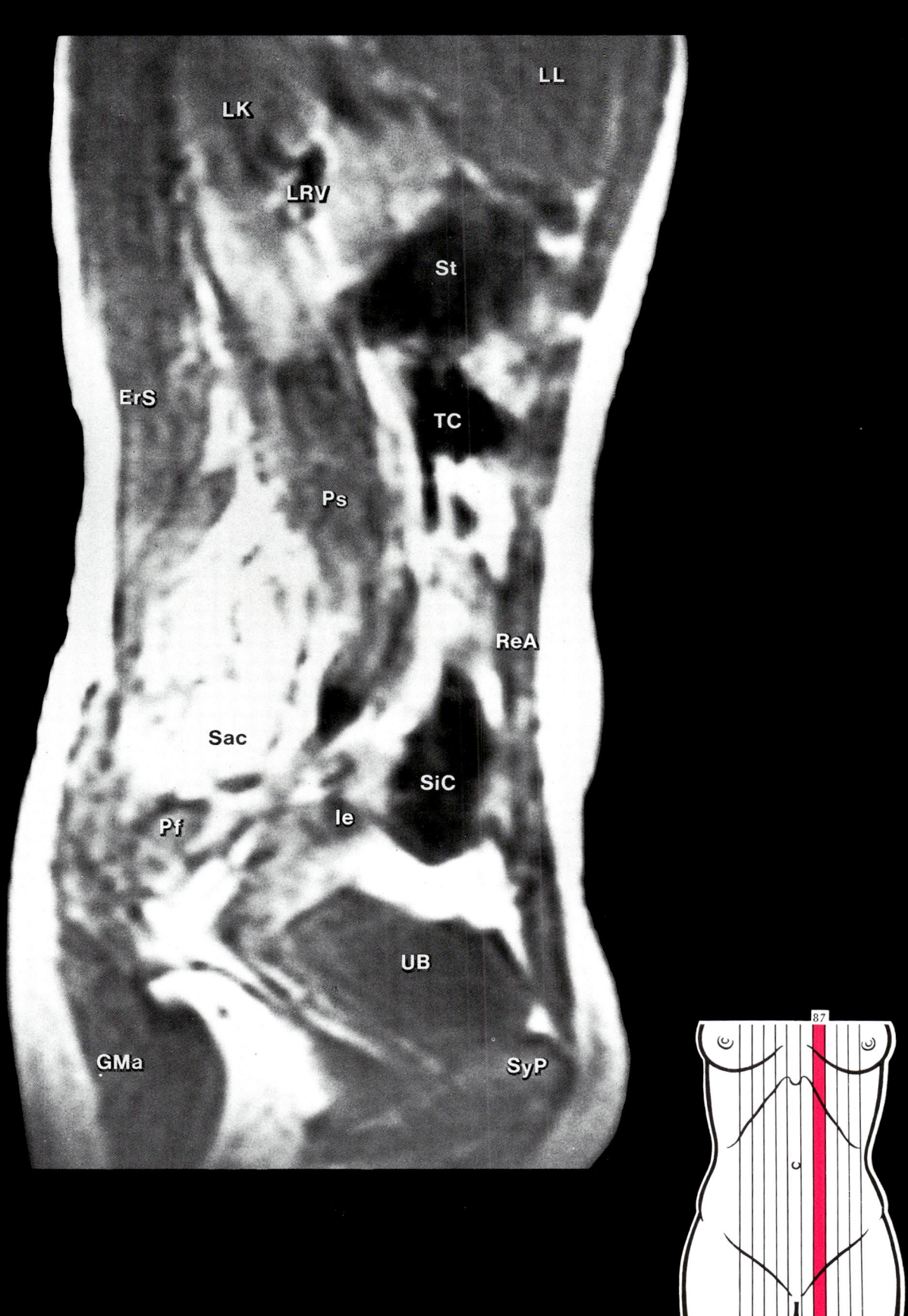

— 193 —

Plate 88. Sagittal ABDOMEN and PELVIS-female

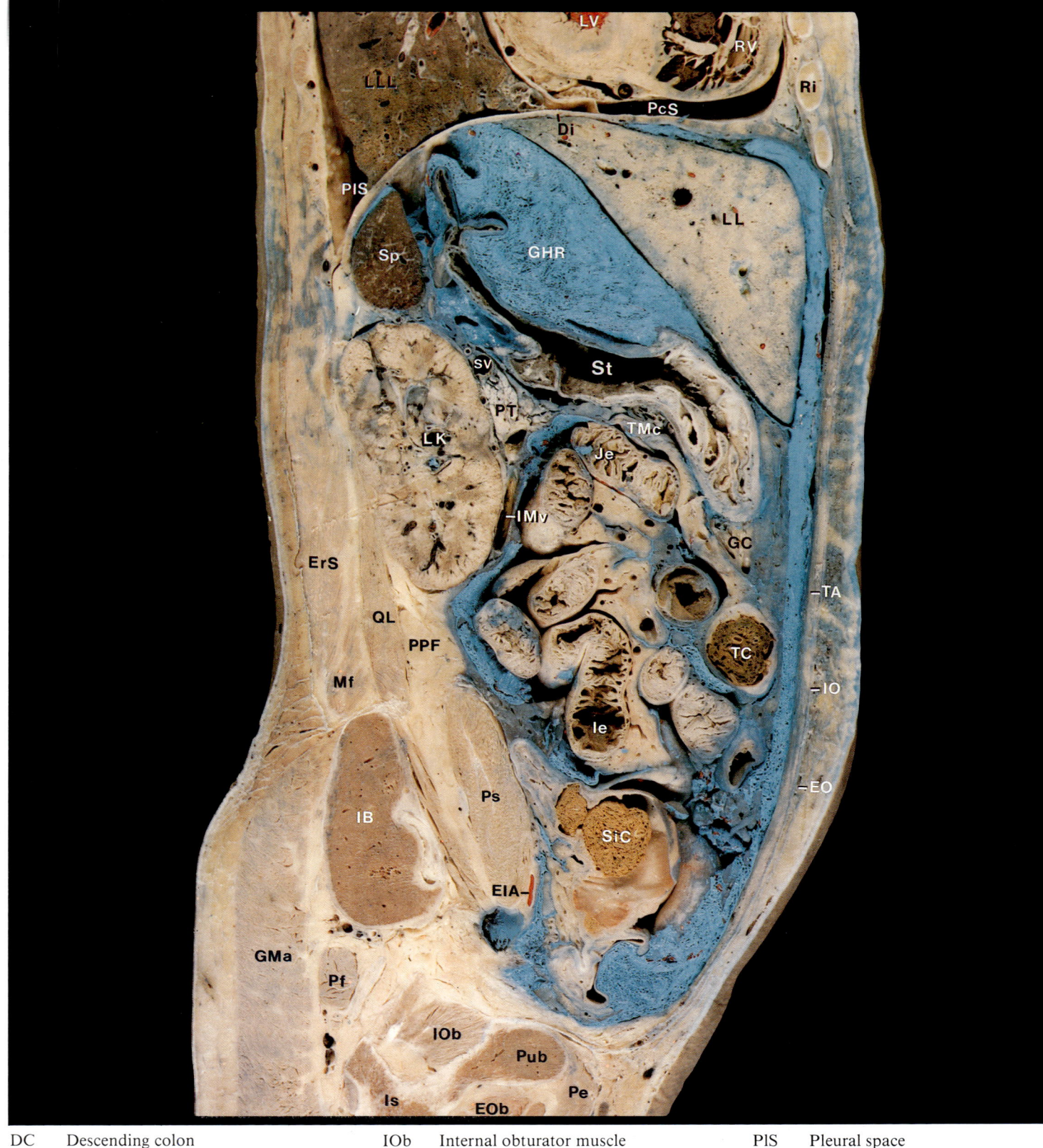

DC	Descending colon	IOb	Internal obturator muscle	PlS	Pleural space
Di	Diaphragm	Is	Ischium	Ps	Psoas muscle
EIA	External iliac artery	Je	Jejunum	Pub	Pubic bone
EO	External oblique muscle	LK	Left kidney	QL	Quadratus lumborum muscle
EOb	External obturator muscle	LL	Left lobe of liver	RV	Right ventricle of heart
ErS	Erector spinae muscle	LLL	Left lower lobe of lung	SV	Splenic vein
GC	Gastrocolic ligament	LV	Left ventricle of heart	SiC	Sigmoid colon
GHR	Gastrohepatic recess	Mf	Multifidus muscle	Sp	Spinalis muscle
GMa	Gluteus maximus muscle	PPF	Posterior pararenal fat	St	Stomach
IB	Iliac bone	PT	Pancreas, tail	SV	Splenic vein
Ie	Ileum	PcS	Pericardial space	TA	Transversus abdominis muscle
IMv	Internal mammary vessel	Pe	Pectineus muscle	TC	Transverse colon
IO	Internal oblique muscle	Pf	Piriformis muscle	TMc	Transverse mesocolon

— 194 —

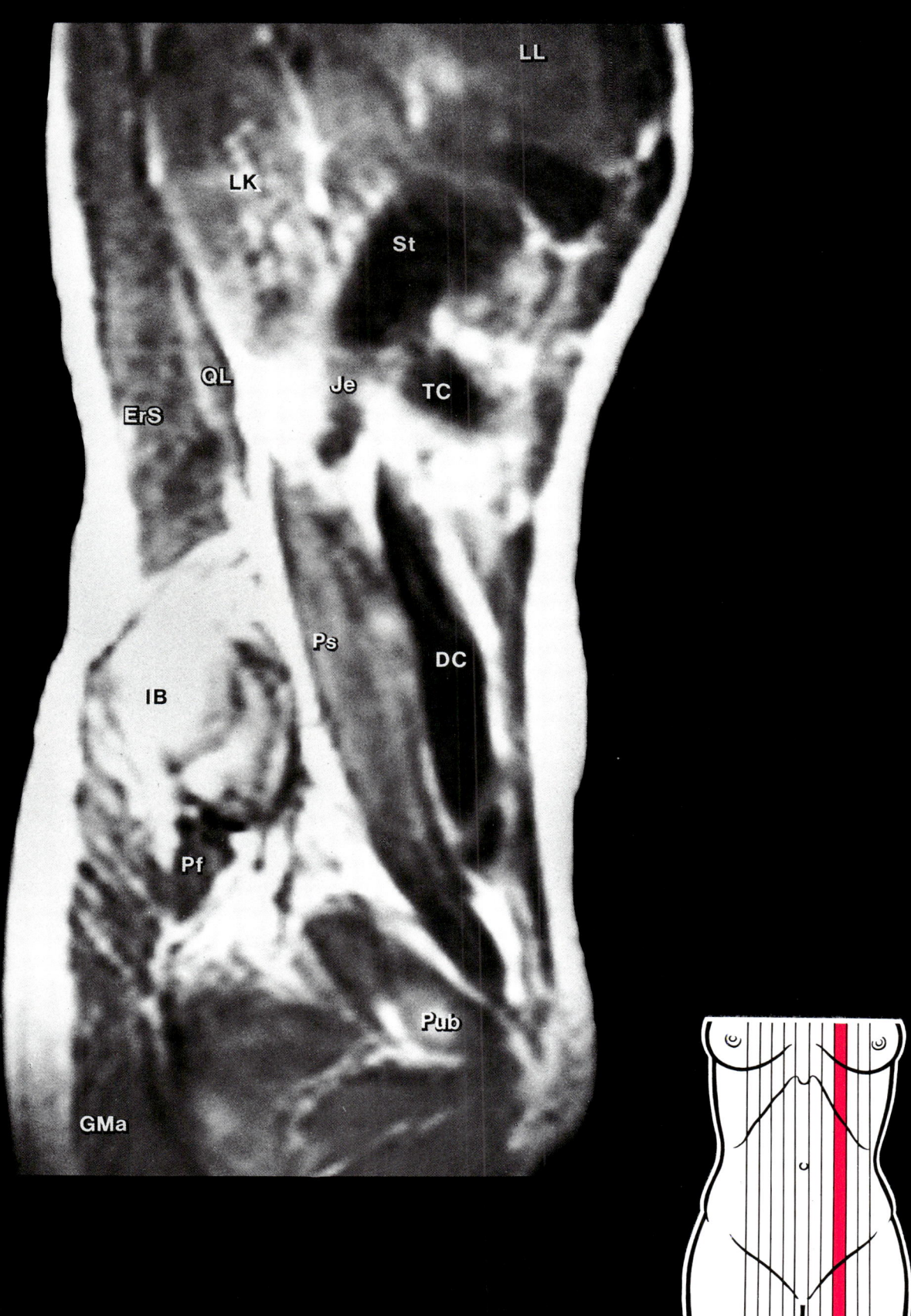

Plate 89. SAGITTAL ABDOMEN AND PELVIS-FEMALE

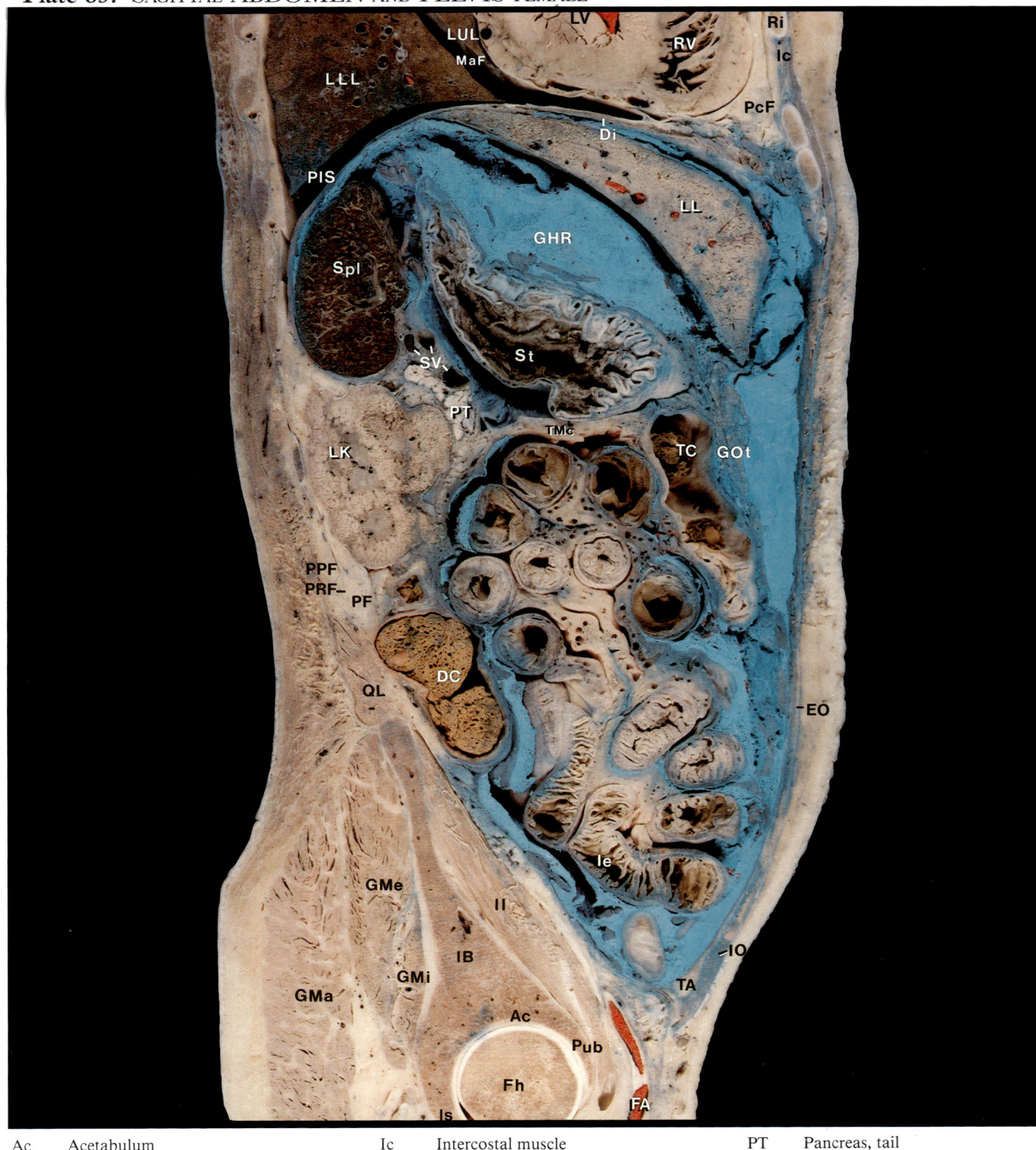

Ac	Acetabulum	Ic	Intercostal muscle	PT	Pancreas, tail
DC	Descending colon	Ie	Ileum	PcF	Pericardial fat
Di	Diaphragm	Il	Iliacus muscle	PlS	Pleural space
EO	External oblique muscle	Is	Ischium	Pub	Pubic bone
FA	Femoral artery	LK	Left kidney	QL	Quadratus lumborum muscle
Fh	Femur, head	LL	Left lobe of liver	RV	Right ventricle of heart
GHR	Gastrohepatic recess	LLL	Left lower lobe of lung	Ri	Rib
GMa	Gluteus maximus muscle	LUL	Left upper lobe of lung	SV	Splenic vein
GMe	Gluteus medius muscle	LV	Left ventricle of heart	Spl	Spleen
GMi	Gluteus minimus muscle	MaF	Major fissure	St	Stomach
GOt	Greater omentum	PF	Perirenal fat	TA	Transversus abdominis muscle
IB	Iliac bone	PPF	Posterior pararenal fat	TC	Transverse colon
IO	Internal oblique muscle	PRF	Posterior renal fascia	TMc	Transverse mesocolon

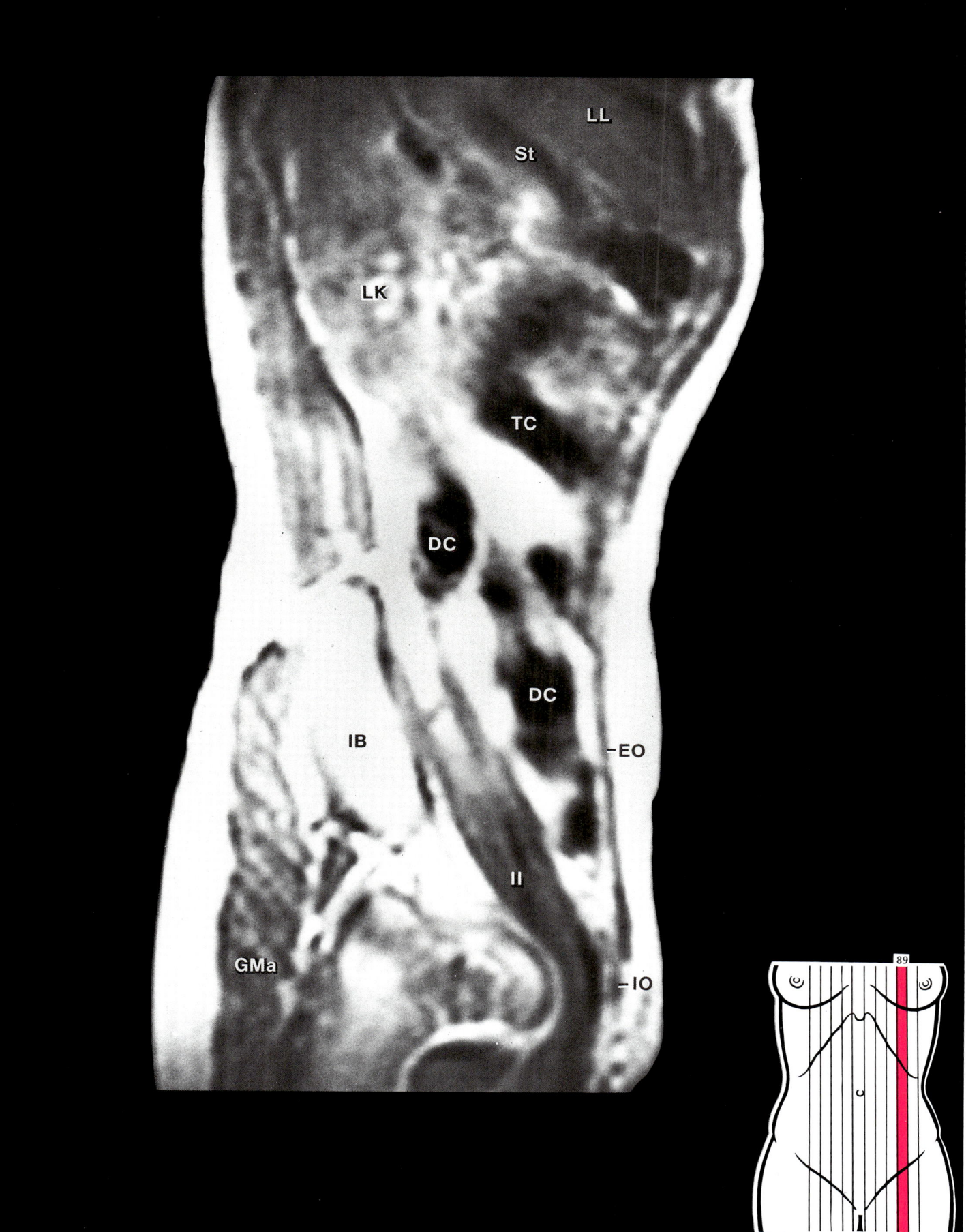

Plate 90. Sagittal ABDOMEN AND PELVIS-female

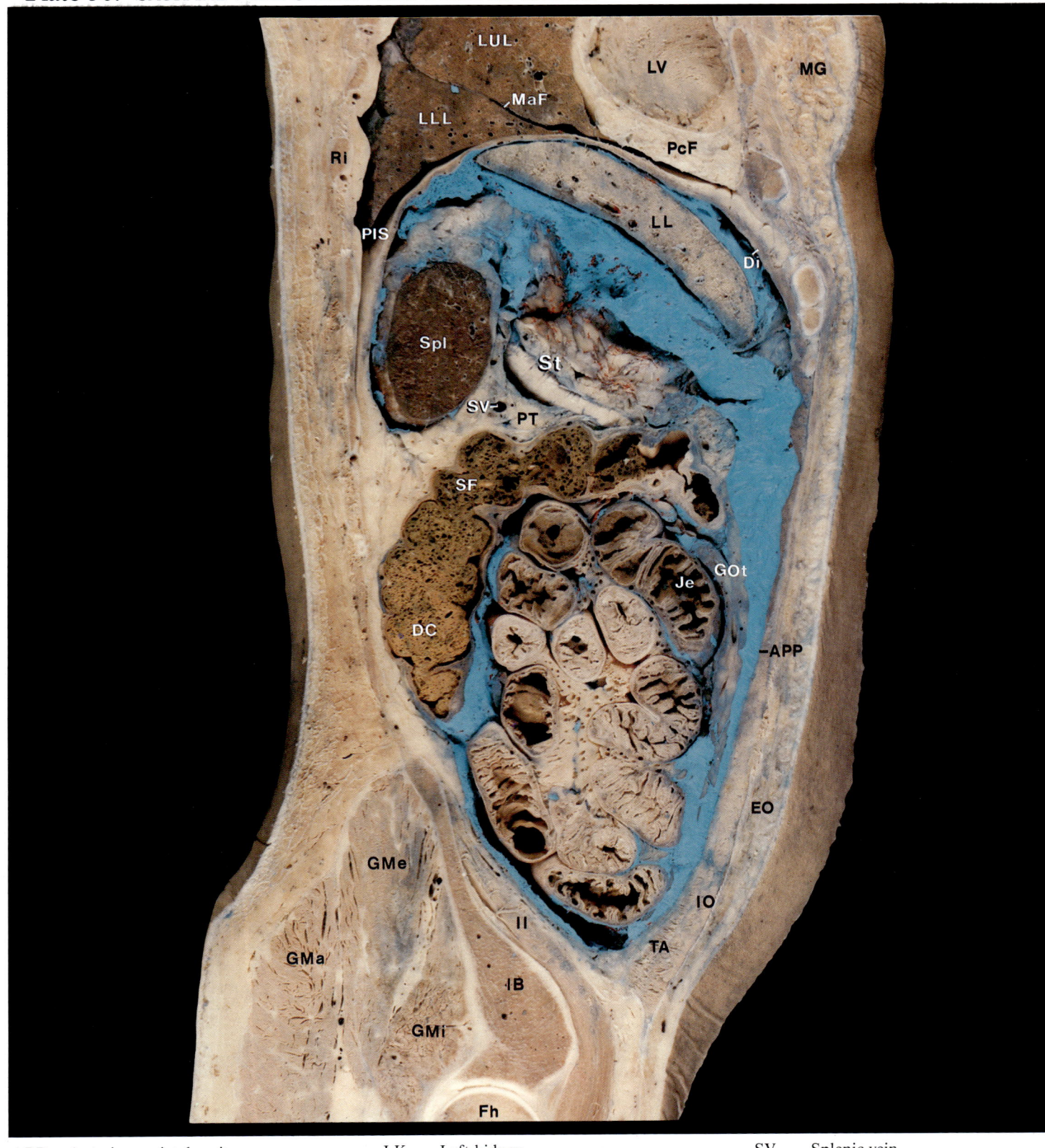

APP	Anterior parietal peritoneum	LK	Left kidney	SV	Splenic vein
DC	Descending colon	LL	Left lobe of liver	Spl	Spleen
Di	Diaphragm	LLL	left lower lobe of lung	St	Stomach
EO	External oblique muscle	LUL	Left upper lobe of lung	TA	Transversus abdominis muscle
Fh	Femur, head	LV	Left ventricle of heart		
GMa	Gluteus maximus muscle	MG	Mammary gland		
GMe	Gluteus medius muscle	MaF	Major fissure		
GMi	Gluteus minimus muscle	PT	Pancreas, tail		
GOt	Greater omentum	PcF	Pericardial fat		
IB	Iliac bone	PlS	Pleural space		
IO	Internal oblique muscle	QL	Quadratus lumborum muscle		
Il	Iliacus muscle	Ri	Rib		
Je	Jejunum	SF	Splenic flexure		

— 199 —

INDEX

Acetabulum	寬骨臼	관골구	Ac	162, 166, 196
Acoustic nerve	聽神經	청신경	AN	20, 54
Adductor minimus muscle	內轉小筋	내전소근	AMi	172~176
Adductor brevis muscle	內轉短筋	내전단근	AB	170~176, 184
Adductor longus muscle	內轉長筋	내전장근	AL	170~176
Adductor magnus muscle	內轉大筋	내전대근	AMa	174~176, 184
Ambient cistern	周圍大槽	주위대조	AmC	14, 54
Amygdala	扁桃核	편도핵	Amy	52
Angular gyrus	角回	각회	Ang	6~8, 58~60, 72
Anterior cerebral artery	前腦動脈	전뇌동맥	ACA	16, 43~50
Anterior chamber of globe	眼球前房	안구전방	ACG	18
Anterior clinoid process	前床突起	전상돌기	ACP	48
Anterior commissure of larynx	喉頭前聯合	후두전연합	ACo	34, 50
Anterior pararenal space	前腎傍腔	전신방강	APS	134, 138~144
Anterior parietal peritoneum	前壁側腹膜	전벽측복막	APP	182, 198
Anterior renal fascia	前腎膜	전신막	ARF	124~144
Anterior sacroiliac ligament	前薦腸骨靱帶	전천장골인대	ASL	150
Anterior scalene muscle	前斜角筋	전사각근	AS	30~40
Anteromedial basal segment of lung	前內基底肺分節	전내기저폐분절	AMB	88
Aorta	大動脈	대동맥	Ao	78~94, 102~104, 114~146, 188~192
Aortic valve	大動脈瓣膜	대동맥판막	AV	88, 104
Apical segment of right upper lobe bronchus	右上葉氣管枝尖分節	우상엽기관지첨분절	Ap	80
Appendix	蟲樣突起	충양돌기	Apx	180
Aqueduct of Sylvius	실비우스導水管	실비우스도수관	Aq	64
Archnoid membrane	蜘蛛膜	지주막	Ara	4, 52
Artery	**動脈**	**동맥**		
anterior cerebral artery	前腦動脈	전뇌동맥	ACA	16, 48~50
axillary artery	腋窩動脈	액와동맥	AxA	78~80
basilar artery	腦底動脈	뇌저동맥	BA	16, 52, 64~66
common carotid artery	總頸動脈	총경동맥	CCA	30~40, 54~56
common hepatic artery	總肝動脈	총간동맥	CHA	126
common iliac artery	總腸骨動脈	총장골동맥	CIA	148~152, 184~192
deep circumflex iliac artery	深腸骨回旋動脈	심장골회선동맥	DCIA	160
deep femoral artery	深大腿動脈	심대퇴동맥	DFA	170~176
external carotid artery	外頸動脈	외경동맥	ECA	24, 28~32
external iliac artery	外腸骨動脈	외장골동맥	EIA	150~162, 180~182, 194
femoral artery	大腿動脈	대퇴동맥	FA	164~168, 172~176, 196
gastroduodenal artery	胃十二指腸動脈	위십이지장동맥	GDA	128
hepatic artery	肝動脈	간동맥	HA	118, 124~126, 184, 188
inferior epigastric artery	下腹壁動脈	하복벽동맥	IEA	150~152, 162
inferior gluteal artery	下臀動脈	하둔동맥	IGA	160~164
inferior mesenteric artery	下腸間膜動脈	하장간막동맥	IMA	144~148
inferior phrenic artery	下橫隔動脈	하횡격동맥	InPA	114~122, 126
inferior vesical artery	下膀胱動脈	하방광동맥	IVA	160~162
innominate artery	無名動脈	무명동맥	InA	78, 100~102
intercostal artery	肋間動脈	늑간동맥	IcA	104, 108 116~118, 192
internal carotid artery	內頸動脈	내경동맥	ICA	16~32, 50~54
internal iliac artery	內腸骨動脈	내장골동맥	IIA	150~158, 182
internal pudendal artery	內陰動脈	내음동맥	IPA	164
lateral femoral circumflex artery	外側大腿骨廻旋動脈	외측대퇴골회선동맥	LFCA	168, 172~174
left anterior descending branch of left coronary artery	左冠狀動脈 左前下行枝	좌관상동맥 좌전하행지	LAD	86~90
left circumflex artery	左廻旋動脈	좌회선동맥	LCx	90~92
left common carotid artery	左總頸動脈	좌총경동맥	LCCA	78, 104
left coronary artery	左冠狀動脈	좌관상동맥	LCA	84~88, 104~108
left descending pulmonary artery	左下行肺動脈	좌하행폐동맥	LDPA	84
left gastric artery	左胃動脈	좌위동맥	LGA	114, 118~124
left pulmonary artery	左肺動脈	좌폐동맥	LPA	82, 86, 104~106
left renal artery	左腎動脈	좌신동맥	LRA	132~138, 192

left subclavian artery	左鎖骨下動脈	좌쇄골하동맥	LScA	104~108
main pulmonary artery	主肺動脈	주폐동맥	MPA	82~84
middle cerebral artery	中大腦動脈	중대뇌동맥	MCA	14~16, 48
obturator artery	閉鎖動脈	폐쇄동맥	ObA	162~166
pericallosal artery	腦梁周圍動脈	뇌량주위동맥	PcA	10, 14, 50, 64
posterior cerebral artery	後大腦動脈	후대뇌동맥	PCA	16, 52~54
right coronary artery	右冠狀動脈	우관상동먁	RCA	88~92, 102
right descending pulmonary artery	右下行肺動脈	우하행폐동맥	RDPA	84~86, 98~100
right hepatic artery	右肝動脈	우간동맥	RHA	122
right pulmonary artery	右肺動脈	우폐동맥	RPA	88, 100~104
right renal artery	右腎動脈	우신동맥	RRA	132~136
right subclavian artery	右鎖骨下動脈	우쇄골하등맥	RScA	98
splenic artery	脾動脈	비동맥	SA	102, 124~126, 190~192
subclavian artery	鎖骨下動脈	쇄골하동댁	ScA	40, 78
superficial femoral artery	淺大腿動脈	천대퇴동댁	SFA	170~172
superior cerebellar artery	上小腦動脈	상소뇌동맥	SCA	53
superior gluteal artery	上臀動脈	상둔동맥	SGA	152~160
superior mesenteric artery	上腸間膜動脈	상장간막동맥	SMA	130~144, 188
vertebral artery	椎骨動脈	추골동맥	VA	20, 24~40, 54
Aryepiglottic fold	披裂喉頭蓋雛壁	피열후두개추벽	AEF	32
Arytenoid	披裂軟骨	피열연골	Ar	34
Ascending colon	上行結腸	상행결장	AC	130~154
Atlantoaxial joint	環椎軸椎關節	환추축추관절	AAJ	26, 54~56
Atlas	環椎	환추	Atl	54~58
Axillary artery	腋窩動脈	액와동맥	AxA	78~80
Axillary vein	腋窩靜脈	액와정맥	AxV	80
Axis	軸椎	축추	Ax	26, 54, 58
Azygoesophageal recess	奇靜脈食道陷凹	기정맥식도함요	AER	90
Azygos vein	奇靜脈	기정맥	Az	80~94, 100, 114~118, 122~130
Base of tongue	舌底	설저	BT	28~30, 52~54
Basilar artery	腦底動脈	뇌저동맥	BA	16, 52, 64~66
Biceps brachii muscle	上腕二頭筋	상완이두근	BB	80
Biceps femoris muscle	大腿二頭筋	대퇴이두근	BF	168, 174
Body of fornix	腦弓體部	뇌궁체부	BoF	50
Brachial plexus	上腕神經叢	상완신경총	BPx	38~40, 108
Brachium pontis	中小腦莖	중소뇌경	BP	16, 54, 66~68
Bronchus	氣管枝	기관지		
apical segment of right upper lobe bronchus	右上葉氣管枝尖分節	우상엽기관지첨분절	Ap	80
bronchus intermedius bronchus	中間氣管枝	중간기관지	BI	82~84
left lower lobe bronchus	左下葉氣管枝	좌하엽기관지	LLLB	84~86, 106
left main bronchus	左主氣管枝	좌주기관지	LMB	82, 102~104
left upper lobe bronchus	左上葉氣管枝	좌상엽기관지	LULB	106
lingular segmental bronchus	舌小葉氣管枝	설소엽기관지	LSB	84
right lower lobe bronchus	右下葉氣管枝	우하엽기관지	RLLB	84~86, 98
right main bronchus	右主氣管枝	우주기관지	RMB	98~100
right middle lobe bronchus	右中葉氣管枝	우중엽기관지	RMLB	86, 98
superior segment of left lower lobe bronchus	左下葉氣管枝上分節	좌하엽기관지상분절	SLLB	84
Bronchus intermedius	中間氣管枝	중간기관지	BI	82~84
Buccinator muscle	頰筋	협근	Bu	24~26, 46~48
Bulbocavernous urethra	球海綿體尿道	구해면체요도	BCU	172
C3 vertebral body	第三頸椎體	제 3 경추체	C3	28, 56
C3-4 intervertebral disc	第三, 四頸椎體間板	제 3-4 경추체간판	C3-4	30
C4 vertebral body	第四頸椎體	제 4 경추체	C4	32
C4-5 intervertebral disc	第四, 五頸椎體間板	제 4-5 경추체간판	C4-5	34
C5 vertebral body	第五頸椎體	제 5 경추체	C5	36
C6 vertebral body	第六頸椎體	제 6 경추체	C6	38~40
Calcarine sulcus	鳥距溝	오거구	CaS	10, 56~60, 66~68
Calcification of lung	肺石灰化	폐석회화	Cal	84
Carina	氣管分岐部	기관분지부	Car	80
Carotid canal	頸動脈管	경동맥관	CaC	20
Cartilage	軟骨	연골	Ca	86, 92~94, 104~106, 114~140
Caudate lobe of liver	尾狀葉	미상엽	CL	102, 118~122, 188~190
Caudate nucleus	尾狀核	미상핵	CN	50

Caudate nucleus, body	尾狀核體	미상핵체	CNb	6, 10
Caudate nucleus, head	尾狀核頭	미상핵두	CNh	10~14, 48~52, 66~68
Caudate process of caudate lobe	尾狀葉尾狀突起	미상엽미상돌기	CPC	122
Cavernous sinus	海綿洞	해면동	CSi	16, 50
Cavum septum pellucidum	透明中隔腔	투명중격강	CSP	14, 48
Cecum	盲腸	맹장	Ce	154~156, 180
Celiac axis	腹腔動脈軸	복강동맥축	CA	102, 126~128, 188~190
Central sulcus	中央溝	중앙구	CnS	6~12, 52~54, 68~70
Centrum ovale	卵圓中心	난원중심	CnO	6
Cerebellar hemisphare	小腦半球	소뇌반구	CbH	12~16, 20~22, 54~60, 64~72
Cerebellar tonsil	小腦扁桃	소뇌편도	CbT	16, 56, 64~66
Cerebellar vermis	小腦蟲部	소뇌충부	CbV	12~16, 56~60, 64
Cerebellum	**小腦**	**소뇌**		
cerebellar hemisphere	小腦半球	소뇌반구	CbH	12~16, 20~22, 54~60, 64~72
cerebellar tonsil	小腦扁桃	소뇌편도	CbT	16, 56, 64~66
cerebellar vermis	小腦蟲部	소뇌충부	CbV	12~16, 56~60, 64
cerebellopontine angle cistern	小腦橋角槽	소뇌교각조	CPAC	16, 20, 54
falx cerebelli	小腦鎌	소뇌겸	FCb	14, 60
inferior cerebellar peduncle	下小腦莖	하소뇌경	ICbP	56
superior cerebellar cistern	上小腦槽	상소뇌조	SCC	10, 56, 66
superior cerebellar artery	上小腦動脈	상소뇌동맥	SCA	52
tentorium cerebelli	小腦天幕	소뇌천막	Ten	8~14, 54~60
Cerebellopontine angle cistern	小腦橋角槽	소뇌교각조	CPAC	16, 20, 54
Cerebral aqueduct	大腦導水管	대뇌도수관	Aq	14, 54
Cerebral peduncle	腦脚	뇌각	CP	14, 66~68
Choroid	脈絡叢	맥락총	Ch	18
Choroid plexus of lateral ventricle	腦側室脈絡叢	뇌측실맥락총	ChP	10, 54~56, 68
Choroidal fissure	脈絡裂	맥락열	ChF	14
Cingulate gyrus	帶狀回	대상회	Cg	4~12, 46~56, 64~68
Cingulate sulcus	帶狀回溝	대상회구	CiS	48, 54, 66
Circular sulcus of insula	島皮質圓形溝	도피질원형구	CSI	10~14, 48~50
Cistern	**槽**	**조**		
ambient cistern	周圍槽	주위조	AmC	14, 54
cerebellopontine angle cistern	小腦橋角槽	소뇌교각조	CPAC	15, 20, 54
pre-pontine cistern	腦橋前槽	뇌교전조	PrPC	16
quadrigeminal cistern	四丘槽	사구조	QC	12~14
superior cerebellar cistern	上小腦槽	상소뇌조	SCC	10, 56, 66
suprasellar cistern	Turkey鞍上槽	터키안상조	SuSC	16
Claustrum	帶狀核	대상핵	Cla	12~14, 48~50
Clavicle	鎖骨	쇄골	Cl	38~40, 78, 98~100, 106~108
Clitoris, crus	陰核脚部	음핵각부	ClCr	186
Cloquet canal	Cloquet管	클로케관	ClC	18
Coccygeus muscle	尾骨筋	미골근	Cge	164~166
Coccyx	尾骨	미골	Coc	164~170
Collateral sulcus	側副溝	측부구	CoS	50~52, 56~58
Colliculi (quadrigeminal plate)	小丘	소구	Col	14, 54, 64
Colon	結腸	결장	Co	120~136, 150
Column of fornix	腦弓柱	뇌궁주	CF	12~14, 64
Commissure of fornix	腦弓接合線	뇌궁접합선	CoF	54
Common bile duct	總輸膽管	총수담관	CBD	126~130, 186
Common carotid artery	總頸動脈	총경동맥	CCA	30~40, 54~56
Common hepatic artery	總肝動脈	총간동맥	CHA	126
Common hepatic duct	總肝膽管	총간담관	CHD	122~124
Common iliac artery	總腸骨動脈	총장골동맥	CIA	148~152, 184~192
Common iliac vein	總腸骨靜脈	총장골정맥	CIV	148~152, 184~192
Coracobrachialis muscle	烏口上腕筋	오구상완근	CoB	78~80
Cornea	角膜	각막	Cor	18
Corona radiata	放線冠	방선관	CR	8~10, 50, 68
Coronary sinus	冠狀靜脈洞	관상정맥동	CS	86~94, 102, 190
Corpus callosum, body	腦梁體	뇌량체	CCb	10~12, 48~52, 64~68
Corpus callosum, genu	腦梁膝	뇌량슬	CCg	8~10, 14, 64
Corpus callosum, rostrum	腦梁吻	뇌량문	CCr	14
Corpus callosum, splenium	腦梁板	뇌량판	CCs	8~10, 54, 64, 68
Corpus cavernosum	海綿體	해면체	CCa	168, 172
Costomediastinal recess	肋骨縱隔洞窩	늑골종격동와	CMR	86
Costotransverse articulation	肋橫突起關節	늑횡돌기관절	CTA	86
Costovertebral articulation	肋椎關節	늑추관절	CVA	86

English	漢字	한글	Abbr.	Pages
Cribriform plate	篩狀板	사상판	CrP	46
Cricoid cartilage	輪狀軟骨	윤상연골	CrC	34~36
Crista galli	雞冠	계관	CG	16, 44~46
Crus of fornix	腦弓脚	뇌궁각	CrF	54
Crus penis	陰莖脚	음경각	CPe	172
Cuneus	楔狀葉	설상엽	Cun	6~10, 58~60, 64
Cystic duct	囊胞管	낭포관	CD	124
Deep cervical lymph node	深頸淋巴節	심경림프절	DCN	54
Deep circumflex iliac artery	深腸骨回旋動脈	심장골회선동맥	DCIA	156, 160
Deep femoral artery	深大腿動脈	심대퇴동맥	DFA	170~176
Deltoid muscle	三角筋	삼각근	De	36~40, 78~80
Dentate ligament	齒狀靭帶	치상인대	DL	32
Dentate nucleus	齒狀核	치상핵	DN	14~16, 56~58, 66~68
Descending colon	下行結腸	하행결장	DC	126~154, 176, 194~198
Diaphragm	橫隔膜	횡격막	Di	94, 98, 102~108, 114~122, 126, 180~184, 190~198
Diaphragmatic crus	橫隔膜脚部	횡격막각부	DiCr	100, 186~190
Digastric muscle	二腹筋	이복근	DG	30
Digastric muscle, anterior belly	二腹筋前腹	이복근전복	DGa	48~50
Digastric muscle, posterior belly	二腹筋後腹	이복근후복	DGp	24~28, 54~56
Diploic space	板間腔	판간강	DS	6
Diploic vein	板間靜脈	판간정맥	DV	4
Douglas pouch	Douglas窩	더글라스와	DP	186
Ductus deferens	精管	정관	DD	160, 166
Duodenal bulb	十二指腸球	십이지장구	DB	122~128, 186
Duodenum	**十二指腸**	**십이지장**		
duodenal bulb	十二指腸球	십이지장구	DB	122~128, 186
first portion of duodenum	十二指腸第一部	십이지장제 1 부	D1	124, 128~132
fourth portion of duodenum	十二指腸第四部	십이지장제 4 부	D4	124~142, 188~192
second portion of duodenum	十二指腸第二部	십이지장제 2 부	D2	130~134, 184
third portion of duodenum	十二指腸第三部	십이지장제 3 부	D3	136~142, 186
Dura mater	硬腦膜	경뇌막	DM	4~6, 44~46, 82, 92~94
Epicardium	心外膜	심외막	Ec	92~94
Epidural venous plexus	硬膜外靜脈叢	경막외정맥총	EPV	40
Epiglottis	喉頭蓋	후두개	Ep	30~32, 54
Erector spinae muscle	脊柱起立筋	척주기립근	ErS	100, 104, 182~194
Esophagus	食道	식도	Es	34~40, 78~94, 100, 114, 188~190
Ethmoid sinus	篩骨洞	사골동	ES	18~20, 44~46
Eustachian tube	耳管	이관	ET	22
Eustachian tube orifice	耳管口	이관구	ETO	50
External auditary canal	外耳道	외이도	EAC	20, 54
External capsule	外被膜	외피막	EC	12~14, 48~52
External carotid artery	外頸動脈	외경동맥	ECA	24, 28~32
External iliac artery	外腸骨動脈	외장골동맥	EIA	150~162, 180~182, 194
External iliac vein	外腸骨靜脈	외장골정맥	EIV	154~162, 182
External jugular vein	外頸靜脈	외경정맥	EJV	30~40
External oblique muscle	外斜筋	외사근	EO	118~154, 180, 194~198
External obturator muscle	外閉鎖筋	외폐쇄근	EOb	168~170, 182~184, 192
External sphincter ani	外肛門括約筋	외항문괄약근	ESA	172
Extrapericardial fat	心膜外脂肪	심막외지방	EPE	94, 100~102, 106~108
Extreme capsule	極被膜	극피막	ExC	12~14, 48~50
Eyeball	眼球	안구	Ey	18, 44
Facet joint of spine	脊椎小面關節	척추소면관절	FJ	32, 36, 102
Falciform ligament	鎌狀靭帶	겸상인대	FaL	118
Falx cerebelli	小腦鎌	소뇌겸	FCb	14, 60
Falx cerebri	大腦鎌	대뇌겸	FC	4~16, 44~48, 56~60
Fascia	**筋膜**	**근막**		
anterior renal fascia	前腎膜	전신막	ARF	124~144
fascia lata	大腿筋膜	대퇴근막	FLa	164~166, 172
lateroconal fascia	外錐筋膜	외추근막	LCoF	126~134, 138~144
obturator fascia	閉鎖筋膜	폐쇄근막	ObF	162
pelvic fascia	骨盤筋膜	골반근막	PeF	162
posterior renal fascia	後腎膜	후신막	PRF	124~146, 196
temporalis fascia	側頭筋膜	측두근막	TF	18~20

tensor fascia lata	大腿筋膜張筋	대퇴근막장근	TFL	160~162, 166~176
Fascia lata	大腿筋膜	대퇴근막	FLa	164~166, 172
Fat	**脂肪**	**지방**		
extrapericardial fat	心膜外脂肪	심막외지방	EPF	94, 100~102, 106~108
mesenteric fat	腸間膜脂肪	장간막지방	MeF	122, 128~148, 180, 186
omental fat	大網脂肪	대망지방	OF	114~124, 168~172
pericardial fat	心外膜脂肪	심외막지방	PcF	114~116, 196~198
perirenal fat	腎周圍脂肪	신주위지방	PF	98, 104, 120~134, 138, 142~144, 148 182
posterior pararenal fat	後腎傍脂肪	후신방지방	PPF	132~148, 180, 194~196
subepicardial fat	心膜下脂肪	심막하지방	SEF	84, 108
Femoral artery	大腿動脈	대퇴동맥	FA	164~168, 172~176, 196
Femoral nerve	大腿神經	대퇴신경	FN	150, 154~160, 166, 184
Femoral vein	大腿靜脈	대퇴정맥	FV	164~172, 176
Femur	大腿骨	대퇴골	Fe	172~176
Femur, head	大腿骨頭	대퇴골두	Fh	162~166, 180, 196~198
Femur, neck	大腿頸部	대퇴경부	Fn	168~170
First portion of duodenum	十二指腸第一部	십이지장제1부	D1	124, 128~132
Fissure for ligamentum venosum	靜脈靭帶裂	정맥인대열	FLV	115~120
Flocculus	片葉	편엽	Fl	54, 68
Fourth portion of duodenum	十二指腸第四部	십이지장제4부	D4	124~142, 188~192
Frontal lobe	前頭葉	전두엽	FL	4~16, 44~48
Frontal sinus	前頭洞	전두동	FS	16
Galea aponeurotica	帽狀腱膜	모상건막	GAp	4~6
Gall bladder	膽囊	담낭	GB	122~130, 182~184
Gasselian ganglion	三叉神經節	삼차신경절	GaG	18
Gastrocolic ligament	胃結腸間膜	위결장막	GC	194
Gastroduodenal artery	胃十二指腸動脈	위십이지장동맥	GDA	128
Gastroesophageal junction	胃食道連結部	위식도연결부	GEJ	102, 116, 190
Gastrohepatic recess	胃肝陷凹	위간함요	GHR	106~108, 194~196
Genioglossus muscle	頤舌筋	이설근	GG	30~32, 48~50
Geniohyoid muscle	頤舌骨筋	이설골근	GH	48
Gland	**腺**	**선**		
left adrenal gland	左副腎	좌부신	LAd	84, 102, 124~138, 192
mammary gland	乳腺	유선	MG	108, 180, 198
parotid gland	耳下腺	이하선	PG	22~28, 48~50, 54
parotid gland, deep lobe	耳下腺深葉	이하선심엽	PGd	22~26, 48
pineal gland	松果腺	송과선	PnG	54, 64
pituitary gland	腦下垂體	뇌하수체	PtG	16, 50
right adrenal gland	右副腎	우부신	RAd	96, 122~128
sublingual gland	舌下腺	설하선	SLG	48
submandibular gland	下顎下腺	하악하선	SMG	28~32, 50~52
thyroid gland	甲狀腺	갑상선	ThG	36~40, 104
Glenohumeral joint	上腕關節	상완관절	GHJ	78
Globus pallidus	淡蒼球	담창구	GP	12~14, 50~52, 66~68
Gluteus maximus muscle	大臀筋	대둔근	GMa	150~176, 180~184, 192~198
Gluteus medius muscle	中臀筋	중둔근	GMe	146~166, 180, 196~198
Gluteus minimus muscle	小臀筋	소둔근	GMi	146, 152~162, 180, 196~198
Gluteus minimus tendon	小臀腱	소둔건	GMT	164
Gracilis muscle	薄筋	박근	Gr	174~176
Greater omentum	大網	대망	GOt	188~190, 196~198
Greater trochanter	大轉子	대전자	GT	164~170
Greater wing of sphenoid	蝶形骨大翼	접형골대익	GWS	18
Gyrus	**回**	**회**		
angular gyrus	角回	각회	Ang	6~8, 58~60, 72
cingulate gyrus	帶狀回	대상회	Cg	4~12, 46~56, 64~68
inferior frontal gyrus	下前頭回	하전두회	IFg	8~14, 44~50, 72
inferior temporal gyrus	下側頭回	하측두회	ITg	12~16, 50~60, 70~72
lateral occipital gryus	外側後頭回	외측후두회	LOg	10, 70
lateral occipito-temporal gyrus	外側後側頭回	외측후측두회	LOTg	50, 54~60, 70
lingual gyrus	舌回	설회	Lg	56~58
medial occipito-temporal gyrus	內側後側頭回	내측후측두회	MOTg	12, 60, 64, 68
middle frontal gyrus	中前頭回	중전두회	MFg	4~14, 44~50, 70
middle temporal gyrus	中側頭回	중측두회	MTg	8~16, 48~56, 60, 72
orbital gyrus	眼窩回	안와회	Og	16, 44~46
parahippocampal gyrus	副海馬回	부해마회	PHg	12~16, 50~54, 68
postcentral gyrus	中心後回	중심후회	Pog	4~12, 52, 66~72

English	漢字	한글	Abbr.	Pages
precentral gyrus	中心前回	중심전회	Prg	4~12, 52~54, 66~72
rectal gyrus	直回	직회	Rg	16, 44~48
superior frontal gyrus	上前頭回	상전두회	SFg	4~14, 44~52, 64~68
superior temporal gyrus	上側頭回	상측두회	STg	10~16, 48~56, 68~72
supramarginal gyrus	縁上回	연상회	SMg	6~8, 54~56, 72
transverse temporal gyrus	橫側頭回	횡측두회	TTg	10
Hard palate	硬口蓋	경구개	HP	24, 46
Heart	**心臟**	**심장**		
aortic valve	大動脈瓣膜	대동맥판막	AV	88, 104
left atrial appendage of heart	左心房耳	좌심방이	LAA	84, 106
left atrium of heart	左心房	좌심방	LA	84~90, 100~104, 192
left ventricle of heart	左心室	좌심실	LV	86~94, 104~108, 192~198
mitral valve	僧帽瓣	승모판	MV	88~90, 104
right atrial appendage of heart	右心房耳	우심방이	RAA	84~88, 100
right atrium of heart	右心房	우심방	RA	88~92, 98~100
right ventricle of heart	右心室	우심실	RV	86~94, 102~108, 190~196
tricuspid valve	三尖瓣	삼첨판	TV	90, 102~104
Hemiazygos vein	半奇靜脈	반기정맥	HzV	84, 90~94, 102, 114~126, 130
Hepatic artery	肝動脈	간동맥	HA	118, 124~126, 184, 188
Hepatic flexure of colon	肝結腸曲	간결장곡	HF	120, 180~182
Hepatic vein	肝靜脈	간정맥	HV	98~100, 120, 186
Hapatorenal recess	肝腎陷凹	간신함요	HRR	180~182
Hippocampal sulcus	海馬溝	해마구	HS	52
Hippocampus	海馬	해마	Hi	12~14, 52
Humerus	上腕骨	상완골	Hu	78~80
Humerus, head	上腕骨頭	상완골두	Hh	36
Hyoglossus muscle	舌骨舌筋	설골설근	HG	28~32, 50~52
Hyoid bone	舌骨	설골	HB	32, 54
Hypopharynx	下咽頭	하인두	HPh	30~32
Hypothalamus	視床下部	시상하부	Hp	12~14, 52
Ileum	回腸	회장	Ie	136~144, 148, 154, 180~196
Iliac bone	腸骨	장골	IB	146~160, 180~182, 194~198
Iliacus muscle	腸骨筋	장골근	Il	146~156, 180~182, 196~198
Iliocostalis lumborum muscle	腸肋腰筋	장늑요근	ICL	150~156
Iliocostalis muscle	腸肋筋	장늑근	IlC	78~82, 114~148
Iliofemoral ligament	腸大腿骨靭帶	장대퇴골인대	IFL	152
Iliopsoas muscle	腸腰筋	장요근	IP	158~172
Inferior cerebellar peduncle	下小腦莖	하소뇌경	ICbP	56
Inferior epigastric artery	下腹壁動脈	하복벽동맥	IEA	150~152, 162
Inferior frontal gyrus	下前頭回	하전두회	IFg	8~14, 44~50, 72
Inferior gemellus muscle	下雙子筋	하쌍자근	IG	166
Inferior gluteal artery	下臀動脈	하둔동맥	IGA	160~164
Inferior gluteal vein	下臀靜脈	하둔정맥	IGV	160, 166~172
Inferior mesenteric artery	下腸間膜動脈	하장간막동맥	IMA	144~146
Inferior mesenteric vein	下腸間膜靜脈	하장간막정맥	IMV	194
Inferior parietal lobule	下頭頂小葉	하두정소엽	IPLo	54~60, 70
Inferior phrenic artery	下橫隔膜動脈	하횡격막동맥	InPA	114~122, 126
Inferior pulmonary ligament	下肺靭帶	하폐인대	IPL	92, 182
Inferior rectus muscle	下直筋	하직근	IR	44~46
Inferior temporal gyrus	下側頭回	하측두회	ITg	12~16, 50~60, 70~72
Inferior turbinate	下鼻介骨	하비개골	IT	22, 44~48
Inferior vena cava	下大靜脈	하대정맥	IVC	84, 92~94, 100, 114~148, 186
Inferior vesical artery	下膀胱動脈	하방광동맥	IVA	160~162
Infraspinatus muscle	棘下筋	극하근	IfS	78~82
Infratemporal fossa	側頭下窩	측두하와	ITF	48, 52
Inguinal ligament	鼠蹊靭帶	서혜인대	Ing	180
Innominate artery	無名動脈	무명동맥	InA	78, 100~102
Insula	島	도	In	10~14, 48~52
Intercostal artery	肋間動脈	늑간동맥	IcA	104, 108, 116, 192
Intercostal muscle	肋間筋	늑간근	Ic	78, 82, 92, 98, 196
Intercostal vein	肋間靜脈	늑간정맥	IcV	84, 88, 92~94, 104, 108, 116~118
Interhemispheric fissure	半球間裂	반구간열	IHF	4, 10~16, 44~48
Internal auditory canal	內耳管	내이관	IAC	20
Internal capsule, anterior limb	內被膜前肢	내피막전지	ICa	12~14, 48~50, 68
Internal capsule, genu	內被膜膝	내피막슬	ICg	66

English	漢字	한글	Abbr.	Pages
Internal capsule, posterior limb	內被膜後肢	내피막후지	ICp	12, 52, 68
Internal carotid artery	內頸動脈	내경동맥	ICA	16~32, 50~54
Internal cerebral vein	內大腦靜脈	내대뇌정맥	ICV	10~12, 52~54
Internal iliac artery	內腸骨動脈	내장골동맥	IIA	150~158, 182
Internal iliac vein	內腸骨靜脈	내장골정맥	IIV	154~158, 182, 192
Internal jugular vein	內頸靜脈	내경정맥	IJV	20~40, 54
Internal mammary vessel	內乳房血管	내유방혈관	IMv	80, 86~88, 92~94
Internal oblique muscle	內腹斜筋	내복사근	IO	136~156, 160, 180, 194~198
Internal obturator muscle	內閉鎖筋	내폐쇄근	IOb	162~170, 182~184, 192~194
Internal occipital protuberance	內後頭隆起	내후두융기	IOP	16
Internal pudendal artery	內陰動脈	내음동맥	IPA	164
Internal pudendal vessel	內陰血管	내음혈관	IPv	165~170
Internal sphincter ani	內肛門括約筋	내항문괄약근	ISA	172
Internal urethral opening	內尿道孔	내요도공	IUO	164
Interosseous sacroiliac ligament	骨間薦腸靭帶	골간천장인대	IoSL	150
Intersublobar septum	小葉間中隔	소엽간중격	ISS	92
Interventricular septum	心室中隔	심실중격	IVS	90~92, 106~108
Intervertebral disc	脊椎間板	척추간판	IVD	56, 100~102, 186~190
Intervertebral foramen	脊椎間孔	척추간공	IVF	32, 38
Intraparietal sulcus	頭頂內溝	두정내구	IPS	55
Intrinsic muscle of tongue	舌自體筋	설자체근	ImT	28, 32
Ischial spine	坐骨棘	좌골극	IsS	164
Ischial tuberosity	坐骨粗面	좌골조면	IsT	168~172
Ischiocavernosus muscle	坐骨海綿體筋	좌골해면체근	Isc	172
Ischiorectal fossa	坐骨直腸窩	좌골직장와	IRF	168~172, 182~184
Ischium	坐骨	좌골	Is	172, 184, 194~196
Jejunum	空腸	공장	Je	122~146, 180~182, 186~191, 194, 198
Joint, articulation	**關節**	**관절**		
atlantoaxial joint	環椎軸椎關節	환추축추관절	AAJ	26, 54~56
costotransverse articulation	肋橫突起關節	늑횡돌기관절	CTA	86
costovertebral articulation	肋椎關節	늑추관절	CVA	86
facet joint of spine	脊椎小面關節	척추소면관절	FJ	32, 36, 102
glenohumeral joint	上腕關節	상완관절	GHJ	78
Luschka joint	Luschka 關節	루시카관절	LJ	32
sacroiliac joint	薦腸關節	천장관절	SIJ	150~156
temporomandibular joint	側頭下顎骨關節	측두하악골관절	TMJ	20
Jugular foramen	頸靜脈孔	경정맥공	JF	20, 54
L1 vertebral body	第一腰椎體	제 1 요추체	L1	124~130, 186
L1-2 intervertebral disc	第一, 二腰椎間板	제 1-2 요추간판	L1-2	130~132
L2 vertebral body	第二腰椎	제 2 요추	L2	130, 134
L2-3 intervertebral disc	第二, 三腰椎間板	제 2-3 요추간판	L2-3	136
L3 vertebral body	第三腰椎	제 3 요추	L3	138~140, 190
L3-4 intervertebral disc	第三, 四腰椎間板	제 3-4 요추간판	L3-4	138
L4 vertebral body	第四腰椎體	제 4 요추체	L4	144~146
L4-5 intervertebral disc	第四, 五腰椎間板	제 4-5 요추간판	L4-5	146
L5 vertebral body	第五腰椎體	제 5 요추체	L5	148, 186~188
L5-S1 intervertebral disc	第五腰椎, 第一薦椎間板	제 5 요추-제 1 천추 간판	L5-S1	150~152
Lamina	板	판	Lm	30~34
Lamina papyracea	紙板	지판	LmP	18, 22, 44~46
Lateral femoral circumflex artery	外側大腿骨廻旋動脈	외측대퇴골회선동맥	LFCA	168, 172~174
Lateral geniculate body	外側膝狀體	외측슬상체	LGB	14
Lateral occipital gyrus	外側後頭回	외측후두회	LOg	10, 70
Lateral occipito~temporal gyrus	外側後側頭回	외측후측두회	LOTg	50, 54~60, 70
Lateral pterygoid muscle	外側翼突筋	외측익돌근	LPm	20, 22, 50~52
Lateral rectus muscle	外側直筋	외측직근	LR	18, 44~46
Lateral sinus	側靜脈洞	측정맥동	LS	14, 58~60
Lateral ventricle, antrum	側腦室洞	측뇌실동	LVa	10, 54, 68
Lateral ventricle, body	側腦室體部	측뇌실체부	LVb	6~10, 52
Lateral ventricle, frontal horn	側腦室前頭角	측뇌실전두각	LVf	10~14, 48, 64
Lateral ventricle, occipital horn	側腦室後頭角	측뇌실후두각	LVo	8~10, 56
Lateral ventricle, temporal horn	側腦室側頭角	측뇌실측두각	LVt	14~16, 52, 68~70
Lateroconal fascia	外錐筋膜	외추근막	LCoF	126~134, 138~144
Latissimus dorsi muscle	廣背筋	광배근	LtD	82~94, 114~142
Left adrenal gland	左副腎	좌부신	LAd	84, 104, 124~128, 192

Left anterior descending branch of left coronary artery	左冠狀動脈左前下行枝	좌관상동맥좌전하행지	LAD	86~90
Left atrial appendage of heart	左心房耳	좌심방이	LAA	84, 106
Left atrium of heart	左心房	좌심방	LA	84~90, 100~104, 192
Left circumflex artery	左廻旋動脈	좌회선동맥	LCx	90~92
Left common carotid artery	左總頸動脈	좌총경동맥	LCCA	78, 104
Left coronary artery	左冠狀動脈	좌관상동맥	LCA	84~88, 104~108
Left descending pulmonary artery	左下行肺動脈	좌하행폐동맥	LDPA	84
Left diaphragmatic crus	左橫隔膜脚	좌횡격막각	LC	114~138, 142
Left gastric artery	左胃動脈	좌위동맥	LGA	114, 118~124
Left gastric vein	左胃靜脈	좌위정맥	LGV	122~124
Left hepatic vein	左肝靜脈	좌간정맥	LHV	102~104, 114~118, 188~192
Left inferior pulmonary vein	左下肺靜脈	좌하폐정맥	LIPV	86~88, 104
Left innominate vein	左無名靜脈	좌무명정맥	LIV	78, 100~106
Left kidney	左腎	좌신	LK	120, 124~144, 192~198
Left lobe of liver	肝左葉	간좌엽	LL	102~108, 114~128, 186~198
Left lower lobe bronchus	左下葉氣管枝	좌하엽기관지	LLLB	84~86, 106
Left lower lobe of lung	左肺下葉	좌폐하엽	LLL	80~94, 104~108, 114~120, 194~198
Left main bronchus	左主氣管枝	좌주기관지	LMB	82, 102~104
Left portal vein	左門脈	좌문맥	LPV	104, 118, 186
Left pulmonary artery	左肺動脈	좌폐동맥	LPA	82, 86, 104~106
Left renal artery	左腎動脈	좌신동맥	LRA	132~138, 192
Left renal vein	左腎靜脈	좌신정맥	LRV	132~138, 186~192
Left subclavian artery	左鎖骨下動脈	좌쇄골하동맥	LScA	104~108
Left subclavian vein	左鎖骨下靜脈	좌쇄골하정맥	LScV	104~108
Left superior pulmonary vein	左上肺靜脈	좌상폐정맥	LSPV	82~84, 104~106
Left upper lobe bronchus	左上葉氣管枝	좌상엽기관지	LULB	106
Left upper lobe of lung	左肺上葉	좌폐상엽	LUL	78~84, 88~92, 104~108, 196~198
Left ventricle of heart	左心室	좌심실	LV	86~94, 104~108, 192~198
Lens	水晶體	수정체	Le	18
Lesser omentum	小網	소망	LOt	116, 120, 188~190
Lesser sac	小囊	소낭	LSa	188~190
Levator ani muscle	肛門擧筋	항문거근	LeA	164~172
Levator palati muscle	口蓋擧筋	구개거근	LP	22, 52
Levator scapularis muscle	肩胛擧筋	견갑거근	LeS	28~34, 38~40
Ligament	**靱帶**	**인대**		
anterior sacroiliac ligament	前薦腸骨靱帶	전천장골인대	ASL	150
dentate ligament	齒狀靱帶	치상인대	DL	32
falciform ligament	鎌狀靱帶	겸상인대	FaL	128
fissure for ligamentum venosum	靜脈靱帶裂	정맥인대열	FLV	116~120
gastrocolic ligament	胃大腸靱帶	위대장인대	GC	194
iliofemoral ligament	腸大腿骨靱帶	장대퇴골인대	IFL	162
inferior pulmonary ligament	下肺靱帶	하폐인대	IPL	92, 182
inguinal ligament	鼠蹊靱帶	서혜인대	Ing	180
interosseous sacroiliac ligament	骨間薦腸靱帶	골간천장인대	IoSL	150
ligamentum capitis femoris	大腿骨頭靱帶	대퇴골두인대	LCF	162
ligamentum flavum	黃色靱帶	황색인대	LF	150
ligamentum teres	圓形靱帶	원형인대	LT	186
medial umbilical ligament	內側臍靱帶	내측제인대	MIUL	152
median umbilical ligament	正中臍靱帶	정중제인대	MUL	152
nuchal ligament	項靱帶	항인대	NL	36, 40
sacrospinous ligament	薦骨脊椎間靱帶	천골척추간인대	SSL	162
vocal ligament	聲帶	성대	VoL	34
Ligamentum capitis femoris	大腿骨頭靱帶	대퇴골두인대	LCF	162
Ligamentum flavum	黃色靱帶	황색인대	LF	150
Ligamentum teres	圓形靱帶	원형인대	LT	186
Lingual gyrus	舌回	설회	Lg	56~58
Lingular segmental bronchus	舌小葉氣管枝	설소엽기관지	LSB	84
Liver	**肝**	**간**		
caudate lobe of liver	尾狀葉	미상엽	CL	102, 118~122, 188~190
caudate process of caudate lobe	尾狀葉尾狀突起	미상엽미상돌기	CPC	122
left lobe of liver	肝左葉	간좌엽	LL	102~108, 114~128, 186~198
papillary process of caudate lobe	尾狀葉乳頭突起	미상엽유두돌기	PPC	122
right lobe of liver	肝右葉	간우엽	RL	94, 98, 114~142, 180~184
Long thoracic nerve	長胸神經	장흉신경	LTN	82
Longissimus dorsi muscle	背側最長筋	배측최장근	LgD	80~94, 114~148
Longus colli and capitis muscle	頸長筋, 頭長筋	경장근 및 두장근	LCC	20~40

English	漢字	한글	Abbr.	Pages
Lumbosacral trunk	腰薦骨神經幹	요천골신경간	LST	154
Lung	**肺**	**폐**		
anteromedial basal segment of lung	前內側基底肺分節	전내측기저폐분절	AMB	88
calcification of lung	肺石灰化	폐석회화	Cal	84
left lower lobe of lung	左肺下葉	좌폐하엽	LLL	80~94, 104~108, 114~120, 194~198
left upper lobe of lung	左肺上葉	좌폐상엽	LUL	78~84, 88~90, 104~108, 196~198
posterolateral basal segment of lung	後外側基底肺分節	후외측기저폐분절	PBS	88
right lower lobe of lung	右肺下葉	우폐하엽	RLL	80~94, 98~100, 114~116, 180~186
right middle lobe of lung	右肺中葉	우폐중엽	RML	86~92, 180~182
right upper lobe of lung	右肺上葉	우폐상엽	RUL	78~82, 98~100
Luschka joint	Luschka關節	루시카관절	LJ	32
Lymph node	淋巴節	림프절	LN	78~82, 98~100, 104~106
Main pulmonary artery	主肺動脈	주폐동맥	MPA	82~84, 104
Major fissure	主裂溝	주열구	MaF	82~88, 92, 98~100, 106~108, 180~182, 196~198
Mammary gland	乳腺	유선	MG	108, 180, 198
Mamillary body	乳頭體	유두체	MB	64
Mandible	下顎骨	하악골	Mn	48
Mandible, angle	下顎角	하악각	Mna	28
Mandible, body	下顎體部	하악체부	Mnb	28~32, 46
Mandible, condylar process	下顎關節突起	하악관절돌기	Mnc	20~22, 52
Mandible, ramus	下顎枝	하악지	Mnr	20~26, 48, 52
Manubrium	槌骨	추골	Man	78, 100~104
Massa intermedia	中間質	중간질	MI	52
Massester muscle	咀嚼筋	저작근	Ma	20~28, 52
Mastoid air cells	乳突蜂巢	유돌봉소	MAC	16, 20~22, 54~56
Mastoid tip	乳樣突起端	유양돌기단	MTp	24
Maxilla	上顎骨	상악골	Mx	22~24, 44~46
Maxillary sinus, antrum	上顎洞	상악동	Mxa	18~22, 44~46
Medial occipito-temporal gyrus	內後側頭回	내후측두회	MOTg	12, 60, 64, 68
Medial pterygoid muscle	內翼突筋	내익돌근	MP	22~28, 48~52
Medial rectus muscle	內直筋	내직근	MR	18, 44~46
Medial umbilical ligament	內側臍靱帶	내측제인대	MIUL	152
Median sulcus	正中溝	정중구	MeS	54
Median umbilical ligament	正中臍靱帶	정중제인대	MUL	152
Medulla oblongata	延髓	연수	MO	20, 22, 54~56, 64
Mesenteric fat	腸間膜脂肪	장간막지방	MeF	122, 128~148, 180, 186
Midbrain	中腦	중뇌	Mi	14, 54, 64
Middle cardiac vein	中心臟靜脈	중심장정맥	MCV	102~106, 190
Middle cerebral artery	中大腦動脈	중대뇌동맥	MCA	14~16, 48
Middle cranial fossa	中頭蓋窩	중두개와	MCF	48
Middle frontal gyrus	中前頭回	중전두회	MFg	4~14, 44~50, 70
Middle hepatic vein	中肝靜脈	중간정맥	MHV	94, 114~118
Middle scalene muscle	中斜角筋	중사각근	MS	28~40
Middle temporal gyrus	中側頭回	중측두회	MTg	8~16, 48~60, 72
Middle turbinate	中鼻介骨	중비개골	MT	18~20, 44~48
Minor fissure	小裂溝	소열구	MiF	98
Mitral valve	僧帽瓣	승모판	MV	88~90, 104
Multifidus muscle	多裂筋肉	다열근육	Mf	82, 86~88, 114~156, 182, 192~194
Muscle	**筋肉**	**근육**		
adductor minimus muscle	內轉小筋	내전소근	AMi	172~176
adductor brevis muscle	內轉短筋	내전단근	AB	170~176, 184
adductor longus muscle	內轉長筋	내전장근	AL	170~176
adductor magnus muscle	內轉大筋	내전대근	AMa	174~176, 184
anterior scalene muscle	前斜角筋	전사각근	AS	30~40
biceps brachii muscle	上腕二頭筋	상완이두근	BB	80
biceps femoris muscle	大腿二頭筋	대퇴이두근	BF	168, 174
buccinator muscle	頰筋	협근	Bu	24, 46~48
coccygeus muscle	尾骨筋	미골근	Cge	164~166
coracobrachialis muscle	烏喙腕筋	오훼완근	CoB	78~80
deltoid muscle	三角筋	삼각근	De	36~40, 78~80
digastric muscle	二腹筋	이복근	DG	30
digastric muscle, anterior belly	二腹筋前腹	이복근전복	DGa	48~50
digastric muscle, posterior belly	二腹筋後腹	이복근후복	DGp	24~28, 54~56
erector spinae muscle	脊柱起立筋	척주기립근	ErS	100, 104, 182~194
external oblique muscle	外斜筋	외사근	EO	118~154, 180, 194~198
external obturator muscle	外閉鎖筋	외폐쇄근	EOb	168~170, 182~184, 192

genioglossus muscle	頤舌筋	이설근	GG	30~32, 48~50
geniohyoid muscle	頤舌骨筋	이설골근	GH	48
gluteus maximus muscle	大臀筋	대둔근	GMa	150~176, 180~184, 192~198
gluteus medius muscle	中臀筋	중둔근	GMe	146~166, 180, 196~198
gluteus minimus muscle	小臀筋	소둔근	GMi	146, 152~162, 180, 196~198
gracilis muscle	薄筋	박근	Gr	174~176
hyoglossus muscle	舌骨舌筋	설골설근	HG	28~32, 50~52
iliacus muscle	腸骨筋	장골근	Il	146~156, 180~182, 196~198
iliocostalis lumborum muscle	腸肋腰筋	장늑요근	ICL	150~156
iliocostalis muscle	腸肋筋	장늑근	IlC	78~82, 114~148
iliopsoas muscle	腸腰筋	장요근	IP	158~172
inferior gemellus muscle	下雙子筋	하쌍자근	IG	166
inferior rectus muscle	下直筋	하직근	IR	44~46
infraspinatus muscle	棘下筋	극하근	IfS	78~82
intercostal muscle	肋間筋	늑간근	Ic	78, 82, 98, 196
internal oblique muscle	內斜筋	내사근	IO	136~156, 160, 180, 194~198
internal obturator muscle	內閉鎖筋	내폐쇄근	IOb	162~170, 182~184, 192~194
intrinsic muscle of tongue	舌自體筋	설자체근	ImT	28, 32
ischiocavernosus muscle	坐骨海綿體筋	좌골해면체근	Isc	172
lateral pterygoid muscle	外側翼突筋	외측익돌근	LPm	20, 22, 50~52
lateral rectus muscle	外側直筋	외측직근	LR	18, 44~46
latissimus dorsi muscle	廣背筋	광배근	LtD	84~94, 114~142
levator ani muscle	肛門擧筋	항문거근	LeA	164~172
levator palati muscle	口蓋擧筋	구개거근	LP	22, 52
levator scapularis muscle	肩胛擧筋	견갑거근	LeS	28~30, 34, 38~40
longissimus dorsi muscle	背側最長筋	배측최장근	LgD	80~82, 86~94, 114~148
longus colli and capitis muscle	頸長筋, 頭長筋	경장근 및 두장근	LCC	20~40
masseter muscle	咀嚼筋	저작근	Ma	20~28, 50
medial pterygoid muscle	內側翼突筋	내측익돌근	MP	20~28, 48~52
medial rectus muscle	內側直筋	내측직근	MR	18, 44~46
middle scalene muscle	中斜角筋	중사각근	MS	28~40
multifidus muscle	多裂筋	다열근	Mf	82, 86~88, 114~156, 192~194
mylohyoid muscle	顎舌骨筋	악설골근	MH	30~32, 48~52
obliquus capitis inferior muscle	下頭斜筋	하두사근	OCI	56
obliquus capitis superior muscle	上頭斜筋	상두사근	OCS	58
obturator muscle	閉鎖筋	폐쇄근	Ob	24, 162
palatopharyngeus muscle	口蓋咽頭筋	구개인두근	PPh	24~26
papillary muscle of myocardium	心乳頭筋	심유두근	Pap	106
pectineus muscle	恥骨筋	치골근	Pe	164, 168~176, 182, 194
pectoralis major muscle	大胸筋	대흉근	PMa	78~90, 98~100, 106~108
pectoralis minor muscle	小胸筋	소흉근	PMi	78~82
pharyngeal muscles	咽頭筋	인두근	Ph	24~32, 52
piriformis muscle	梨狀筋	이상근	Pf	158~160, 182~184, 192~194
posterior scalene muscle	後斜角筋	후사각근	PSc	32~36
psoas muscle	腰筋	요근	Ps	128~156, 182~184, 194
quadratus femoris muscle	大腿方形筋	대퇴방형근	QF	168~172
quadratus lumborum muscle	腰方形筋	요방형근	QL	130~146, 180~182, 192~198
rectus abdominis muscle	腹直筋	복직근	ReA	116~162, 184~192
rectus capitis posterior major muscle	大後頭直筋	대후두직근	RCPM	60
rectus capitis posterior minor muscle	小後頭直筋	소후두직근	RCPm	60
rectus femoris muscle	大腿直筋	대퇴직근	RFe	164~176
rhomboideus major muscle	大稜形筋	대능형근	RMa	78~82, 98~100
rhomboideus minor muscle	小稜形筋	소능형근	RMi	36
sartorius muscle	縫工筋	봉공근	Sar	158~176
semispinalis capitis muscle	頭部半棘筋	두부반극근	SSC	26~32, 60
semispinalis cervicalis muscle	頸部半棘筋	경부반극근	SSCe	26~32, 36~40
semispinalis dorsi muscle	背部半棘筋	배부반극근	SSD	78~82, 86~88, 94, 114~122
semitendinosus muscle	半腱狀筋	반건상근	Se	174
serratus anterior muscle	前鋸筋	전거근	SeA	40, 78, 82~92, 114~120
spinalis cervicalis muscle	頸棘筋	경극근	SCe	34~40
spinalis muscle	脊椎棘筋	척추극근	Sp	114~122, 194
splenius capitis muscle	頭部脊椎棘筋	두부척추극근	SpC	26~32, 58, 60
sternocleidomastoid muscle	胸鎖乳突筋	흉쇄유돌근	SCM	24~40, 54~56
styloglossus muscle	柱狀舌筋	주상설근	SG	28, 32, 52
stylohyoid muscle	柱狀舌骨筋	주상설골근	SH	30
styloid muscles	柱狀筋	주상근	Sty	24
subscapularis muscle	肩胛下筋	견갑하근	SbS	36~40, 78~82, 108

superior gemellus muscle	上雙子筋	상쌍자근	SGe	164
superior rectus muscle	上直筋	상직근	SR	44~46
supraspinatus muscle	棘上筋	극상근	SSp	38, 80
temporalis muscle	側頭筋	측두근	Te	16~24, 46~48
tensor palati muscle	口蓋帆張筋	구개범장근	TP	22
teres major muscle	大圓筋	대원근	TMa	80~88
transversus abdominis muscle	腹橫筋	복횡근	TA	128~154, 180, 194~198
trapezius muscle	僧帽筋	승모근	Trp	30~40, 78~88, 98~100, 104~106
triceps brachii muscle	上腕三頭筋	상완삼두근	Tri	80
vastus intermedius muscle	中間廣筋	중간광근	VI	174~176
vastus lateralis muscle	外側廣筋	외측광근	VL	168~172, 176
vastus medialis muscle	內側廣筋	내측광근	VM	174~176
Mylohyoid muscle	顎舌骨筋	악설골근	MH	30~32, 48~52
Nasal cavity	鼻腔	비강	NC	18~20, 44
Nasal septum	鼻中隔	비중격	NS	18~22, 44~46
Nasolacrimal duct	鼻淚管	비루관	NLD	18~20
Nasopharynx	鼻咽頭	비인두	NPh	20~24, 48~52
Nasopharynx, roof	鼻咽頭蓋	비인두개	NPhr	20, 50~52
Nerve	**神經**	**신경**		
2nd cervical nerve	第二頸椎神經	제 2 경추신경	2CN	56
3rd cranial nerve	第三腦神經	제 3 뇌신경	3N	52
5th cranial nerve	第五腦神經	제 5 뇌신경	5N	16~18
acoustic nerve	聽神經	청신경	AN	20, 54
femoral nerve	大腿神經	대퇴신경	FN	150, 154~160, 166, 184
long thoracic nerve	長胸神經	장흉신경	LTN	82
obturator nerve	閉鎖神經	폐쇄신경	ObN	150
optic nerve	視神經	시신경	ON	16~18, 46~48, 64
right phrenic nerve	右橫隔神經	우횡격신경	RPN	92~94
sacral nerve	薦骨神經	천골신경	SaN	150~152
sciatic nerve	坐骨神經	좌골신경	SN	164, 168, 174
spinal nerve ganglion	脊髓神經節	척수신경절	SNG	26, 34, 40
Nuchal ligament	項靱帶	항인대	NL	36, 40
Obliquus capitis inferior muscle	下頭斜筋	하두사근	OCI	56
Obliquus capitis superior muscle	上頭斜筋	상두사근	OCS	58
Obturator artery	閉鎖動脈	폐쇄동맥	ObA	162~166
Obturator fascia	閉鎖筋膜	폐쇄근막	ObF	162
Obturator muscle	閉鎖筋	폐쇄근	Ob	24, 162
Obturator nerve	閉鎖神經	폐쇄신경	ObN	150
Obturator vein	閉鎖靜脈	폐쇄정맥	ObV	162~166
Obturator vessel	閉鎖血管	폐쇄혈관	Obv	172
Occipital bone	後頭骨	후두골	OB	20, 24, 54~56, 60
Occipital lobe	後頭葉	후두엽	OL	6~14, 60, 66~68
Old infarct	舊梗塞	구경색	If	8~12
Olfactory bulb	嗅球	후구	OlB	46
Olfactory gyrus	嗅神經回	후신경회	Olg	66~70
Olfactory tract	嗅索	후삭	OlT	66
Omental fat	大網脂肪	대망지방	OF	114~124, 168~172
Optic canal	視神經管	시신경관	OC	18
Optic chiasm	視神經交叉	시신경교차	OCh	16, 50
Optic nerve	視神經	시신경	ON	16~18, 46~48, 64
Optic radiation	視放射	시방사	OpR	10, 54~56, 68
Optic tract	視索	시색	OpT	52, 66
Orbital gyrus	眼窩回	안와회	Og	16, 44~46
Orbital roof	眼窩蓋	안와개	OR	16
Oropharynx	口咽頭	구인두	OPh	26~28, 50
Outer table of calvarium	頭蓋冠外板	두개관외판	OT	4~6
Palatine tonsil	口蓋扁桃	구개편도	PaT	28
Palatopharyngeus muscle	口蓋咽頭筋	구개인두근	PPh	24~26
Pancreas, body	膵臟體部	췌장체부	PB	120~128, 186~192
Pancreas, head	膵頭	췌두	PH	130
Pancreas, tail	膵尾	췌미	PT	120~122, 126~128, 194~198
Pancreatic duct	膵管	췌관	PD	128~130
Panniculus adiposus	皮下脂肪層	피하지방층	PA	170
Pampiniform plexus	蔓狀靜脈叢	만상정맥총	PaP	166

Papillary muscle of myocardium	心乳頭筋	심유두근	Pap	106
Papillary process of caudate lobe	尾狀葉乳頭突起	미상엽유두돌기	PPC	122
Paracentral lobule	副中心小葉	부중심소엽	Pal	4, 54~56, 64
Parahippocampal gyrus	副海馬回	부해마회	PHg	12~16, 50~54, 68
Paralaryngeal space	副喉頭腔	부후두강	PLS	34
Parapharyngeal space	副咽頭腔	부인두강	PPS	20~34, 50
Parietal lobe	頭頂葉	두정엽	PL	4~10, 52, 56~58
Parietal paritoneum	壁側腹膜	벽측복막	PP	134~138
Parietal pleura	壁側胸膜	벽측흉막	PPl	86
Parieto-occipital sulcus	頭頂後頭溝	두정후두구	POS	6~10, 58~60, 66~68
Parotid gland	耳下腺	이하선	PG	22~28, 48~50, 54
Parotid gland, deep lobe	耳下腺深葉	이하선심엽	PGd	22~28, 48
Pectineus muscle	恥骨筋	치골근	Pe	164,168~176, 182, 194
Pectoralis major muscle	大胸筋	대흉근	PMa	78~90, 98~100, 106~108
Pectoralis minor muscle	小胸筋	소흉근	PMi	78~82
Pedicle	莖	경	Ped	100
Pelvic fascia	骨盤筋膜	골반근막	PeF	162
Pericallosal artery	腦梁周圍動脈	뇌량주위동맥	PcA	10, 14, 50, 64
Pericardial fat	心外膜脂肪	심외막지방	PcF	114~116, 196~198
Pericardial space	心囊腔	심낭강	PcS	80, 84, 88~90, 94, 100~108, 114, 188~190, 194
Pericardium	心外膜	심외막	Pc	82, 86, 90, 94, 114
Perirenal fat	腎周圍脂肪	신주위지방	PF	98, 104, 120~138, 142~144, 148, 182~184, 192, 196
Peritoneal cavity	腹膜腔	복막강	PeC	114~116, 132~134, 140~142, 146~148, 152, 156, 180, 186
Perpendicular plate	垂直板	수직판	PeP	44~46
Pharyngeal muscles	咽頭筋	인두근	Ph	24~32, 52
Pineal gland	松果腺	송과선	PnG	12, 54, 64
Piriformis muscle	梨狀筋	이상근	Pf	158~160, 182~184, 192~194
Pituitary gland	腦下垂體	뇌하수체	PtG	16, 50
Pituitary stalk	腦下垂體梗	뇌하수체경	PtS	16, 50
Planum sphenoidale	蝶形骨平面	접형골평면	PS	48
Pleural space	胸膜腔	흉막강	PlS	78~86, 90~94, 100, 106~108, 114~130 182~184, 192~198
Pleuropericardial space	胸心膜腔	흉심막강	PlPS	82~88
Pons	腦橋	뇌교	Po	16, 54, 64~66
Porta hepatis	肝門脈	간문맥	PoH	118~120
Portal vein	門脈	문맥	PV	98~100, 120~128, 184~188
Postcentral gyrus	中心後回	중심후회	Pog	4~12, 52~54, 66~72
Posterior cerebral artery	後大腦動脈	후대뇌동맥	PCA	16, 52
Posterior pararenal fat	後腎傍脂肪	후신방지방	PPF	132~148, 180, 194~196
Posterior parietal peritoneum	後壁側腹膜	후벽측복막	PPP	182
Posterior renal fascia	後腎膜	후신막	PRF	124~146, 196
Posterior scalene muscle	後斜角筋	후사각근	PSc	32~36
Posterolateral basal segment of lung	後外側基底肺分節	후외측기저폐분절	PBS	88
Pre-pontine cistern	腦橋前槽	뇌교전조	PrPC	16
Precentral gyrus	中心前回	중심전회	Prg	4~12, 50~54, 66~72
Precuneus	楔前部	설전부	Prc	4~6, 56~60, 64
Prevertebral space	脊椎前腔	척추전강	PVS	32
Prostate	前立腺	전립선	Pr	166~172
Psoas muscle	腰筋	요근	Ps	128~156, 182~184, 192~194
Pterygoid plate	翼突板	익돌판	PtP	20~24, 48
Pterygopalatine fossa	翼突口蓋窩	익돌구개와	PPf	20, 48
Pubic bone	恥骨	치골	Pub	166~170, 182~184, 194~196
Pudendal plexus	外陰部叢	외음부총	PPx	164~170
Pulmonary valve	肺動脈瓣	폐동맥판	PV	106
Putamen	被殼	피각	Pu	12~14, 48~52, 68
Pyloric canal of stomach	胃幽門	위유문	PC	126
Pyramid	錐體	추체	Py	20
Pyramis vermis	蟲部錐體	충부추체	PyV	56~60
Quadratus femoris muscle	大腿方形筋	대퇴방형근	QF	168~172
Quadratus lumborum muscle	腰方形筋	요방형근	QL	132~146, 180~182, 192~198
Quadrigeminal cistern	四丘槽	사구조	QC	12~14
Rectal gyrus	直回	직회	Rg	16, 44~48, 64

Rectum	直腸	직장	Rt	156~170, 186~190
Rectus abdominis muscle	腹直筋	복직근	ReA	116~162, 184~192
Rectus capitis posterior major muscle	大後頭直筋	대후두직근	RCPM	60
Rectus capitis posterior minor muscle	小後頭直筋	소후두직근	RCPm	60
Rectus femoris muscle	大腿直筋	대퇴직근	RFe	164~176
Red nucleus	赤核	적핵	RN	14
Renal cortex	腎皮質	신피질	RCx	130, 134, 138, 182
Renal medulla	腎髓質	신수질	RM	130, 134, 182
Renal pelvis	腎盂	신우	RP	134~136, 140~144
Retina	網膜	망막	Re	18
Retromandibular vein	下顎後靜脈	하악후정맥	RMV	22~28
Rhomboideus major muscle	大稜形筋	대능형근	RMa	78~82, 98~100
Rhomboideus minor muscle	小稜形筋	소능형근	RMi	36
Rib	肋骨	늑골	Ri	78~82, 86~88, 92~94, 98~100, 106~108, 114~128, 134~142, 180~182, 194~198
Right adrenal gland	右副腎	우부신	RAd	122~123
Right atrial appendage of heart	右心房耳	우심방이	RAA	84~88, 100
Right atrium of heart	右心房	우심방	RA	88~92, 98~100
Right coronary artery	右冠狀動脈	우관상동맥	RCA	88~92, 102
Right descending pulmonary artery	右下行肺動脈	우하행폐동맥	RDPA	84~86, 98~100
Right diaphragmatic crus	右橫隔膜脚	우횡격막각	RC	114~138, 142
Right hepatic artery	右肝動脈	우간동맥	RHA	122
Right hepatic vein	右肝靜脈	우간정맥	RHV	94, 98~100, 114~120, 184
Right inferior pulmonary vein	右下肺靜脈	우하폐정맥	RIPV	86~88
Right innominate vein	右無名靜脈	우무명정맥	RIV	78, 98~100
Right kidney	右腎	우신	RK	98, 126~144, 180~184
Right lobe of liver	肝右葉	간우엽	RL	94, 98, 114~142, 180, 184
Right lower lobe bronchus	右下葉氣管枝	우하엽기관지	RLL3	84~86, 98
Right lower lobe of lung	右肺下葉	우폐하엽	RLL	80~94, 98~100, 114~116, 180~186
Right main bronchus	右主氣管枝	우주기관지	RMB	98~100
Right middle lobe bronchus	右中葉氣管枝	우중엽기관지	RMLB	86, 98
Right middle lobe of lung	右肺中葉	우폐중엽	RML	86~92, 98, 180~182
Right phrenic nerve	右橫隔神經	우횡격신경	RPN	92~94
Right portal vein	右門脈	우문맥	RPV	82, 114~124, 128, 182
Right pulmonary artery	右肺動脈	우폐동맥	RPA	88, 100~104
Right renal artery	右腎動脈	우신동맥	RRA	132~136, 184
Right renal vein	右腎靜脈	우신정맥	RRV	132~136, 184
Right subclavian artery	右鎖骨下動脈	우쇄골하동맥	RScA	98
Right superior pulmonary vein	右上肺靜脈	우상폐정맥	RSPV	82~84, 98
Right upper lobe of lung	右肺上葉	우폐상엽	RUL	78~82, 98~100
Right ventricle of heart	右心室	우심실	RV	86~94, 102~108, 190, 194~196
Root of penis	陰莖根	음경근	RPe	168~172
Rosenmüller fossa	Rosenmüller 窩	로젠뮬러와	RF	22, 50~52
Sacral nerve	薦骨神經	천골신경	SaN	150~152
Sacroiliac joint	薦腸關節	천장관절	SIJ	150~156
Sacrospinous ligament	薦骨脊椎間靱帶	천골척추간인대	SSL	162
Sacrum	薦骨	천골	Sac	150~162, 182~186, 192
Sartorius muscle	縫工筋	봉공근	Sar	158~176
Scapula	肩胛骨	견갑골	Sca	36~40, 78~88, 102, 108
Sciatic nerve	坐骨神經	좌골신경	SN	164, 168, 174
Sclera	鞏膜	공막	Scl	18
Scrotum	陰囊	음낭	Scr	174~176
Second portion of duodenum	十二指腸第二部	십이지장제2부	D2	130~134, 184
Seminal vesicle	精囊	정낭	SVe	164
Semispinalis capitis muscle	頭部半棘筋	두부반극근	SSC	26~32, 60
Semispinalis cervicalis muscle	頸部半棘筋	경부반극근	SSCe	26~32, 36~40
Semispinalis dorsi muscle	背半棘筋	배반극근	SSD	78~82, 86~88, 94, 114~122
Semitendinosus muscle	半腱狀筋	반건상근	Se	174~176
Septum pelludicum	透明中隔	투명중격	SPe	10~12, 48~52
Serratus anterior muscle	前鋸筋	전거근	SeA	40, 78, 82~92, 114~120
Sigmoid colon	S狀結腸	S상결장	SiC	140~156, 182~194
Sigmoid sinus	S形洞	S형동	SS	16, 22, 54~56
Soft palate	軟口蓋	연구개	SP	24~26, 48~52
Spermatic cord	精索	정색	SCo	156, 160~172
Sphenoid sinus	蝶形骨洞	접형골동	SpS	18, 48~50
Spinal cord	脊髓	척수	SC	26~40, 56~60, 82, 90~94, 100~102, 114~130

English	Hanja	Korean	Abbr	Pages
Spinal nerve ganglion	脊髓神經神經節	척수신경신경절	SNG	26, 34, 40
Spinalis cervicalis muscle	頸棘筋	경극근	SCe	34~40
Spinalis muscle	脊椎棘筋	척추극근	Sp	114~122, 194
Spleen	脾臟	비장	Spl	106~108, 114~130, 134, 196~198
Splenic artery	脾動脈	비동맥	SA	102, 124~126, 190~192
Splenic flexure of colon	脾結腸曲	비결장곡	SF	198
Splenic vein	脾靜脈	비정맥	SV	120~128, 190~198
Splenius capitis muscle	頭部脊椎棘筋	두부척추극근	SpC	26~32, 58~60
Sternocleidomastoid muscle	胸鎖乳突筋	흉쇄유돌근	SCM	24~40, 54~56
Sternum	胸骨	흉골	Stn	82~92, 102, 114
Stomach	胃	위	St	104~108, 114~130, 190, 194~198
Stomach, antrum	胃前庭部	위전정부	StA	120~128, 188, 192
Straight sinus	直靜脈洞	직정맥동	StS	10, 32, 58~60
Styloglossus muscle	莖突舌筋	경돌설근	SG	28, 32, 52
Stylohyoid muscle	莖突舌骨筋	경돌설골근	SH	30
Styloid muscle	莖突筋	경돌근	Sty	24
Styloid process	莖狀突起	경상돌기	Stp	22~24
Subarachnoid space	蜘蛛膜下腔	지주막하강	SAS	26, 28
Subclavian artery	鎖骨下動脈	쇄골하동맥	ScA	40, 78
Subclavian vein	鎖骨下靜脈	쇄골하정맥	ScV	78~80
Subdural space	硬膜下腔	경막하강	SDS	4, 10~12, 44
Subepicardial fat	心膜下脂肪	심막하지방	SEF	94, 108
Sublingual gland	舌下腺	설하선	SLG	48
Submandibular gland	下顎下腺	하악하선	SMG	28~32, 50~52
Subscapularis muscle	肩胛下筋	견갑하근	SbS	36~40, 78~82, 108
Substantia nigra	黑質	흑질	SNi	14, 66
Sulcus	溝	구		
calcarine sulcus	鳥距溝	오거구	CaS	56~60
central sulcus	中央溝	중앙구	CnS	6~12, 52~54
cingulate sulcus	帶狀回溝	대상회구	CiS	48, 54
circular sulcus of insula	島皮質圓形溝	도피질원형구	CSI	10~14, 48~52
collateral sulcus	側部溝	측부구	CoS	56~58
hippocampal sulcus	海馬溝	해마구	HS	52
intraparietal sulcus	頭頂內溝	두정내구	IPS	56
median sulcus	正中溝	정중구	MeS	54
parieto-occipital sulcus	頭頂後頭溝	두정후두구	POS	6~10, 58~60
Superficial femoral artery	淺大腿動脈	천대퇴동맥	SFA	170~172
Superior cerebellar cistern	上小腦槽	상소뇌조	SCC	10, 56, 66
Superior cerebellar artery	上小腦動脈	상소뇌동맥	SCA	52
Superior frontal gyrus	上前頭回	상전두회	SFg	4~14, 44~52, 64~68
Superior gemellus muscle	上雙子筋	상쌍자근	SGe	164
Superior gluteal artery	上臀動脈	상둔동맥	SGA	152~160
Superior gluteal vein	上臀靜脈	상둔정맥	SGV	154~160
Superior mesenteric artery	上腸間膜動脈	상장간막동맥	SMA	130~144, 188
Superior mesenteric vein	上腸間膜靜脈	상장간막정맥	SMV	130~144, 190~192
Superior ophthalmic vein	上眼靜脈	상안정맥	SOV	44~48
Superior orbital fissure	上眼窩裂	상안와열	SOF	48
Superior parietal lobule	上頭頂小葉	상두정소엽	SPL	4, 56~60, 66~70
Superior rectus muscle	上直筋	상직근	SR	44~46
Superior sagittal sinus	上矢狀靜脈洞	상시상정맥동	SSS	4, 10, 46, 50, 58~60
Superior segment of left lower lobe bronchus	左下葉氣管枝上分節	좌하엽기관지상분절	SLLB	84
Superior sinus of pericardium	上心膜洞	상심막동	SSP	80
Superior temporal gyrus	上側頭回	상측두회	STg	10~16, 48~56, 68~72
Superior vena cava	上大靜脈	상대정맥	SVC	80~88, 98~100
Supramarginal gyrus	緣上回	연상회	SMg	6~8, 54~56, 72
Suprasellar cistern	Turkey 鞍上槽	터키안상조	SuSC	16
Supraspinatus muscle	棘上筋	극상근	SSp	38, 80
Sylvian fissure	Sylvius 裂	실비우스열	SF	10~14, 48, 52, 56, 70~72
Symphysis pubis	恥骨結合	치골결합	SyP	166. 186~192
T1 vertebral body	第一胸椎體	제 1 흉추체	T1	102
T6 vertebral body	第六胸椎體	제 6 흉추체	T6	102
T7 vertebral body	第七胸椎體	제 7 흉추체	T7	82
T8 vertebral body	第八胸椎體	제 8 흉추체	T8	86
T8-9 intervertebral disc	第八, 九胸椎間板	제 8-9 흉추간판	T8-9	88
T10-11 intervertebral disc	第十, 十一胸椎間板	제 10-11 흉추간판	T10-11	114

English	Chinese	Korean	Abbr.	Pages
T11 vertebral body	第十一胸椎體	제 11 흉추체	T11	114~116
T11-12 intervertebral disc	第十一, 十二 胸椎間板	제 11-12 흉추간판	T11-12	116~118
T12 vertebral body	第十二胸椎體	제 12 흉추체	T12	120~122
T12-L1 intervertebral disc	第十二胸椎, 第一腰椎間板	제 12 흉추-제 1 요추 간판	T12-L1	124
Tegmentum, midrain	中腦被蓋	중뇌피개	Teg	14
Temporal bone	側頭骨	측두골	TB	18~20
Temporal lobe	側頭葉	측두엽	TL	10~18, 48, 56~58, 70
Temporalis fascia	側頭筋膜	측두근막	TF	18~20
Temporalis muscle	側頭筋	측두근	Te	16~24, 46~48
Temporomandibular joint	側頭下顎骨關節	측두하악골관절	TMJ	20
Tensor fascia lata	大腿筋膜張筋	대퇴근막장근	TFL	160~162, 166~176
Tensor palati muscle	口蓋帆張筋	구개범장근	TP	22
Tentorium cerebelli	小腦天幕	소뇌천막	Ten	8~14, 54~60
Teres major muscle	大圓筋	대원근	TMa	80~88
Testis	睾丸	고환	Tes	172~176
Thalamus	視床	시상	Th	12, 52~54, 64~68
Third portion of duodenum	十二指腸第三部	십이지장제 3 부	D3	136~142, 186
Thoracic duct	胸管	흉관	TD	86, 90, 94, 102
Thyroid cartilage	甲狀軟骨	갑상연골	ThC	34
Thyroid cartilage, inferior cornu	甲狀軟骨下角	갑상연골하각	TIC	34
Thyroid gland	甲狀腺	갑상선	ThG	36~40, 104
Tongue	舌	설	To	26, 44~46
Torus tubarius	耳管隆起	이관융기	TT	22, 50
Trachea	氣管	기관	Tr	36~40, 78 100~102
Transverse colon	橫行結腸	횡행결장	TC	116~136, 180~196
Transverse foramen	橫突孔	횡돌공	TrF	34~36
Transverse mesocolon	橫結腸間膜	횡결장간막	TMc	190~196
Transverse process of vertebra	脊椎橫突起	척추횡돌기	TPV	80, 100
Transverse sinus of pericardium	心膜橫洞	심막횡동	TSP	84, 102~104
Transverse temporal gyrus	橫側頭回	횡측두회	TTg	10
Transversus abdominis muscle	腹橫筋	복횡근	TA	128~154, 180, 194~198
Trapezius muscle	僧帽筋	승모근	Trp	30~40, 78~88, 98~100, 104~106
Triceps brachii muscle	上腕三頭筋	상완삼두근	Tri	80
Tricuspid valve	三尖瓣	삼첨판	TV	90, 102~104
Trochanteric bursa	轉子滑液囊	전자활액낭	TrB	164~168
Truncus anterior	前幹	전간	TrA	16, 100
Tuberculum sellae	Turkey 鞍	터키안	TS	16, 48
Tunica vaginalis	鞘膜	초막	TVa	174~176
Uncinate process of pancreas, head	膵臟鉤狀突起	췌장구상돌기	UnP	132~136
Uncus	鉤狀突起	구상돌기	Unc	14~16, 50, 68~70
Ureter	尿管	요관	Ur	132~162, 184, 192
Urethra	尿道	요도	Ua	170~172
Urinary bladder	膀胱	방광	UB	154~166, 186~192
Uterus	子宮	자궁	Ut	186~190
Uvula	口蓋垂	구개수	Uv	26, 52, 58
Vagina	膣	질	Vg	186
Vallecula	谷	곡	Va	30~32, 64
Vas deferens	精管	정관	VD	162~164
Vastus iniermedius muscle	中間廣筋	중간광근	VI	174~176
Vastus lateralis muscle	外側廣筋	외측광근	VL	168~176
Vastus medialis muscle	內側廣筋	내측광근	VM	174~176
Vein	**靜脈**	**정맥**		
axillary vein	腋窩靜脈	액와정맥	AxV	80
azygos vein	奇靜脈	기정맥	Az	80~94, 100, 114~118, 122~130
common iliac vein	總腸骨靜脈	총장골정맥	CIV	148~152, 184~192
diploic vein	板間靜脈	판간정맥	DV	4
external iliac vein	外腸骨靜脈	외장골정맥	EIV	154~162, 182
external jugular vein	外頸靜脈	외경정맥	EJV	30~40
femoral vein	大腿靜脈	대퇴정맥	FV	164~172, 176
hemiazygos vein	半奇靜脈	반기정맥	HzV	84, 90~94, 102~126, 130
hepatic vein	肝靜脈	간정맥	HV	98~100, 120, 186
inferior gluteal vein	下臀靜脈	하둔정맥	IGV	160, 166~172
intercostal vein	肋間靜脈	늑간정맥	IcV	84, 88, 92~94, 104, 108, 116~118
internal cerebral vein	內大腦靜脈	내대뇌정맥	ICV	10~12, 52~54
internal iliac vein	內腸骨靜脈	내장골정맥	IIV	154~158, 182, 192

English	漢字	한글	Abbr	Pages
internal jugular vein	內頸靜脈	내경정맥	IJV	20~40, 54
internal mesentenic vein	下腸間膜靜脈	하장간막정맥	IMV	194
left gastric vein	左胃靜脈	좌위정맥	LGV	122~124
left hepatic vein	左肝靜脈	좌간정맥	LHV	102, 104, 114~118, 188~192
left inferior pulmonary vein	左下肺靜脈	좌하폐정맥	LIPV	86~88
left innominate vein	左無名靜脈	좌무명정맥	LIV	78, 100~106
left portal vein	左門脈	좌문맥	LPV	118, 186
left renal vein	左腎靜脈	좌신정맥	LRV	132~138, 186~192
left subclavian vein	左鎖骨下靜脈	좌쇄골하정맥	LScV	108
left superior pulmonary vein	左上肺靜脈	좌상폐정맥	LSPV	82~84, 104~106
middle cardiac vein	中心靜脈	중심정맥	MCV	102~106, 190
middle hepatic vein	中肝靜脈	중간정맥	MHV	94, 114~118
obturator vein	閉鎖靜脈	폐쇄정맥	ObV	162~166
portal vein	門脈	문맥	PV	98~100, 120~128, 184~188
retromandibular vein	後下顎靜脈	후하악정맥	RMV	24~28
right hepatic vein	右肝靜脈	우간정맥	RHV	94, 98~100, 114~120, 184
right inferior pulmonary vein	右下肺靜脈	우하폐정맥	RIPV	86~88
right innominate vein	右無名靜脈	우무명정맥	RIV	78, 98, 100
right portal vein	右門脈	우문맥	RPV	82, 114~124, 128, 182
right renal vein	右腎靜脈	우신정맥	RRV	132~134, 184
right superior pulmonary vein	右上肺靜脈	우상폐정맥	RSPV	82~84, 98
splenic vein	脾靜脈	비정맥	SV	120~128, 190~198
subclavian vein	鎖骨下靜脈	쇄골하정맥	ScV	78~80
superior gluteal vein	上臀靜脈	상둔정맥	SGV	154~160
superior mesenteric vein	上腸間膜靜脈	상장간막정맥	SMV	130~144, 190~192
superior ophthalmic vein	上眼靜脈	상안정맥	SOV	44~48
vein of Galen	Galen 靜脈	갈렌정맥	VG	56
vertebral vein	椎骨靜脈	추골정맥	VV	56
Ventricle	**腦室**	**뇌실**		
3rd ventricle	第三腦室	제삼뇌실	3V	12~14, 64
4th ventricle	第四腦室	제사뇌실	4V	16, 56, 64
choroid plexus of lateral ventricle	側腦室脈絡叢	측뇌실맥락총	ChP	10, 54~56, 68
lateral ventricle, antrum	側腦室洞	측뇌실동	LVa	10, 54, 68
lateral ventricle, body	側腦室體部	측뇌실체부	LVb	6~10, 52
lateral ventricle, frontal horn	側腦室前頭角	측뇌실전두각	LVf	10~14, 48~52, 64
lateral ventricle, occipital horn	側腦室後頭角	측뇌실후두각	LVo	8~10, 56
lateral ventricle, temporal horn	側腦室側頭角	측뇌실측두각	LVt	14~16, 52, 68~70
Vertebra	**脊椎**	**척추**		
C3 vertebral body	第三頸椎體	제 3 경추체	C3	28, 56
C3-4 intervertebral disc	第三, 四頸椎間板	제 3-4 경추간판	C3-4	30
C4 vertebral body	第四頸椎體	제 4 경추체	C4	32
C4-5 intervertebral disc	第四, 五頸椎間板	제 4-5 경추간판	C4-5	34
C5 vertebral body	第五頸椎體	제 5 경추체	C5	36
C6 vertebral body	第六頸椎體	제 6 경추체	C6	38~40
costovertebral articulation	肋椎關節	늑추관절	CVA	86
intervertebral disc	脊椎間板	척추간판	IVD	56, 100~102, 186~188
intervertebral foramen	脊椎間孔	척추간공	IVF	32, 38
L1 vertebral body	第一腰椎體	제 1 요추체	L1	124~130, 186
L1-2 intervertebral disc	第一, 二腰椎間板	제 1-2 요추간판	L1-2	130~132
L2 vertebral body	第二腰椎體	제 2 요추체	L2	130, 134
L2-3 intervertebral disc	第二, 三腰椎間板	제 2-3 요추간판	L2-3	136
L3 vertebral body	第三腰椎體	제 3 요추체	L3	138~140
L3-4 intervertebral disc	第三, 四腰椎間板	제 3-4 요추간판	L3-4	142
L4 vertebral body	第四腰椎體	제 4 요추체	L4	144~146
L4-5 intervertebral disc	第四, 五腰椎間板	제 4-5 요추간판	L4-5	146
L5 vertebral body	第五腰椎體	제 5 요추체	L5	148, 186~188
L5-S1 intervertebral disc	第五腰椎, 第一薦椎間板	제 5 요추-제 1 천추간판	L5-S1	150~152
prevertebral space	脊椎前腔	척추전강	PVS	32
T1 vertebral body	第一胸椎體	제 1 흉추체	T1	102
T6 vertebral body	第六胸椎體	제 6 흉추체	T6	102
T8 vertebral body	第八胸椎體	제 8 흉추체	T8	86
T8-9 intervertebral disc	第八, 九胸椎間板	제 8-9 흉추간판	T8-9	88
T10-11 intervertebral disc	第十, 十一胸椎間板	제 10-11 흉추간판	T10-11	114
T11 vertebral body	第十一胸椎體	제 11 흉추체	T11	114~116
T11-12 intervertebral disc	第十一, 十二胸椎間板	제 11-12 흉추간판	T11-12	116~118

English	漢字	한글	Abbr.	Pages
T12 vertebral body	第十二胸椎體	제 12 흉추체	T12	102, 120~122, 128
T12-L1 intervertebral disc	第十二胸椎, 第一腰椎間板	제 12 흉추–제 1 요추 간판	T12-L1	124
transverse process of vertebra	脊椎橫突起	척추횡돌기	TPA	80, 100
vertebral artery	椎骨動脈	추골동맥	VA	20, 24~40, 54
vertebral body	脊椎體	척추체	VB	30, 34
vertebral vein	椎骨靜脈	추골정맥	VV	56
Vertebral artery	椎骨動脈	추골동맥	VA	20, 24~40, 54
Vertebral body	脊椎體	척추체	VB	30, 34
Vertebral vein	椎骨靜脈	추골정맥	VV	56
Vitreous	硝子體	초자체	Vi	18
Vocal cord	聲帶	성대	VC	34~36
Vocal ligament	聲帶靱帶	성대인대	VoL	34
Xiphoid process	劍狀突起	검상돌기	XP	114~118
Zygomatic bone	顴骨	관골	ZB	18~20